Sino-Nasal and Olfactory System Disorders

Edited by Thomas Heinbockel and Balwant Singh Gendeh

Published in London, United Kingdom

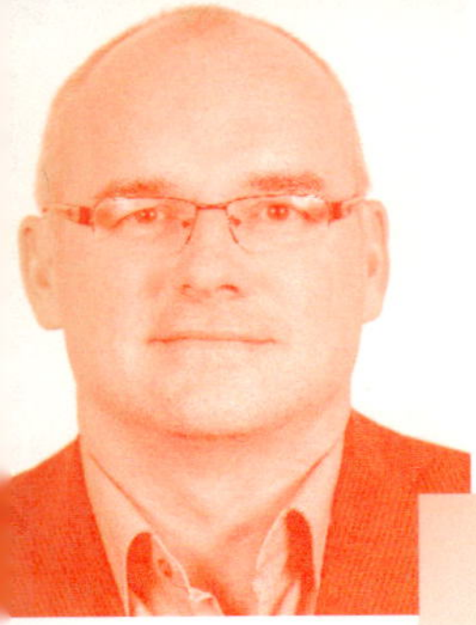
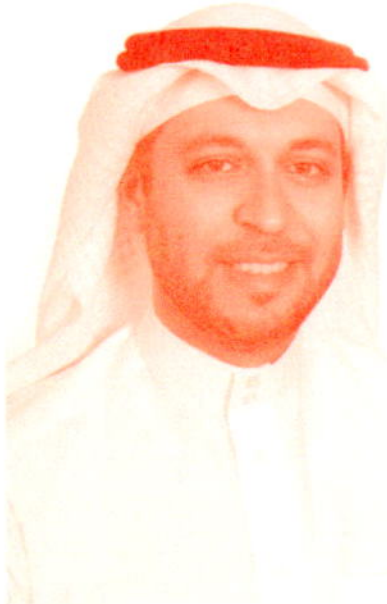
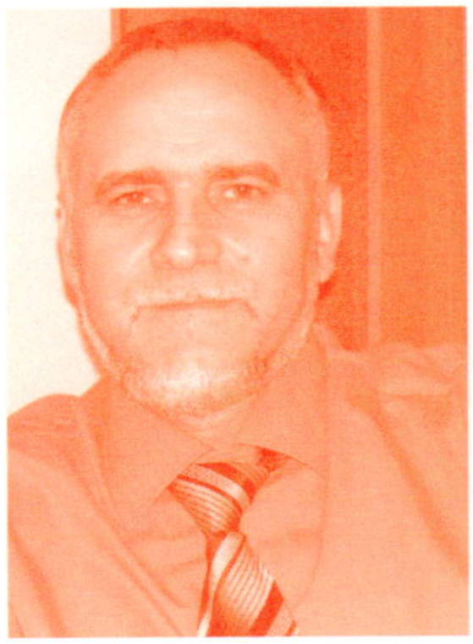
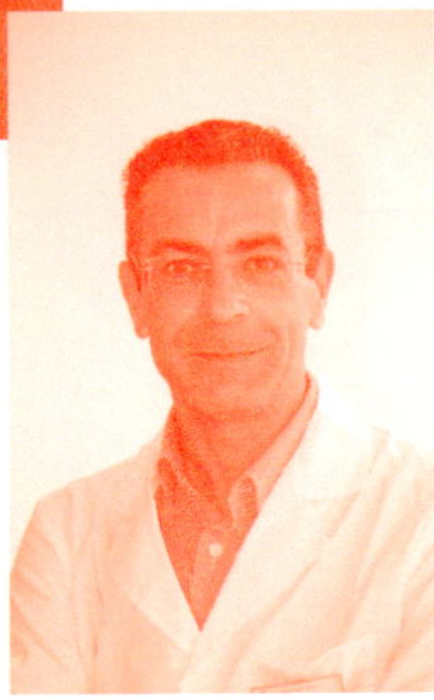
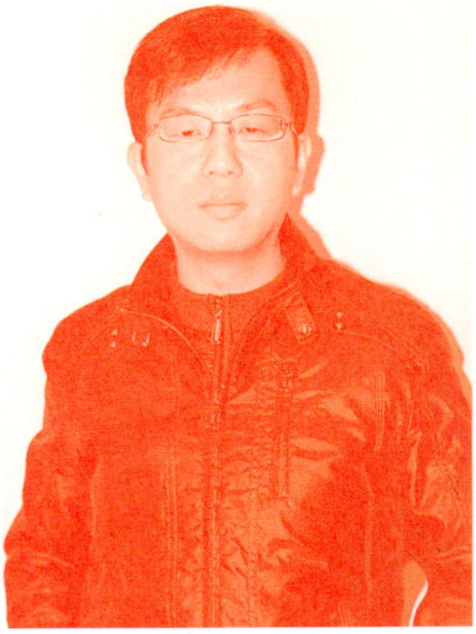
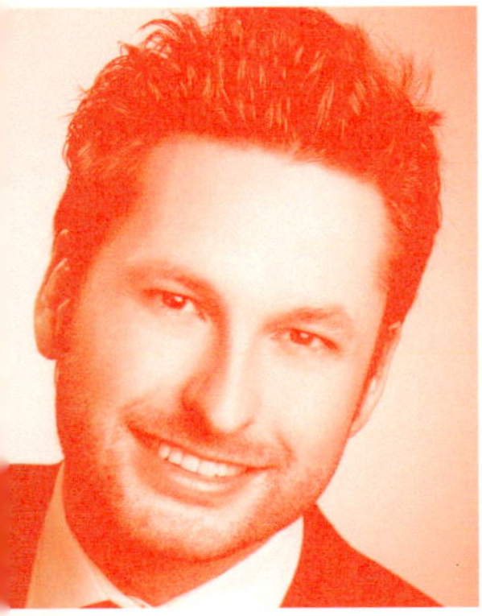
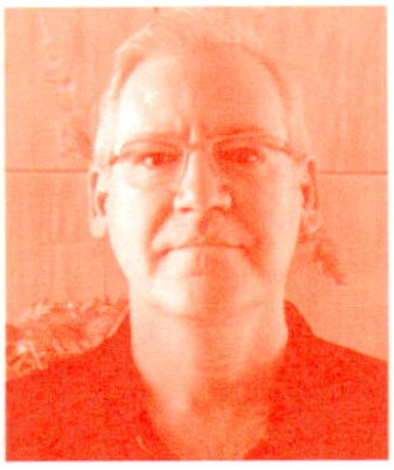

IntechOpen

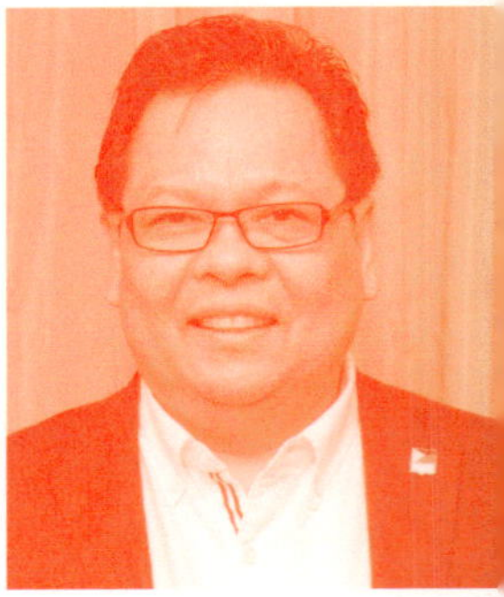
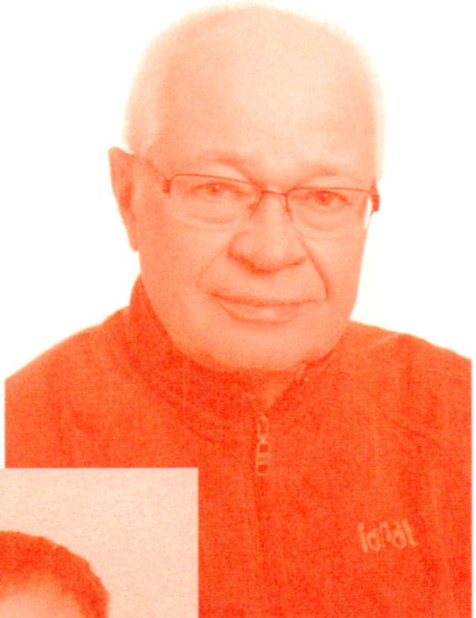
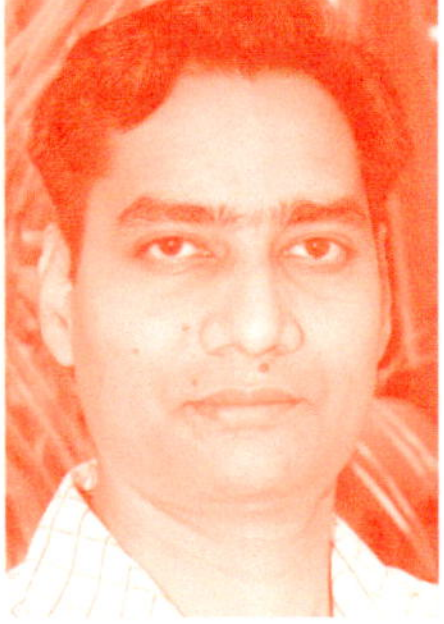
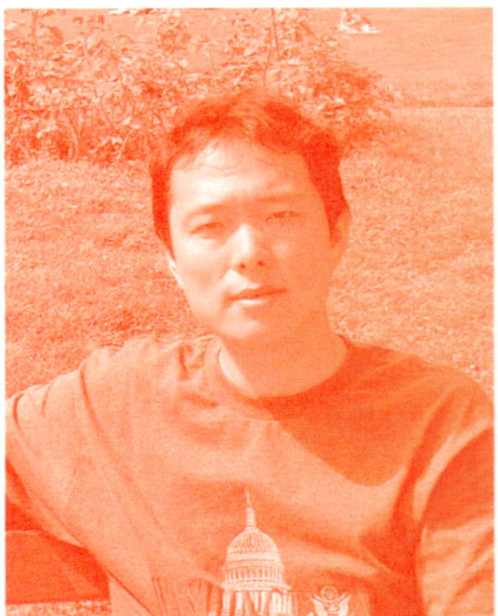
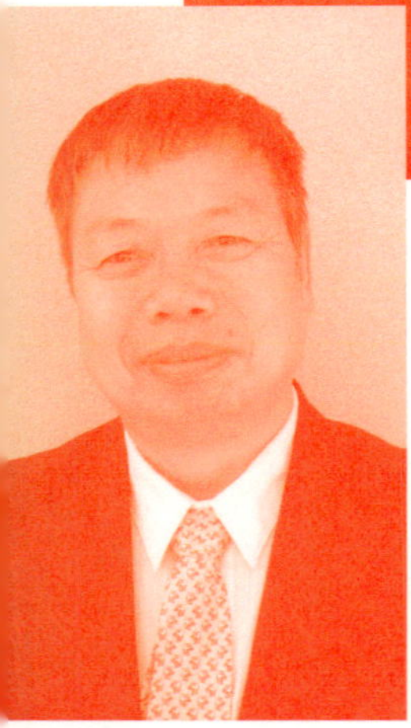
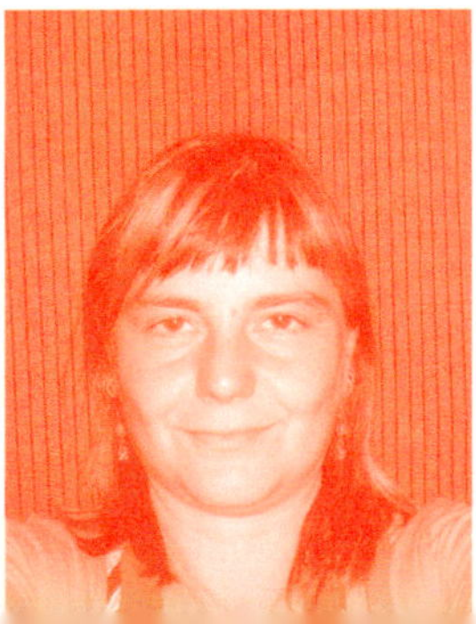

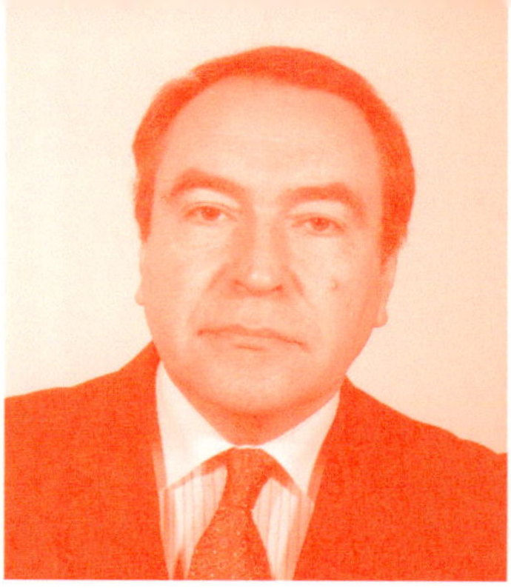
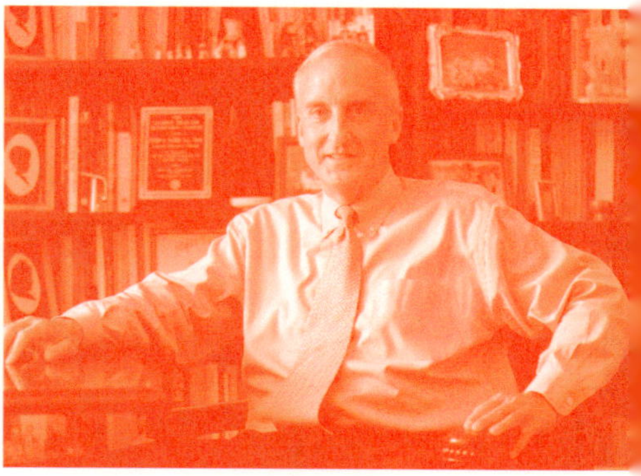
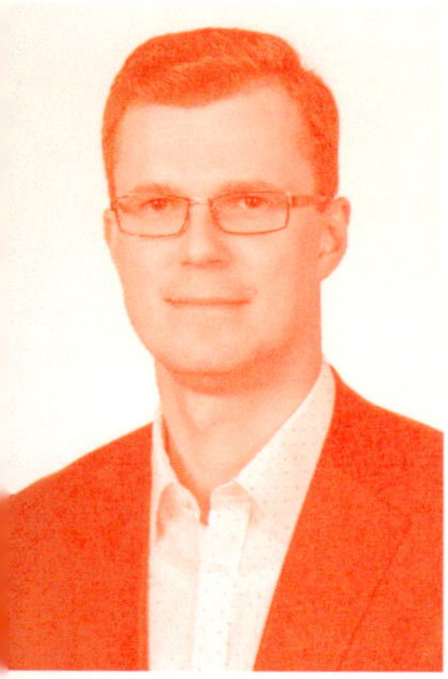
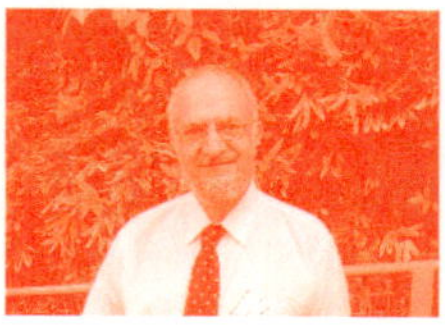
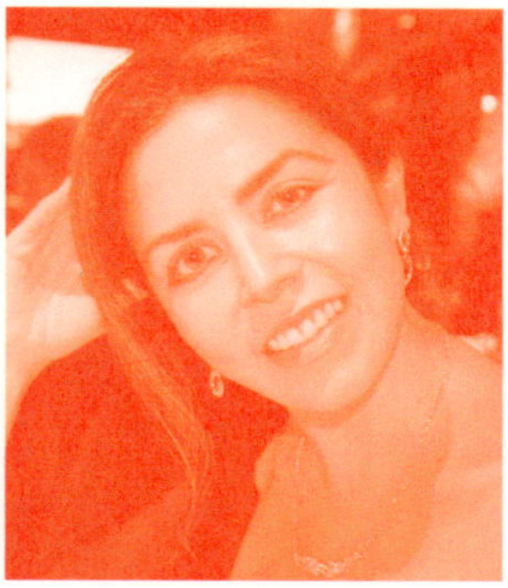

Supporting open minds since 2005

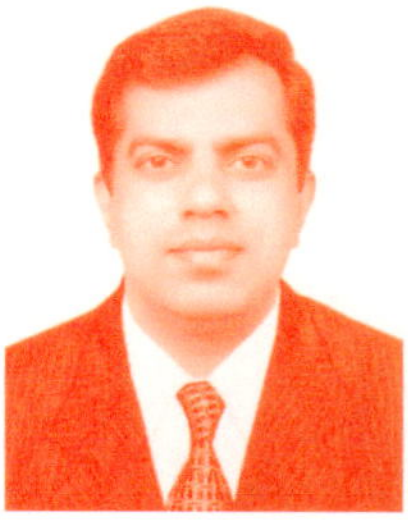
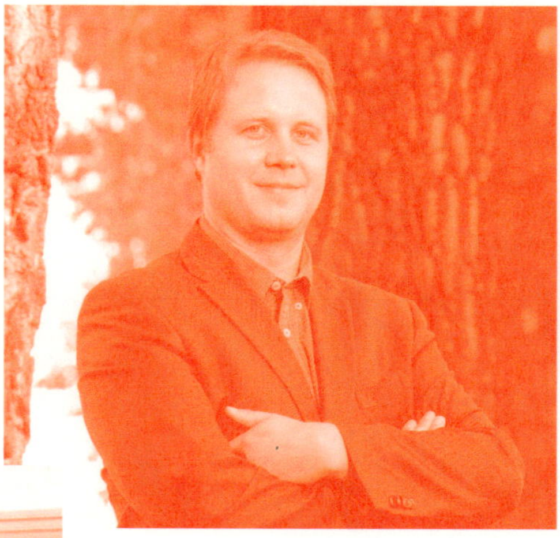
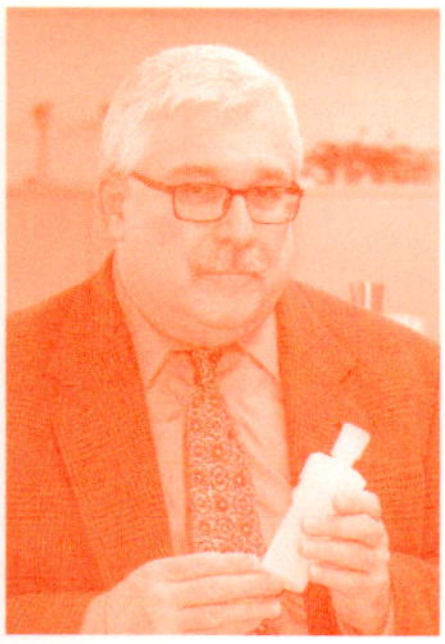
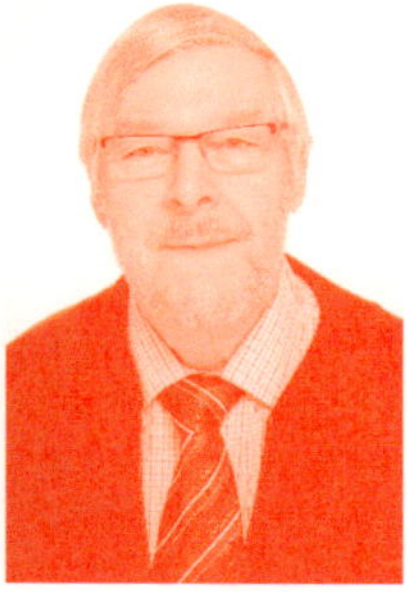
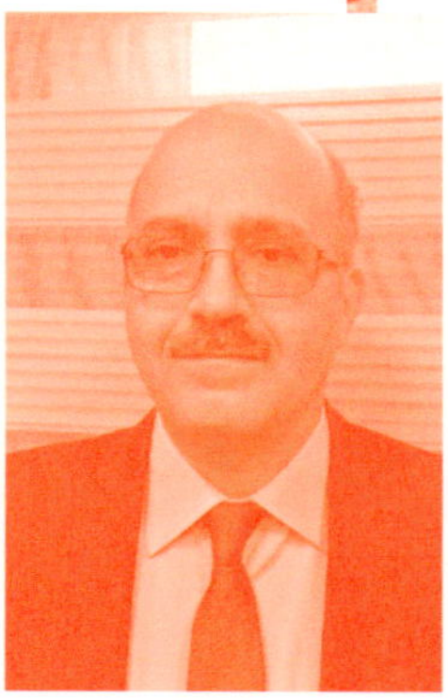
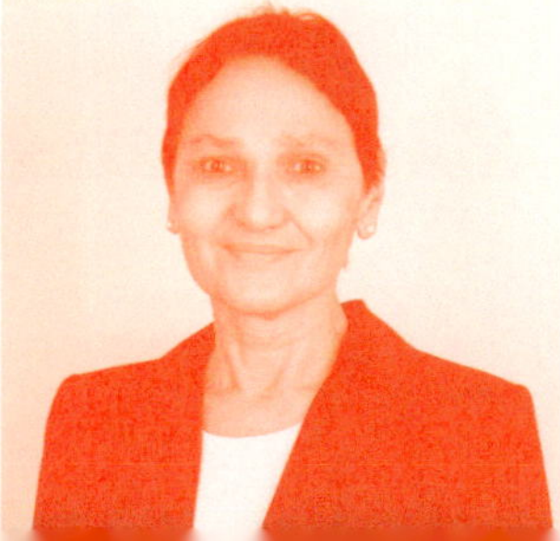
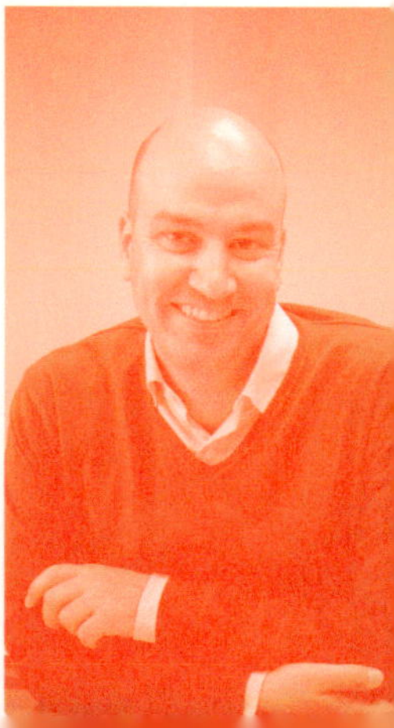

Sino-Nasal and Olfactory System Disorders
http://dx.doi.org/10.5772/intechopen.80149
Edited by Thomas Heinbockel and Balwant Singh Gendeh

Contributors
Motoyasu Honma, Fozia Masood, Philippe Eloy, Mitsuo Tonoike, Assia Belhassan, Samir Chtita, Tahar Lakhlifi, Mohammed Bouachrine, Tanwee Das De, Heidi Beate Eggesbø, Henry Barham, Christian Hall, Harry Zylicz, Yi-Tsen Lin, Seiko Mitachi, Ken Satoh, Kumiko Shimoyama, Makoto Satoh, Takeshi Sugiyama, Thomas Heinbockel, Naina Naina Bhatia-Dey, Balwant Singh Gendeh, C. Fervaille, M.C. Nollevaux, Rajnikant Dixit

First published in London, United Kingdom, 2020 by IntechOpen
IntechOpen is the global imprint of INTECHOPEN LIMITED, registered in England and Wales, registration number: 11086078, 5 Princes Gate Court, London, SW7 2QJ, United Kingdom
Printed in Croatia

British Library Cataloguing-in-Publication Data
A catalogue record for this book is available from the British Library

Additional hard and PDF copies can be obtained from orders@intechopen.com

Sino-Nasal and Olfactory System Disorders
Edited by Thomas Heinbockel and Balwant Singh Gendeh
p. cm.
Print ISBN 978-1-83880-950-8
Online ISBN 978-1-83880-951-5
eBook (PDF) ISBN 978-1-83880-952-2

For EU product safety concerns:
IN TECH d.o.o., Prolaz Marije Krucifikse Kozulić 3, 51000 Rijeka, Croatia, info@intechopen.com or visit our website at intechopen.com.

Meet the editors

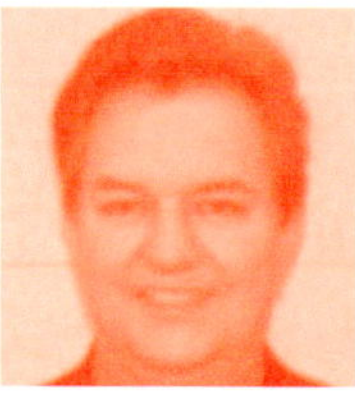

Thomas Heinbockel, Ph.D., is a Professor and Interim Chair in the Department of Anatomy, Howard University College of Medicine, Washington, DC. Dr. Heinbockel's laboratory engages in multidisciplinary research to elucidate organizational principles of neural systems in the brain, specifically the limbic and olfactory system. His research has been directed at understanding brain mechanisms of information processing and their relation to neurological and neuropsychiatric disorders. His laboratory also works on translational projects, specifically, the development of novel anti-epileptic drugs and pharmacotherapeutic treatment options for drug addiction. His laboratory analyzes drug actions at the epi- and genetic level using next-generation sequencing technology. The goal of his studies is to conduct innovative basic and applied research on fundamental biological mechanisms involved in disease conditions (Covid-19, HIV). Dr. Heinbockel studied biology at the Philipps-University, Marburg, Germany. His studies of the brain started during his M.S. thesis work at the Max-Planck-Institute for Behavioral Physiology, Starnberg/Seewiesen, Germany. Subsequently, he completed a Ph.D. in Neuroscience at the University of Arizona, Tucson, Arizona, USA. After graduating, he worked as a Research Associate at the Institute of Physiology, Otto-von-Guericke-University School of Medicine, Magdeburg, Germany. Prior to his arrival at Howard University, Dr. Heinbockel held joint research faculty appointments in the Department of Anatomy & Neurobiology and the Department of Physiology at the University of Maryland School of Medicine, Baltimore, Maryland, USA. He still maintains an adjunct appointment in these departments.

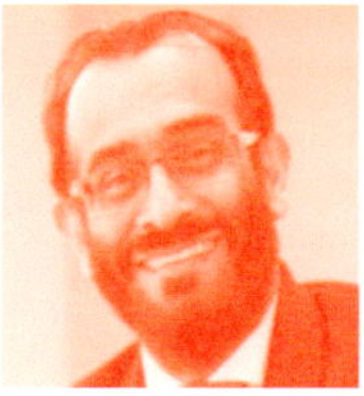

Dr. Balwant Singh Gendeh is a senior consultant ENT surgeon with sub-specialty interest in rhinology (allergy, sinonasal diseases, endoscopic sinus, anterior and ventral skull base surgery, and functional and cosmetic nasal surgery). He was an ENT registrar at the Royal Infirmary, Middlesbrough, United Kingdom in 1993 and subsequently a JW Fulbright scholar at the University of Pittsburgh, USA in 1997. During his Fulbright experience, he also worked at the Hospital of the University of Pennsylvania (HUP), Philadelphia and St Joseph's Hospital, Chicago, USA with sub-specialty interest in rhinology and aesthetic nasal surgery. Dr. BS Gendeh retired as a consultant ENT surgeon at the National University of Malaysia Medical Center (UKMMC) in 2014, and is presently a Visiting Professor at the Department of Otorhinolaryngology-Head and Neck Surgery at UKMMC and is a resident ENT consultant at Pantai Hospital Kuala Lumpur since 2014. Due to his vast contribution to the academia in research and clinical publication, he was elected as a Diploma of Fellowship Academy of Medicine Malaysia (FAMM) in October 2000, International Fellow of the American Academy of Otolaryngology Head and Neck Surgery in April 2004, Fellow of the Academy of Sciences Malaysia (FASc) in April 2016 and as Fellow of Malaysian Scientific Association (FMSA) in September 2017. He has written 94 scientific papers in peer-reviewed journals with more than 470 citations, HI of 13 and editor of 8 books and 7 book chapters.

Contents

Preface

Our chemical senses, smell and taste, are of critical importance in our daily lives and contribute to our personal well-being and safety as well as communication with others. However, it is only when disease or injury impairs their function that we appreciate the relevance of these sensory modalities. During the past three decades, research of the olfactory sense has seen an ever-growing interest in this exciting field of study. This book provides the reader with an overview of the latest developments in sino-nasal and olfactory system disorders and focuses on the most important evidence-based developments in this area. This book addresses disorders, dysfunctions, diseases, and syndromes of our olfactory system ranging from molecular, cellular, and systems to cognitive and behavioral topics. Individual chapters center around recent advances in specific areas of chemosensory pathological conditions, while other chapters focus on technological developments to study the function and dysfunction of our olfactory pathways. All chapters represent recent contributions to the rapidly developing field of sino-nasal and olfactory sciences. Accordingly, this book contains chapters from a variety of topics, written by experts in their respective fields. This book will be a most valuable resource for healthcare professionals and scientists alike. In addition, it will contribute to the training of current and future researchers and, hopefully, will lead us on the path to curing some of the biggest challenges in human health.

The book is divided into two section that address primarily sino-nasal disorders (Section 1) or central olfactory functions and disorders (Section 2). Chapter 1 ('Introductory Chapter: Dysfunction of the Olfactory System & Nasal Disorders') by Thomas Heinbockel and Balwant Gendeh introduces the structures and functions of the nose and olfactory pathway, since they form the basis of dysfunctions of the olfactory system and nasal disorders. Other chapters in Section 1 address 'Imaging in Sino-Nasal Disorders' by Heidi Beate Eggesbo (Chapter 2), 'Sinusitis, Asthma and Headache' by Fozia Masood (Chapter 3), 'Septoplasty: endoscopic and open techniques' by Yi-Tsen Lin (Chapter 4), and 'REAHs and REAH – like: an underdiagnosed lesion often misdiagnosed with nasal polyps' by Philippe Eloy, C Fervaille , and MC Nollevaux (Chapter 5).

Section 2 of the book starts with a chapter on 'Neuro-olfactory regulation and salivary actions: a coordinated event for successful blood-feeding behavior in mosquitoes' by Tanwee Das De and Rajnikant Dixit (Chapter 6). This is followed by Chapter 7 about 'Neurological and Neuropsychiatric Disorders in Relation to Olfactory Dysfunction' by Naina Bhatia-Dey and Thomas Heinbockel. Chapter 8 by Motoyasu Honma addresses 'Cross-Modality Dysfunction between the Visual and Olfactory Systems in Parkinson's Disease'. In Chapter 9, Henry P. Barham, Harry E. Zylicz, and Christian A. Hall discuss 'Cerebrospinal Fluid Leaks and Encephaloceles'. Chapter 10 focusses on 'Optical Fiber-based Sleep Apnea Syndrome Sensor' written by Seiko Mitachi, Ken Satoh, Kumiko Shimoyama, Makoto Satoh, and Takeshi Sugiyama. In Chapter 11, Assia Belhassan, Samir Chtita, Tahar Lakhlifi, and Mohammed Bouachrine review the topic of '2D and 3D-QSRR Studies of Linear Retention Indices for Volatile Alkylated Phenols'. In the final chapter (Chapter 12), Mitsuo Tonoike explains 'Smelling "Zuko", incense rubbing into hands and putting the hands together promote to excite brain'.

We are grateful to IntechOpen for conceiving of this book project and for asking us to serve as editors. Thanks goes to Mia Vulovic at IntechOpen, London, England for guiding us through the publication process and for moving the book ahead in a timely fashion. Thanks are due to all contributors of this book for taking the time to write a chapter proposal, compose their chapter and make the requested revisions. Hopefully, all contributors will continue their nasal and olfactory research with many intellectual challenges in exciting new directions. T.H. would like to thank his wife Dr. Vonnie D.C. Shields, Associate Dean and Professor, Towson University, Towson, MD and their son Torben Heinbockel for the time that he was able to spend working on this book project during the past year. Finally, T.H. is grateful to his parents Erich and Renate Heinbockel for their continuous support and interest in his work over many years.

Thomas Heinbockel, Ph.D.
Professor and Interim Chair,
Department of Anatomy,
Howard University College of Medicine,
Washington, USA

Balwant Singh Gendeh, MD
Pantai Hospital Kuala Lumpur,
Kuala Lumpur, Malaysia

Section 1

Sino-Nasal Disorders

Chapter 1

Introductory Chapter: Dysfunction of the Olfactory System and Nasal Disorders

Thomas Heinbockel and Balwant S. Gendeh

1. Introduction

Our sensory systems are continuously exposed to external stimuli that are processed in the neural pathways of the nervous system in order to maintain bodily homeostasis and to provide appropriate behavioral responses. While some of our senses are more readily recognized for their role in guiding our daily lives and routine behaviors, such as vision and hearing, other senses are noticed primarily when they fail to work or are impaired during disease. This is the case for our chemical senses, taste and smell [1]. Recent estimates suggest that more than 12% of the U.S. population experiences taste or smell (chemosensory) dysfunction [2, 3]. Therefore, it is critical to identify treatments for smell and taste disorders [4]. Olfaction is increasingly acknowledged for its predictive value as an indicator of disorders. Olfactory deficits are evident early on in certain disorders such as Alzheimer's Disease and Parkinson's Disease. More generally, olfactory dysfunction is found in diseases that cause degenerative neuropathology, progressive loss of memory and communication function, normal age-based decline of physiological functions, intellectual challenges, depressive and anxiety disorders, as well as post-traumatic stress disorders. The relevance of olfaction as a predictor of disease has come to the forefront during the Covid-19 pandemic. Many Covid-19 patients experience smell and taste dysfunctions that are not related to blockage of nasal passages as seen in the upper respiratory tract infections [5–8].

2. The olfactory epithelium

This chapter briefly introduces the structures and functions of the nose and olfactory pathway since they form the basis of dysfunctions of the olfactory system and nasal disorders. The nasal passages start with the nostrils or nares separated by a septum. The nasal passages include the vestibule which is the most anterior part of the nasal cavity. The nasal cavity is enclosed by an elastic cartilage and lined by a stratified squamous, keratinized epithelium. The back part of the nasal cavity is lined by the respiratory epithelium, which is a pseudostratified, ciliated, and columnar epithelium. Likewise, this respiratory epithelium is found further down the airways including the trachea and bronchi. Our organ of smell is a specialized epithelium, the olfactory epithelium, which is also a pseudostratified, ciliated, and columnar epithelium. This epithelium covers the superior nasal concha and presents as the olfactory area. Each nasal cavity has an olfactory area in the roof of the nose. The term olfactory mucosa describes the olfactory epithelium and the underlying connective tissue (lamina propria). The olfactory mucosa contains several

IntechOpen

cell types. The olfactory receptor cells in the epithelium are bipolar nerve cells. Their oval nuclei are located in the central one third of the olfactory epithelium. These cells detect smell [9]. The axons of olfactory receptor cells form the olfactory nerve, cranial nerve I. The axons traverse the cribriform plate of the ethmoid bone and project to the ipsilateral olfactory bulb where they target central neurons. Olfactory receptor cells are surrounded and cushioned by the supporting cells. The supporting cells (sustentacular cells) have their nuclei in the upper one third of the epithelium. They have cigar-shaped, elongated nuclei. Olfactory receptor cells are equipped with radiating cilia, whereas the supporting cells have microvilli at their apical surface. The basal cells have their nuclei in the lower one third of the epithelium at the base of the epithelium. They are precursor cells and actively divide after birth to replace olfactory receptor cells. The life span of olfactory receptor cells is 30–60 days. They undergo continuous replacement through the basal stem cell population [10]. Bowman's glands in the connective tissue secrete mucus to prevent constant olfactory stimulation. Bowman's glands have a duct to the surface of the olfactory epithelium. Their secretion produces a fluid environment around the olfactory cilia and may clear the cilia, facilitating the access of new odor substances. In addition, the mucus creates the ionic milieu around the cilia and contains an odorant-binding protein to trap odorants and to bring them to cilia.

The olfactory epithelium in the nose is part of the respiratory system. The primary function of the respiratory system is respiration, that is, the system provides the gas exchange between air and blood, so blood becomes oxygenated. The part of the system involved in gas exchange is the lungs. Another part of the system is a branching system of airways that brings air to and from lungs via the respiratory movements of thoracic walls and diaphragm. This part carries out a second function of the system, which is a somewhat minor function, namely, it humidifies the air, cleans the air, and warms the air. It works more like an air-conditioning system. Along the same line, we can divide the system into two principal regions. The conducting portion includes the parts of the respiratory system that are responsible for supplying the lungs with air: nasal cavities with olfactory areas, nasopharynx, larynx and epiglottis, trachea, bronchi, bronchioles, and terminal bronchioles. The respiratory portion is the site of gas exchange and includes the respiratory bronchioles, alveolar ducts and sacs, and alveoli. The olfactory epithelium is much thicker than the respiratory epithelium, which is found in the nose and the respiratory tract, whereas the olfactory epithelium is found only on the roof of nasal cavity. The respiratory epithelium contains goblet cells that secret a mucus which covers the epithelium and traps dust particles. Goblet cells are absent from the olfactory epithelium.

3. Olfactory receptor cells and transduction

Olfactory receptor cells have a distinct dendritic process that extends to the surface of the epithelium where its tip is expanded into a club-shaped prominence, the olfactory vesicle. This bears cilia, which have the typical 9 + 2 microtubule arrangement for some of their length, but there is a long distal portion, which contains only the two central microtubule fibers. In contrast to cilia in the respiratory epithelium, the olfactory cilia (5–20) are almost immotile, and they are inserted into basal bodies in the olfactory vesicle. It is in the cilia of olfactory receptor cells where olfactory transduction takes place, that is, the conversion of an odor signal into an electrical signal. Odorant molecules bind to olfactory receptor proteins and trigger a signaling cascade that involves G-proteins and leads to the generation of action potentials (nerve impulses). These nerve impulses are sent to the brain, specifically, to the olfactory bulb.

All olfactory receptor proteins are part of a family of G-protein-coupled receptors that are expressed in the olfactory epithelium [11–13]. There are many different odor receptor proteins and genes that encode them, with more than 1000 in the mammalian genome. Not all of these potential odor receptor genes are expressed and functional. The olfactory receptor multigene family consists of around 400 genes in humans and 1400 genes in mice [14–17]. According to an analysis of data derived from the Human Genome Project, humans have approximately 400 functional genes coding for olfactory receptors, and about 600 candidates are pseudogenes [14]. It implies that a human nose has around 400 types of scent receptors or ~ 400 different functional olfactory receptors. This is a large number since the entire human genome has only ~20,000–25,000 genes. It implies that ~2% of our genes are coding for olfactory receptors. Each olfactory receptor cell in the olfactory epithelium expresses only one of these 1000 olfactory receptor genes [18]. The expression of olfactory receptor genes is confined to four different zones of the olfactory epithelium [19–21]. Olfactory receptor cells that express the same olfactory receptor are found in only one of the four zones and they project to the same glomerulus in the olfactory bulb. The cells are randomly distributed in a given zone.

Olfactory receptor cells respond to several different odor-causing chemicals. Each receptor cell type can respond to more than one odorant. A given odorant can activate one or more receptor cells. Different types of receptor cells can respond not only to the same but also to different odorants. When an odorant ligand binds to a receptor protein, these proteins initiate a G-protein mechanism, which uses cyclic AMP (cAMP) or inositol triphosphate (IP3) as a second messenger [22]. The intracellular messengers open sodium and calcium channels, which results in depolarization of the receptor membrane that then triggers an action potential.

4. The olfactory pathway

The olfactory pathway starts with olfactory receptor neurons in the olfactory epithelium that send their axons to the ipsilateral olfactory bulb. There, they make synaptic contacts with central neurons in spherical structures, the olfactory glomeruli (2000 per bulb in the mouse). In the olfactory bulb, sensory information is processed in olfactory glomeruli. Each glomerulus is a discrete anatomical and functional unit and serves as an anatomical address dedicated to collecting and processing of specific molecular features about the olfactory environment conveyed to it by olfactory receptor cell axons expressing specific olfactory receptor proteins [23–25]. Thus, the glomeruli in the olfactory bulbs are organized chemotopically [26, 27], analogous to visuotopy, in visual systems, and tonotopy, in auditory systems. Olfactory information is extensively processed at the level of the glomeruli through feedforward and feedback inhibition and modulation provided by centrifugal neurons. Information is subsequently conveyed to higher-order olfactory center such as the olfactory cortex in vertebrates.

Olfactory receptor cells in the olfactory epithelium that have the same type of olfactory receptor, that is, they express the same olfactory receptor gene (1 of ~1000), send their axons to the same glomerulus (1 of 2000) in the olfactory bulb. This is an example of sensory axons converging on one glomerulus in the brain. In the olfactory bulb, olfactory receptor cell axons synapse on mitral/tufted cells. Glomerular mitral/tufted cells process odor signals coming from the nasal olfactory epithelium. The central neurons in the olfactory bulb, such as the mitral and tufted cells, project to higher olfactory centers. Twenty to 50 neurons output neurons (mitral/tufted cells), innervate each glomerulus, and project out of the olfactory bulb. Mitral cells that innervate different glomeruli typically respond to different types of odorants. A given odorant can activate mitral cells in several or many glomeruli. Odorant identity can be encoded through a combination of olfactory receptors, where each olfactory receptor detects one molecular feature of the odorant. Mitral and tufted cells send their axons through the lateral olfactory tract to the olfactory cortex, which includes the anterior olfactory nucleus, the piriform cortex, parts of the amygdala, the olfactory tubercle, and parts of the entorhinal cortex. From the amygdala, olfactory information is passed on to the hypothalamus and from the entorhinal cortex to the hippocampus. Olfactory information can be sent to the orbitofrontal cortex through the thalamus from olfactory cortical areas, except the anterior olfactory nucleus. Centrifugal fibers that originate outside of the olfactory bulb project to the olfactory bulb from the basal forebrain (horizontal limb of the diagonal band) and midbrain (locus coeruleus and raphe). The functional significance is a possible modulation of olfactory processing during different behavioral states.

Olfactory disorders and dysfunctions have received attention because they can result in serious problems, such as our inability to smell warning odors (fire, gas) and an impaired ability to taste food through retronasal stimulation of olfactory receptors [3]. Anosmia (loss of smell) and hyposmia (diminished smell) result from a number of etiologies. Specific anosmia refers to lowered sensitivity to a specific odorant and general anosmia denotes complete lack of olfactory sensation. Dysosmia (distorted smell) and phantosmia (phantom smells) may accompany these conditions. Cacosmia refers to olfactory hallucinations of repugnant smells.

5. Olfaction and gustation

Olfaction and gustation are our chemical senses and share a number of similarities and differences. Both senses extract information from the chemical stimuli in the environment, respond to a wide array of chemicals, and use G-protein-coupled receptors. However, in taste, this transduction mechanism is limited to sweet, bitter, and umami, whereas salty and sour use other signaling mechanisms. Receptor cells in olfaction and gustation show strong adaptation during continued stimulation and they undergo turnover and replacement throughout life. Both chemical senses provide important information for our survival and play a role in food selection and protect us from ingesting toxins. One difference between the two sensory systems is the fact that olfactory receptor cells are neurons and taste receptor cells are modified epithelial cells. Our understanding of the coding of taste qualities is better than that of odor quality. While olfactory stimuli evoke many sensations, no clear odor qualities have been described. The success of the perfume industry tells about the importance of olfactory stimuli as social cues.

Acknowledgements

This work was supported in part by grants from the National Science Foundation (NSF IOS-1355034) to Thomas Heinbockel.

Conflict of interest

The authors declare that there is no conflict of interests regarding the publication of this chapter.

Author details

Thomas Heinbockel* and Balwant S. Gendeh
Department of Anatomy, Howard University College of Medicine, Washington, DC, USA

*Address all correspondence to: theinbockel@howard.edu

References

[1] Souder E, Yoder L. Olfaction: The neglected sense. The Journal of Neuroscience Nursing. 1992;**24**(5): 273-280. DOI: 10.1097/01376517-199210000-00009

[2] Hoffman HJ, Rawal S, Li CM, Duffy VB. New chemosensory component in the U.S. National Health and nutrition examination survey (NHANES): First-year results for measured olfactory dysfunction. Reviews in Endocrine & Metabolic Disorders. 2016;**17**:221-240

[3] Ruggiero GF, Wick JY. Olfaction: New understandings, diagnostic applications. The Consultant Pharmacist. 2016;**31**(11):624-632. DOI: 10.4140/TCP.n.2016.624

[4] Mainland JD, Barlow LA, Munger SD, Millar SE, Vergara MN, Jiang P, et al. Identifying treatments for taste and smell disorders: Gaps and opportunities. Chemical Senses. 2020:bjaa038. DOI: 10.1093/chemse/bjaa038

[5] Pellegrino R, Cooper KW, Di Pizio A, Joseph PV, Bhutani S, Parma V. Corona viruses and the chemical senses: past, present, and future. Chemical Senses. 2020:bjaa031. DOI: 10.1093/chemse/bjaa031

[6] Parma V, Ohla K, Veldhuizen MG, et al. More than smell - COVID-19 is associated with severe impairment of smell, taste, and chemesthesis. Chemical Senses. 2020:bjaa041. DOI: 10.1093/chemse/bjaa041

[7] Cooper KW, Brann DH, Farruggia MC, Bhutani S, Pellegrino R, Tsukahara T, et al. Di Pizio a COVID-19 and the chemical senses: Supporting players take center stage. Neuron. 2020;**107**(2):219-233. DOI: 10.1016/j.neuron.2020.06.032

[8] Brann DH, Tsukahara T, Weinreb C, Lipovsek M, Van den Berge K, Gong B, et al. Non-neuronal expression of SARS-CoV-2 entry genes in the olfactory system suggests mechanisms underlying COVID-19-associated anosmia. Science Advances. 2020;**6**(31):eabc5801. DOI: 10.1126/sciadv.abc5801

[9] Bushdid C, Magnasco MO, Vosshall LB, Keller A. Humans can discriminate more than 1 trillion olfactory stimuli. Science. 2014;**343**:1370-1372. DOI: 10.1126/science.1249168

[10] Sokpor G, Abbas E, Rosenbusch J, Staiger JF, Tuoc T. Transcriptional and epigenetic control of mammalian olfactory epithelium development. Molecular Neurobiology. 2018;**55**(11): 8306-8327. DOI: 10.1007/s12035-018-0987-y

[11] Young JM, Friedman C, Williams EM, Ross JA, Tonnes-Priddy L, Trask BJ. Different evolutionary processes shaped the mouse and human olfactory receptor gene families. Human Molecular Genetics. 2002;**5**:535-546

[12] Axel R. Scents and sensibility: A molecular logic of olfactory perception (Nobel lecture). Angewandte Chemie (International Ed. in English). 2005;**44**(38):6110-6127. DOI: 10.1002/anie.200501726

[13] Buck LB. Unraveling the sense of smell (Nobel lecture). Angewandte Chemie (International Ed. in English). 2005;**44**(38):6128-6140. DOI: 10.1002/anie.200501120

[14] Gilad Y, Lancet D. Population differences in the human functional olfactory repertoire. Molecular Biology and Evolution. 2003;**20**(3):307-314

[15] Niimura Y. Evolutionary dynamics of olfactory receptor genes in chordates:

Interaction between environments and genomic contents. Human Genomics. 2009;**4**(2):107-118

[16] Mainland JD, Keller A, Li YR, Zhou T, Trimmer C, Snyder LL, et al. The missense of smell: Functional variability in the human odorant receptor repertoire. Nature Neuroscience. 2013;**17**(1):114-120. DOI: 10.1038/nn.3598

[17] Hayden S, Teeling EC. The molecular biology of vertebrate olfaction. The Anatomical Record. 2014;**297**:2216-2226. DOI: doi.org/10.1002/ar.23031

[18] Buck L, Axel R. A novel multigene family may encode odorant receptors: A molecular basis for odor recognition. Cell. 1991;**65**(1):175-187

[19] Ressler KJ, Sullivan SL, Buck LB. A zonal organization of odorant receptor gene expression in the olfactory epithelium. Cell. 1993;**73**(3):597-609. DOI: 10.1016/0092-8674(93)90145-g

[20] Buck LB. Receptor diversity and spatial patterning in the mammalian olfactory system. Ciba Foundation Symposium. 1993;**179**: 51-64; discussion 64-7, 88-96. DOI: 10.1002/9780470514511.ch4

[21] Sullivan SL, Ressler KJ, Buck LB. Odorant receptor diversity and patterned gene expression in the mammalian olfactory epithelium. Progress in Clinical and Biological Research. 1994;**390**:75-84

[22] Zufall F, Munger SD. From odor and pheromone transduction to the organization of the sense of smell. Trends in Neurosciences. 2001;**24**(4):191-193. DOI: 10.1016/s0166-2236(00)01765-3

[23] Buck LB. Information coding in the vertebrate olfactory system. Annual Review of Neuroscience. 1996;**19**:517-544

[24] Buonviso N, Chaput MA. Response similarity of odors in olfactory bulb output cells presumed to be connected to the same glomerulus: Electrophysiological study using simultaneous single-unit recordings. Journal of Neurophysiology. 1990;**63**(3):447-454

[25] Mombaerts P. Targeting olfaction. Current Opinion in Neurobiology. 1996;**6**(4):481-486

[26] Sharp FR, Kauer JS, Shepherd GM. Local sites of activity-related glucose metabolism in rat olfactory bulb during olfactory stimulation. Brain Research. 1975;**98**(3):596-600

[27] Friedrich RW, Korsching SI. Combinatorial and chemotopic odorant coding in the zebrafish olfactory bulb visualized by optical imaging. Neuron. 1997;**18**(5):737-752

Chapter 2

Imaging in Sinonasal Disorders

Heidi Beate Eggesbø

Abstract

Computed tomography (CT) is the "working horse" in sinonasal imaging and should always be the first choice. Magnetic resonance imaging (MRI) is complementary to CT when complications to rhinosinusitis or neoplasm are suspected. Imaging of the paranasal sinuses is common due to stuffy nose. In order to correct interpretation, proper imaging technique as well as knowledge of bony anatomy and variants and mucosal incidental findings are of outmost importance. Acute rhinosinusitis is very common and does not need imaging unless complications are suspected. In chronic rhinosinusitis, a CT examination is needed to find the cause and site of the mucociliary obstruction and to rule out other causes as odontogenic and fungal sinusitis and neoplasms.

Keywords: paranasal sinuses, computed tomography, magnetic resonance imaging, retention cysts, polyps, mucocele, pyocele, rhinosinusitis, odontogenic sinusitis, fungal sinusitis, neoplasms, systemic diseases

1. Introduction

Computed tomography (CT) is the "working horse" in sinonasal imaging and should always be the first choice. Magnetic resonance imaging (MRI) is complementary to CT when complications to rhinosinusitis or neoplasm are suspected.

Imaging of the paranasal sinuses is common due to stuffy nose. In order to correct interpretation, proper imaging technique as well as knowledge of bony anatomy and variants and mucosal incidental findings are of outmost importance.

Imaging should be performed when the stuffy nose and rhinosinusitis do not heal despite medical therapy. Acute rhinosinusitis (ARS) is usually self-limiting, and imaging is only indicated when complications are suspected.

In chronic rhinosinusitis, a CT examination is needed to find the cause and site of the mucociliary obstruction and to rule out other causes as odontogenic and fungal sinusitis and neoplasms.

2. Imaging techniques

Imaging of the paranasal sinuses should always start with CT. CT delineates both bony anatomy and possible sinonasal opacifications.

Odontogenic pathology in the upper jaw often involves the maxillary sinuses. Hence, it is of outmost importance that the upper jaw teeth are included in the image volume and that this area is included in the radiological report [1].

Post-processing of the CT images usually include only reconstruction with bone algorithm in three planes. However, in case of opacification, soft tissue algorithm offers important details of the sinus content [2].

IntechOpen

Reconstruction with bone algorithm should be done with slices no thicker than 1 mm. Thin slices are important for evaluation of periapical tooth lucencies as seen in odontogenic sinusitis and for erosion and destruction of bone in case of malignant disorders.

Additional reconstruction with soft tissue algorithm, with 2.5-mm-thick slices, may be extremely valuable and mandatory in case of soft tissue pathology inside or outside the sinus walls. In the case of pyocele or allergic fungal sinusitis, the attenuation usually is higher than mucus [3], and a fungus ball (mycetoma) has typical scattered microcalcifications that are better presented on soft tissue algorithm. In the case of invasive fungal sinusitis, this can be diagnosed by obliteration of the fat planes outside the sinus walls that is best seen on soft tissue algorithm.

Magnetic resonance imaging (MRI) is complementary to CT when complications to infection and neoplasms must be assessed.

Low-dose CT (<20 mAs), without intravenous contrast medium, usually will be sufficient for "screening." However, if complications or malignant disease are suspected, CT should be performed with at least 50 mAs and with intravenous contrast medium administration.

3. Retention cysts and polyps

Retention cysts, mucinous or serous, are common findings and appear as smooth, convex soft tissue masses from the mucosal lining (**Figure 1a** and **b**) and should not be mistaken as fluid (**Figure 2**). The floor of the maxillary sinus is the most common site for retention cysts.

Mucinous retention cysts are due to obstruction of a mucinous gland, while serous retention cysts are caused by accumulation of fluid in the submucosal layer. Hence, they are not "true" cysts and therefore are also referred to as pseudocysts [4]. Retention cysts have no clinical significance and usually show no significant change in size by time [5].

Odontogenic cysts may mimic retention cysts. However, CT with bone algorithm and thin slices may reveal a tiny, peripheral calcification that will differentiate these from retention cysts (**Figure 3a** and **b**).

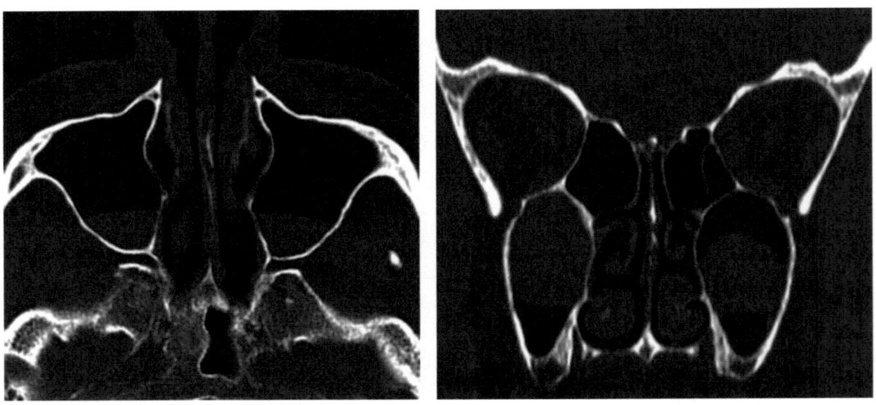

(a) (b)

Figure 1.
(a) Axial CT shows maxillary sinus retention cyst bilaterally from the posterior wall with dome-shaped appearance with upward convexity. (b) Coronal CT clearly reveals the cystic appearance.

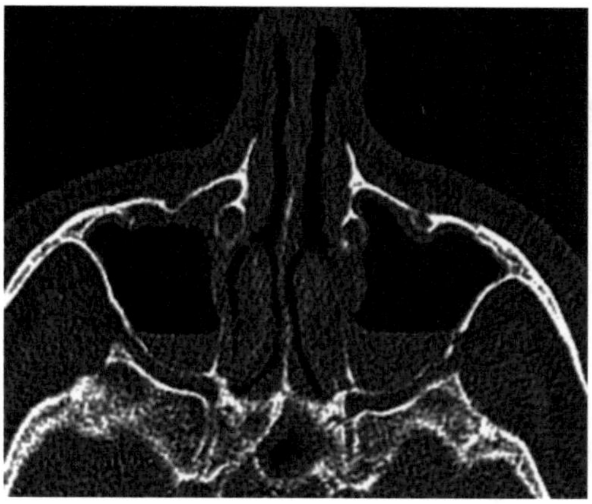

Figure 2.
Axial CT demonstrates bilateral maxillary sinus fluid. In contrast to retention cysts, fluid has upward concavity due to the fluid that settles along the sinus walls.

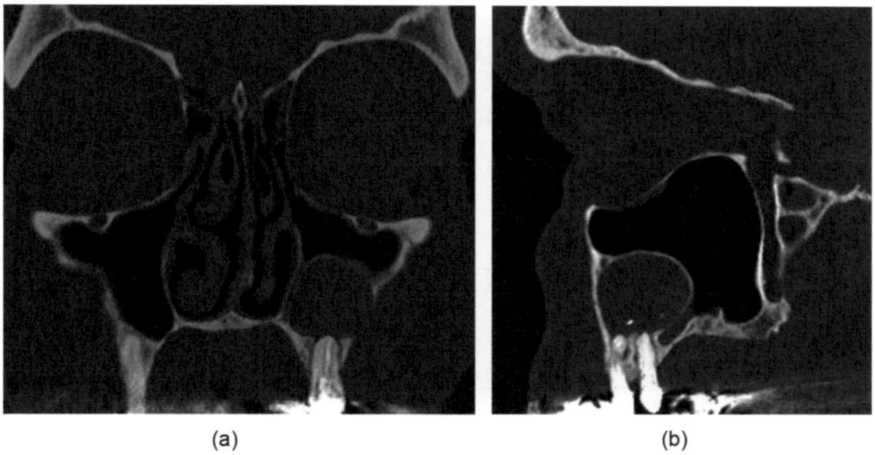

Figure 3.
(a) Coronal CT and (b) sagittal CT show an odontogenic cyst with characteristic peripheral calcification. Odontogenic cysts may persist, despite dental treatment.

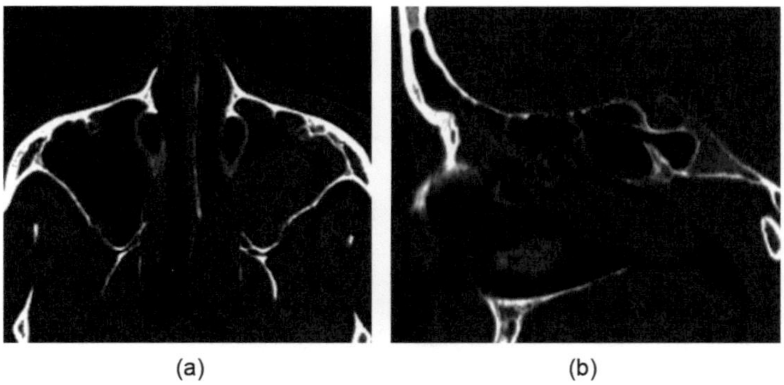

Figure 4.
(a) Coronal CT and (b) sagittal CT reveal a large pseudocyst growing out of the left maxillary sinus into the nasal cavity and choana forming an antrochoanal polyp.

When more fluid is accumulated in the retention cysts, they may grow out of the maxillary sinus through the ethmoid infundibulum or the accessory maxillary ostium into the nasal cavity and choana and then be referred to as an antrochoanal polyp [4] (**Figure 4a** and **b**).

Pseudocysts are often referred to as a polyp in the radiological report. However, polyps contain more fibrous connective tissue than pseudocyst and tend to be more fibrotic. Hence polyps can surgically be removed intact, but not pseudocysts [4]. Pseudocysts may also rupture spontaneously or traumatically, causing unilateral rhinorrhea [6].

4. Acute rhinosinusitis and complications

Acute rhinosinusitis (ARS), defined as symptoms less than 4 weeks, is the most common disease of the paranasal sinuses. Fluid is often an incidental finding at CT (**Figure 2**) and should not be misinterpreted as ARS. Mucosal thickening and air bubbles in the opacification can be interpreted as ARS, if clinical symptoms harmonize [7] (**Figure 5a** and **b**).

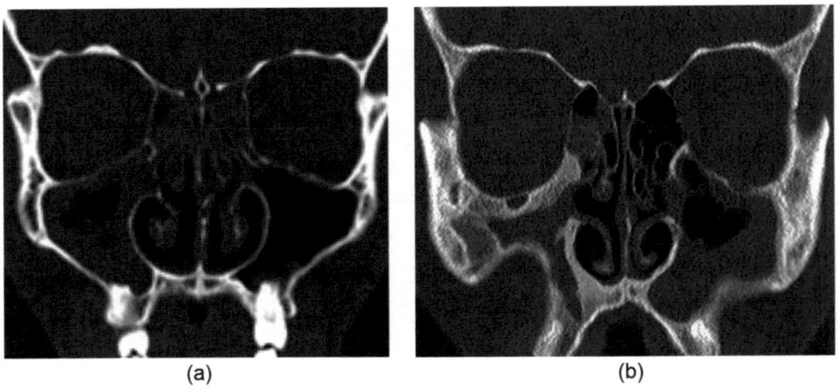

Figure 5.
(a) Coronal CT shows right-sided maxillary opacification with air bubbles consistent with acute rhinosinusitis. (b) Coronal CT shows thick, sclerotic right maxillary sinus walls that indicate a long-standing infection. In addition, the sinus walls are retracted due to a vacuum effect, referred to as sinus silent syndrome. In the left maxillary sinus, the opacification contains air bubbles consistent with an active bacterial infection.

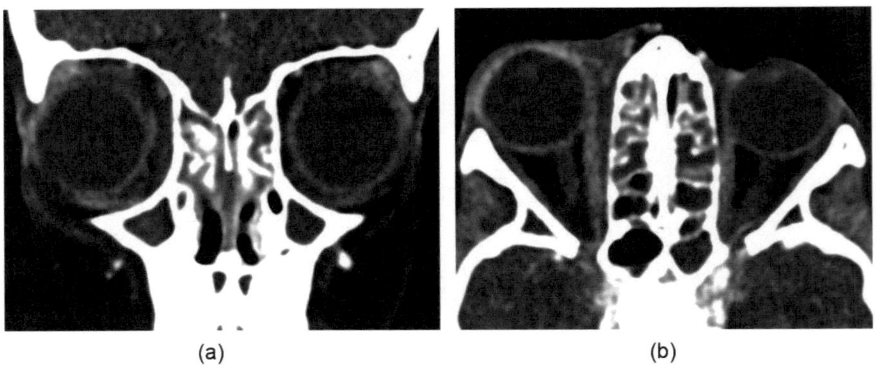

Figure 6.
(a) Coronal and (b) axial CT of a 6-year-old boy with complication to acute rhinosinusitis. The infection has spread through the thin lamina papyracea on the right side, and there is stranding of the fat preseptal and postseptal (intraorbital), consistent with phlegmon. Notice also the marked proptosis of the affected side and slightly lateral displacement of the medial rectus muscle.

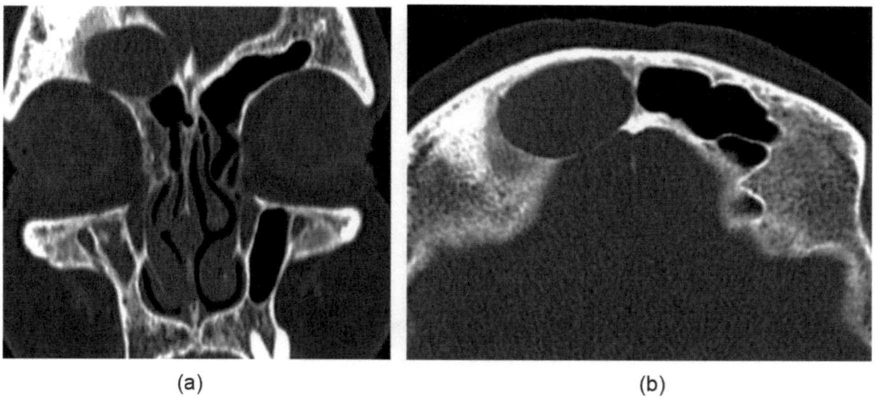

Figure 7.
(a) Coronal CT in a patient with granulomatosis with polyangiitis shows a frontal sinus mucocele/pyocele due to obstruction of the frontal recess. By time remodelling of bone may cause erosion into the orbit. (b) Axial CT demonstrates erosion of the posterior sinus wall and risk of intracranial involvement.

In acute rhinosinusitis, imaging is only indicated when complications are suspected. Extra-sinonasal spread of infection is rare but needs urgent treatment. Children are at most risk. Intraorbital spread from ethmoid and frontal ARS is the most common complication and may present as cellulitis, subperiosteal or intraorbital phlegmon and abscess, and lateral displacement of the medial rectus muscle (**Figure 6a** and **b**). The clinical presentation may be forward protrusion of the eyeball, proptosis [8–10].

Intracranial spread is most commonly seen in frontal and ethmoid ARS and presents as complications that include epidural and brain abscesses, subdural empyema, meningitis, and cavernous sinus thrombosis [11].

Mucocele and pyocele if not treated may also erode into the orbit and cranial cavity by time (**Figure 7a** and **b**) or erode the anterior frontal bone resulting in a subcutaneous abscess, referred to as Pott's puffy tumor.

A recent study has focused on the intake of ibuprofen in children as a risk factor for developing orbital and intracranial complications of ARS [12].

5. Chronic rhinosinusitis and complications

An underlying odontogenic infection is reported to be the cause in up to 40% of chronic rhinosinusitis (CRS). In addition, several other conditions may mimic rhinosinusitis and challenge the radiological interpretation.

Five distinct radiological inflammatory patterns have been described, each with a different therapeutic course and surgical options [13], where the first three are caused by obstruction of the mucociliary flow. Obstruction of the maxillary sinus drainage is the most common. The level of obstruction is at the ostium and the thin ethmoid infundibulum and referred to as infundibular pattern. Obstruction of the middle meatus, the common drainage way for the frontal, anterior ethmoid, and maxillary sinuses, will cause obstruction of ipsilateral sinuses and is referred to as ostiomeatal (from ostium and meatus) complex (OMC) pattern. Less common is obstruction of the sphenoethmoidal recess that drains the posterior ethmoid and sphenoid sinuses. The two last patterns are sinonasal polyposis and incidental findings.

Surgical intervention of mucociliary obstruction is referred to as functional endoscopic sinus surgery (FESS). Functional refers to the widening of the natural ostia. For the infundibular and OMC inflammatory pattern, FESS includes uncinectomy (removing the uncinate process), opening the ethmoid infundibulum, and making a larger opening to the antrum (maxillary sinus) referred to as media-antrostomy.

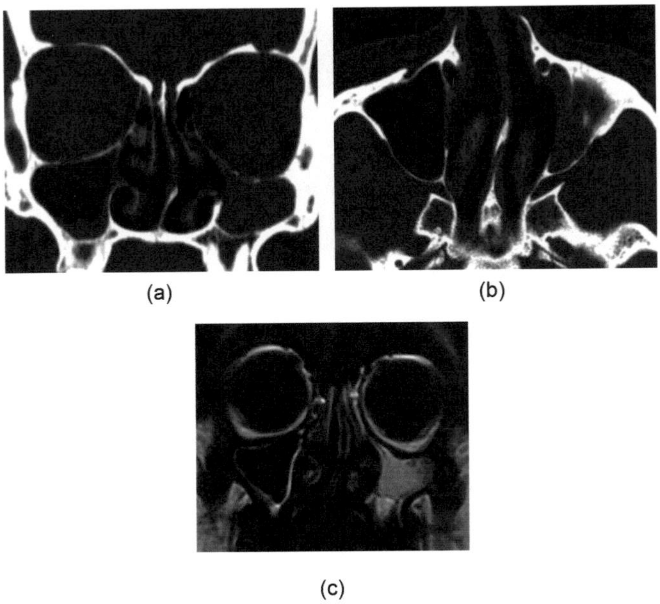

Figure 8.
(a) Coronal CT and (b) axial CT demonstrate a left-sided hypoplastic maxillary sinus with a retracted posterior fontanelle (lateral nasal wall) that mimic chronic rhinosinusitis. (c) On coronal MRI with T2 sequence, the sinus content is equal to mucus. There is no bowing of the sinus walls as typical for mucocele.

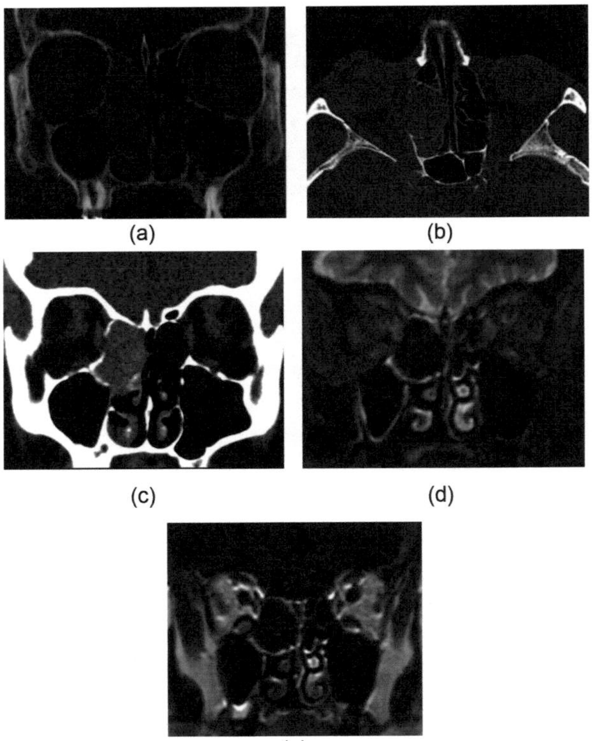

Figure 9.
(a) Coronal CT and (b) axial CT with bone algorithm and (b) with soft tissue algorithm demonstrate a pyocele (superinfected mucocele). (c) Coronal CT with soft tissue algorithm shows high attenuation more characteristic for a pyocele than a mucocele. (d) Coronal MRI T2 with fat suppression shows characteristic signal void of the pyocele. (e) Coronal MRI T1 with gadolinium shows contrast medium enhancement only in the peripheral mucosal lining.

Sometimes ethmoidectomy also is performed during FESS. Therefore, the course of the anterior ethmoid artery should be included in the radiological report.

Complications to CRS are bone thickening (sclerosis, osteitis, neo-osteogenesis), demineralization and erosion of bone, and a negative sinus pressure that can cause infoldings of the sinus walls, referred to as silent sinus syndrome (**Figure 5b**), which may result in larger orbit and cause enophthalmos and diplopia.

Hypoplastic maxillary sinus with retracted posterior fontanelle (**Figure 8a–c**) may mimic silent sinus syndrome but usually has no clinical impact despite the mucus-filled sinus (**Figure 8c**).

In addition, retracted posterior fontanelle should not be confused with a mucocele that remodels and expands the sinus. A bacterial superinfection of a mucocele will result in a pyocele. A pyocele has characteristic CT and MR findings compared to a mucocele (**Figure 9a–e**).

6. Odontogenic sinusitis

Odontogenic sinusitis should be suspected when maxillary sinusitis does not heal [14, 15]. This is especially in the case of unilateral CRS (**Figure 10a** and **b**), but odontogenic infection may also be the source of bilateral CRS. Before referring to FESS, due to maxillary sinus opacification, odontogenic maxillary sinusitis must be ruled out. FESS in odontogenic cases may induce more inflammation and osteitis [1]. Odontogenic sinusitis and sinonasal complications of dental disease or treatment represent a heterogeneous group of conditions that often require multidisciplinary care [17].

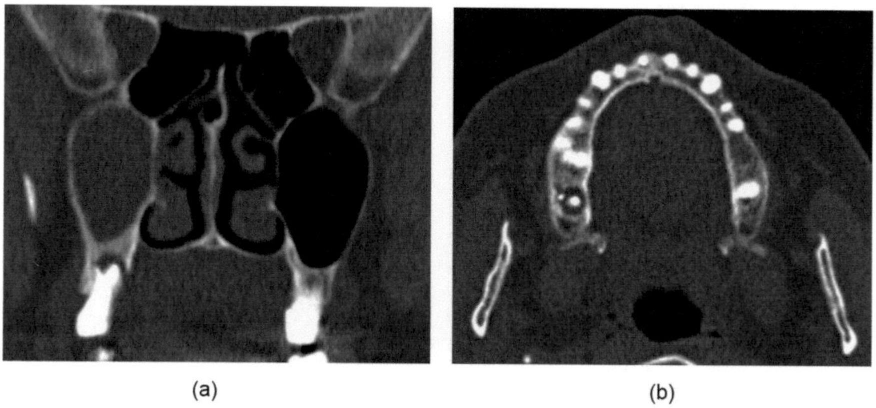

Figure 10.
(a) Coronal CT and (b) axial CT reveal periapical lucency around a molar tooth [16] consistent with odontogenic infection as the cause of sinusitis. The sclerotic maxillary sinus walls indicate a long-standing infection.

7. Fungal sinusitis

Fungal sinusitis can be noninvasive, which includes fungus ball (mycetoma) (**Figure 11a–c**) and allergic fungal sinusitis (**Figure 12a–d**), or invasive with an acute, chronic, or granulomatous course [16].

Invasive fungal sinusitis is revealed by fungal deposits outside the sinus walls that obliterate the fat plane. The sinus wall usually is sclerotic and intact, and the spread of fungus is by the vessels through the bone (**Figure 13a–d**). Demineralization and erosion of the lateral nasal wall is usually seen when the maxillary sinus is involved. Invasive fungal sinusitis is most common in immunocompromised patients.

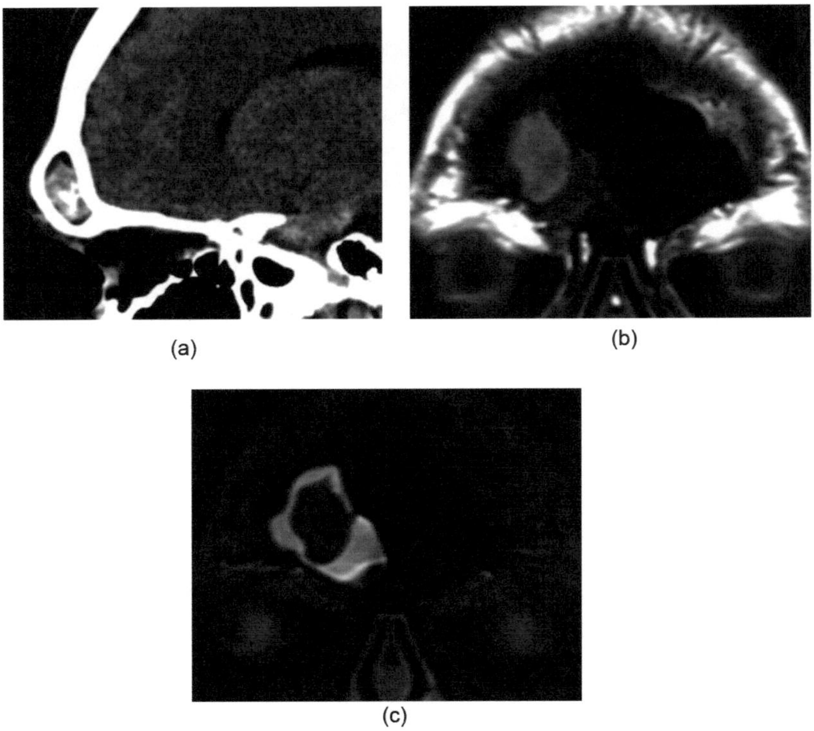

Figure 11.
(a) Sagittal CT shows scattered calcifications in the frontal sinus opacification consistent with a fungus ball (mycetoma). (b) Coronal MRI T1 shows the central fungus ball as high signal surrounded by low signal from edematous thickened mucosal lining, while (c) coronal MRI T2 shows fungus ball with low signal, surrounded by high signal mucosal lining. The low signal is explained by the by the iron and manganese contents in the fungi.

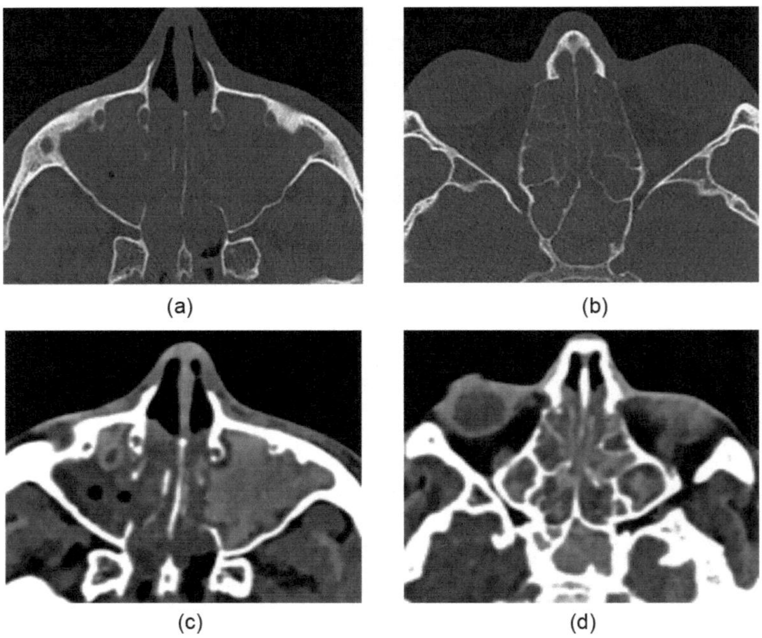

Figure 12.
Axial CT at the level of the (a) maxillary and (b) ethmoid sinuses shows panopacification. Reconstruction, with soft tissue algorithm (c) and (d), shows high attenuation in all sinuses, which is typical for allergic fungal sinusitis. Slightly thickened, sclerotic sinus walls indicate a long-standing condition.

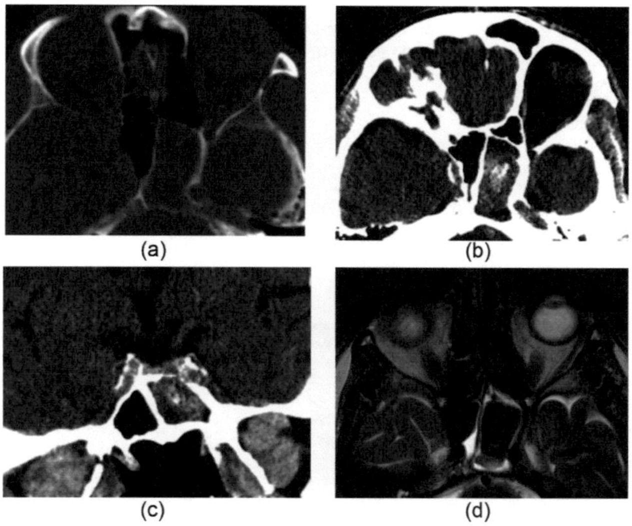

Figure 13.
A 53-year-old man, who presented with diplopia. (a) Axial CT with bone algorithm was reported as chronic sphenoid sinusitis. The patient did not improve on antibiotic treatment. (b) A new examination with cerebral CT and reconstruction with soft tissue algorithm revealed scattered calcifications in the opacification and (c) erosion of the thickened, sclerotic bone, consistent with invasive fungal infection to the cavernous sinus and hence possible affection of the cranial nerves 3, 4, 5, and 6 that pass through the cavernous sinus. (d) Axial MRI with T2 sequence shows fungi with low signal surrounded by mucosal lining with high signal.

8. Systemic diseases

Several systemic diseases have sinonasal manifestations [18]. One of these is granulomatosis with polyangiitis (GPA) (formerly Wegener's granulomatosis), with a prevalence of 10–25/100,000. Age group mostly affected is 50–70 years. Oral and sinonasal manifestations are seen in 85%.

Both extensive bone osteoneogenesis (osteitis) and destructions seen in GPA imaging are used to assess disease activity even though little is known about CT or

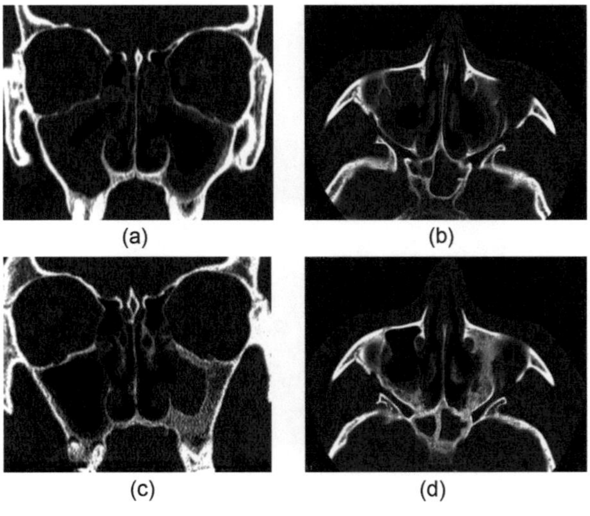

Figure 14.
(a) Coronal CT and (b) axial CT in granulomatosis with polyangiitis show status after bilateral endoscopic sinus surgery (media-antrostomy). The bone is thickened due to chronic osteitis. Notice small peripheral rim of osteoneogenesis along the lining of the left maxillary sinus. (c) Coronal CT and (d) axial CT, follow-up CT 5 years later, demonstrate extensive bilateral osteitis of the maxillary and sphenoid sinuses. Notice also the small periapical lucencies around the roots of the right upper molar, often seen in patients with granulomatosis with polyangiitis.

MRI findings that may indicate poor prognosis [19]. Sinonasal surgery in GPA is debated [20] and may cause increased osteoneogenesis (**Figure 14a–c**).

9. Neoplasms

Osteoma is one of the most common benign neoplasms in the paranasal sinuses (**Figure 15a** and **b**), followed by fibrous dysplasia (**Figure 16a–c**) and inverted papillomas (IP) (**Figure 17a–c**).

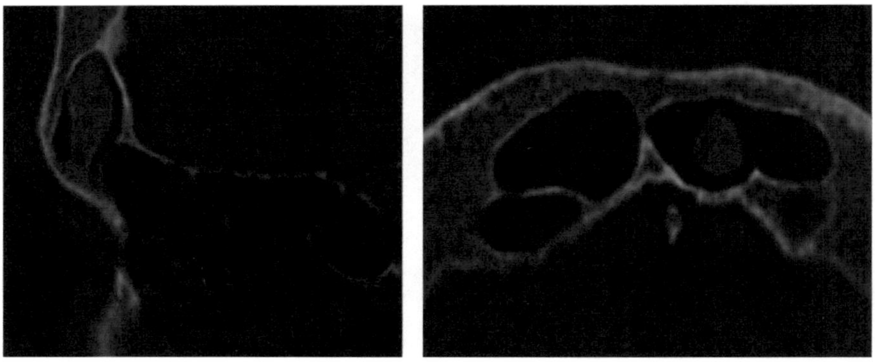

(a) (b)

Figure 15.
(a) Sagittal and (b) axial CT of an osteoma in the frontal sinus. Unless obstruction of the mucociliary drainage, osteomas have no clinical impact.

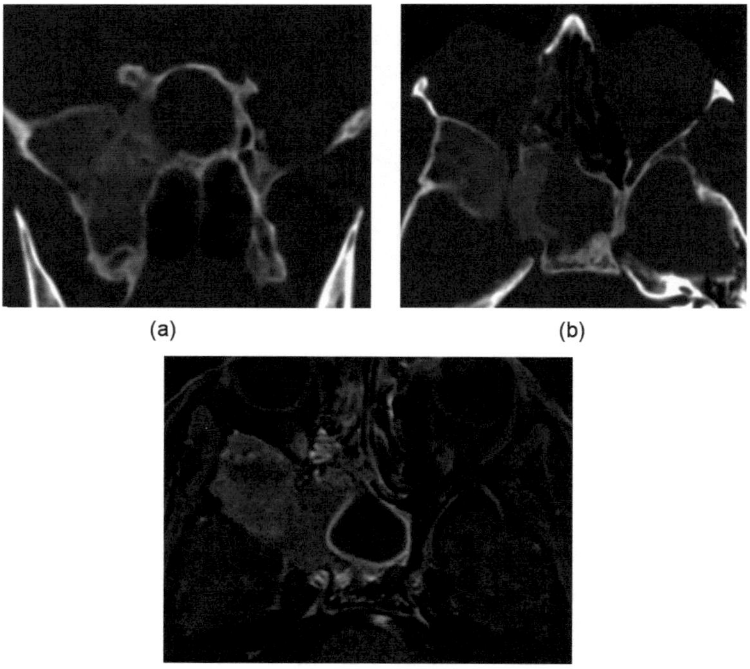

(a) (b) (c)

Figure 16.
(a) Coronal CT and (b) axial CT demonstrate fibrous dysplasia, in the right sphenoid bone. The bone has characteristic "ground glass" appearance and encircles the foramen rotundum and the Vidian canal. In addition, the sphenoethmoid recess is obstructed and mucus entrapped in the right sphenoid sinus, with bowing of the sinus walls typical for mucocele and pyocele. (c) Axial MRI with T1 with gadolinium shows contrast medium enhancement limited to the mucosal lining. The low signal in the sinus is consistent with a mucocele.

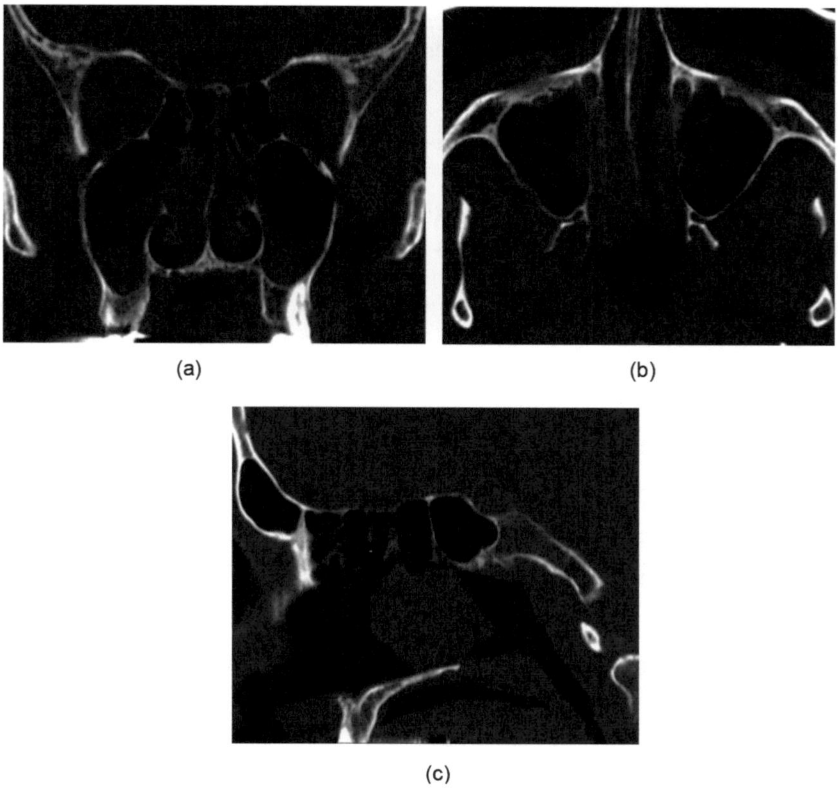

Figure 17.
(a) Coronal, (b) axial, and (c) sagittal CT of an inverted papilloma originating from the ethmoid sinus and filling the middle part of the nasal cavity and choana. The site of origin often shows hyperkeratosis. In this case the origin could be from beneath the ethmoid cells that shows slight keratosis at the sagittal CT.

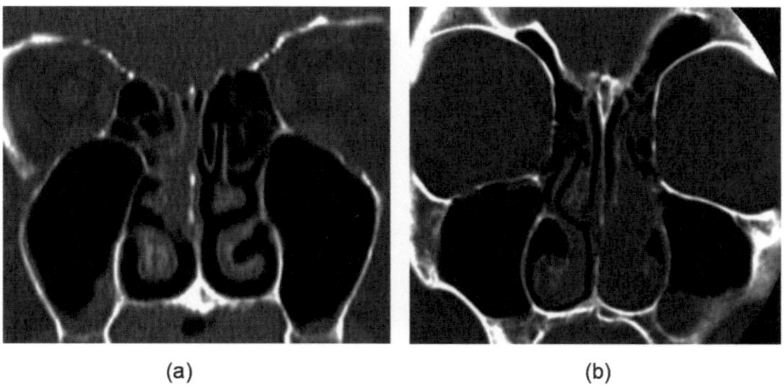

Figure 18.
(a) Coronal CT shows a tiny polyp in the right nasal cavity. Histopathology revealed olfactory neuroblastoma. (b) Coronal CT shows a polyp in the left nasal cavity, where histology revealed acinic cell carcinoma, which is a malignant salivary gland tumor. Malignancy in solitary polyps in the nasal cavity must always be ruled out.

IP is reported to be up to 5% of sinonasal tumors. Age group affected is 40–70 years, with a male preponderance. IP derives from the respiratory mucosa. The characteristic growth pattern with mucosal infoldings into the stroma is the origin to the name inverted. In most cases IP originates from the ethmoid sinuses and middle meatus [21]. Etiology is not confirmed, but a viral infection has been postulated as a cause [22].

Though initially benign, the recurrence rate is up to 25%, and malignant transformation is common, especially in smokers.

IP may display characteristic hyperkeratosis at CT from where the IP origin in the sinus wall. Radiological reporting of the attachment site is important for complete surgical resection [23] (**Figure 17a–c**).

Malignant sinonasal tumors are rare, and squamous cell carcinomas are the most common (80%). Rarer malignant sinonasal neoplasms are adenocarcinoma, olfactory neuroblastoma (**Figure 18a**), salivary gland tumors (**Figure 18b**), chondrosarcoma, B- and T-cell lymphoma, and mucosal malignant melanoma.

Juvenile nasopharyngeal angiofibroma is a benign tumor in adolescent males that arises from testosterone-sensitive cells in the pterygoid plates [24].

10. Conclusion

Imaging of sinonasal disorders shows a wide specter of diseases. However, the most common cause to unilateral CRS is odontogenic infection.

Odontogenic infection, pyocele, and fungal sinusitis are very often not in the list of the radiologist's differential diagnoses and often due to wrong CT imaging technique.

Sinonasal malignancy is rare but should always be in mind, especially in unilateral disease.

Conflict of interest

The author declares no conflict of interest.

Author details

Heidi Beate Eggesbø
Division of Radiology and Nuclear Medicine, Oslo University Hospital, Oslo, Norway

*Address all correspondence to: h.b.eggesbo@medisin.uio.no

References

[1] Whyte A, Boeddinghaus R. Imaging of odontogenic sinusitis. Clinical Radiology. 2019;**74**(7):503-516

[2] Madani G, Beale TJ. Sinonasal inflammatory disease. Seminars in Ultrasound, CT, and MR. 2009;**30**(1):17-24

[3] Osguthorpe JD. Adult rhinosinusitis: Diagnosis and management. American Family Physician. 2001;**63**(1):69-76

[4] Gardner DG. Pseudocysts and retention cysts of the maxillary sinus. Oral Surgery, Oral Medicine, and Oral Pathology. 1984;**58**(5):561-567

[5] Wang JH, Jang YJ, Lee BJ. Natural course of retention cysts of the maxillary sinus: Long-term follow-up results. The Laryngoscope. 2007;**117**(2):341-344

[6] Hoang JK, Smith EC, Barboriak DP. Ruptured maxillary retention cyst: Cause of unilateral rhinorrhea after trauma. AJNR. American Journal of Neuroradiology. 2009;**30**(6):1121-1122

[7] Eggesbo HB. Radiological imaging of inflammatory lesions in the nasal cavity and paranasal sinuses. European Radiology. 2006;**16**(4):872-888

[8] Chandler JR, Langenbrunner DJ, Stevens ER. The pathogenesis of orbital complications in acute sinusitis. The Laryngoscope. 1970;**80**(9):1414-1428

[9] Sharma PK, Saikia B, Sharma R. Orbitocranial complications of acute sinusitis in children. The Journal of Emergency Medicine. 2014;**47**(3):282-285

[10] Nguyen VD, Singh AK, Altmeyer WB, Tantiwongkosi B. Demystifying orbital emergencies: A pictorial review. Radiographics. 2017;**37**(3):947-962

[11] Kou YF, Killeen D, Whittemore B, Farzal Z, Booth T, Swift D, et al. Intracranial complications of acute sinusitis in children: The role of endoscopic sinus surgery. International Journal of Pediatric Otorhinolaryngology. 2018;**110**:147-151

[12] Nicollas R, Moreddu E, Le Treut-Gay C, Mancini J, Akkari M, Mondain M, et al. Ibuprofen as risk-factor for complications of acute anterior sinusitis in children. European Annals of Otorhinolaryngology, Head and Neck Diseases. 2019

[13] Harnsberger HR, Babbel RW, Davis WL. The major obstructive inflammatory patterns of the sinonasal region seen on screening sinus computed tomography. Seminars in Ultrasound, CT, and MR. 1991;**12**(6):541-560

[14] Vestin Fredriksson M, Ohman A, Flygare L, Tano K. When maxillary sinusitis does not heal: Findings on CBCT scans of the sinuses with a particular focus on the occurrence of odontogenic causes of maxillary sinusitis. Laryngoscope Investigative Otolaryngology. 2017;**2**(6):442-446

[15] Ganguly R, Ramesh A. Odontogenic sinusitis: An underdiagnosed condition. Journal of the Massachusetts Dental Society. 2014;**63**(1):46-47

[16] Gavito-Higuera J, Mullins CB, Ramos-Duran L, Sandoval H, Akle N, Figueroa R. Sinonasal fungal infections and complications: A pictorial review. Journal of Clinical Imaging Science. 2016;**6**:23

[17] Saibene AM, Collura F, Pipolo C, Bulfamante AM, Lozza P, Maccari A, et al. Odontogenic rhinosinusitis and sinonasal complications of dental disease or treatment: Prospective validation of a classification and

treatment protocol. European Archives of Oto-Rhino-Laryngology. 2019;**276**(2):401-406

[18] Eggesbo HB. Imaging Rhinosinusitis. Rijeka: IntechOpen; 2011

[19] Holme SS, Moen JM, Kilian K, Haukeland H, Molberg O, Eggesbo HB. Development of CT-based methods for longitudinal analyses of paranasal sinus osteitis in granulomatosis with polyangiitis. BMC Medical Imaging. 2019;**19**(1):13

[20] Pagella F, Canzi P, Matti E, Giourgos G, Caporali R, Cavagna L. Sinonasal surgery in Wegener's granulomatosis: Is it time to go on? The Laryngoscope. 2011;**121**(12):2717-2718; author reply 9-20

[21] Khandekar S, Dive A, Mishra R, Upadhyaya N. Sinonasal inverted papilloma: A case report and mini review of histopathological features. Journal of Oral and Maxillofacial Pathology. 2015;**19**(3):405

[22] Wang MJ, Noel JE. Etiology of sinonasal inverted papilloma: A narrative review. World Journal of Otorhinolaryngology—Head and Neck Surgery. 2017;**3**(1):54-58

[23] Makihara S, Kariya S, Naito T, Uraguchi K, Matsumoto J, Noda Y, et al. Attachment-oriented endoscopic surgical management for inverted papillomas in the nasal cavity and paranasal sinuses. Auris, Nasus, Larynx. 2019;**46**(5):748-753

[24] Eggesbo HB. Imaging of sinonasal tumours. Cancer Imaging. 2012;**12**:136-152

Chapter 3

Sinusitis, Asthma and Headache

Fozia Masood

Abstract

Sinusitis is the infection of sinuses. Sinuses are four hollow cavities in face which are connected to nasal pathways to help moisten, warm and filter the air which we breathe in. Sinuses get irritated due to bacteria, virus and allergens. It is often associated with asthma and headache. Pressure in the sinuses is built by over production of mucous and leads to sinus headache. Asthma gets severe with the sinusitis as both are related to sino-nasal pathway. Treatment includes steroids, nasal decongestants, antibiotics and to avoid allergens which not only reduce the symptoms of asthma but also sinusitis. Acute sinusitis may turn into chronic sinusitis including narrowing of nasal passages, deviated septum and lumps in the nose (polyp). It can be treated with surgical procedures. The only way to prevent sinusitis is by precaution and medication. Post nasal drip may also associate with asthma causing bronchial constriction.

Keywords: sinusitis, sinus headache, sinus asthma, post nasal drip, treatment, factors, prevention

1. Introduction

Sinusitis is swelling or an inflammation of the tissue lining of the sinuses. Sinuses are hollow cavities anatomically located within the cheekbone, around the eyes and behind the nose. Physiologically sinuses are filled with air and contain mucous which helps in moisten, warm and filter the inhaled air. Pathophysiologically, when the sinuses get blocked by the mucous, viruses and bacteria can grow and cause infection in sinuses [1].

1.1 Types of sinusitis

There are basis four types of sinusitis or rhino sinusitis.

1.1.1 Acute sinusitis

Sudden onset with cold-like symptoms (runny and stuffy nose, fever, facial pain). It may last for 2–4 weeks.

1.1.2 Sub-acute sinusitis

It is usually the continuation of acute sinusitis which may last up to 12 weeks.

1.1.3 Recurrent acute sinusitis

It happens several times per year. Four or more episodes of acute sinusitis for 7 days in 1 year of period.

1.1.4 Chronic sinusitis

Persistent symptoms of sinusitis for 12 weeks or longer [1].

1.2 Etiology, prevalence and epidemiology

Sinusitis is the inflammation of facial sinuses. Different factors may contribute in sinusitis. Sinusitis may develop by the combination of environmental and host factors. Acute sinusitis is more common in occurrence as compared to chronic sinusitis. High prevalence of sinusitis is in the Midwest, south and among women. Sinusitis more often affects children younger than 15 years of age and adults 25–64 years of age. Common cause of sinusitis is viruses and mostly they are self-limiting. About 90% of the population who get cold also have viral sinusitis. Not only patients suffering with cold have sinusitis elements but atopic patients may also develop sinusitis. Risk factors causing sinusitis are viruses, bacteria, fungi, allergens, irritants (dander, polluted air, smoke, dust mites) [2].

Other risk factors for sinusitis may involve: anatomic defects such as septal deviations, polyps, conchae bullosa, other trauma and fractures involving the sinuses or the facial area surrounding them. Rhinitis medicamentosa, toxic rhinitis, nasal cocaine abuse, barotrauma, foreign bodies. Patients with nasogastric or nasotracheal tubes. Body positioning, intensive care unit (ICU) patients due to prolonged supine positioning that compromises muco-ciliary clearance. Impaired mucous transport from diseases such as cystic fibrosis, ciliary dyskinesia. Immunodeficiency from chemotherapy, HIV, diabetes mellitus, etc. Prolonged oxygen use due to drying of mucosal lining [3].

1.3 Histopathology

Histopathology is the examination of pathological condition of tissues. Histopathology of respiratory track reveals incidents 1% of viruses, 3% *Streptococcus pneumoniae*, 6% anaerobes, 2% *Streptococcus pyogenes*, 2% *Moraxella*, 21% *Haemophilus influenza* 21%, anaerobes and 4% *Staphylococcus aureus*. In case of chronic sinusitis 20% *S. aureus*, 20%, 4% *S. pneumoniae*, 3% anaerobes, 16% multiple organisms. About 2–7% are fungal incidences in which most common is Aspergillus seen in immunocompromised patients [4].

1.4 Pathophysiology of sinusitis

There are four sinuses in the facial area around the nose i.e. frontal sinus, maxillary sinus, sphenoid sinus and ethmoid sinus. Most commonly sinusitis develops by the attack of viruses on the upper respiratory track followed by edema and inflammation of nasal lining. This inflammation leads to thick mucus production that obstructs the paranasal sinuses due to which immunity is disturbed and bacterial infection appear at once. Allergic rhinitis may proceed in to sinusitis due to ostial obstruction. Cilia get immobilized due to heavy nasal mucous discharge which further block the drainage. That give the opportunity to the bacteria to enter into sinuses by coughing or by nose blowing. Bacterial sinusitis develop after the viral attack on the upper respiratory track, symptoms of sino nasal disease may get worse in 5 days or become persistent in 10 days [5].

1.5 Clinical presentation of symptoms

Major symptoms shown by sinusitis patients are pain or pressure on face, nasal obstruction, hyposmia, nasal and post nasal purulence, facial congestion and fullness, fever. Minor symptoms of sino nasal disease include malaise, headache, cough, dental pain, headache, halitosis, otalgia, fatigue [6, 7].

1.6 Physical examination and lab findings

Physical examination is performed after the topical decongestant.

- Physical examination include looking for the facial swelling, looking for the periorbital edema, post nasal drip, cervical adenopathy and pharyngitis.
- Anterior rhinoscopy shows mucous crusting, obstructive polyps, mucosal edema, frank purulence and other anatomical defects.
- Press the forehead and cheeks for deep tenderness.
- Transillumination of the sinuses are also performed.
- Five important predicators of sinusitis include 1. Abnormal sinus transillumination, 2. Maxillary dental pain, 3. Colored nasal discharge, 4. Poor response to nasal decongestants and anti-histamines, 5. Mucopurulent seen on examination.

Overall examination of the patient is more valid then to observe single parameter to confirm the sinusitis [8].

1.7 Evaluation of lab findings

For the acute sinusitis no laboratory tests are recommended in emergency departments because for the acute sinusitis diagnosis is clinically. For the diagnosis of maxillary, frontal, sphenoid sinusitis plain sinus X-ray is most accurate. In contrast plain X-ray is not suitable for the evaluation of ostiomeatal complex or anterior ethmoid cells, which are the originating cell for sino nasal diseases. Positive lab test on plain films for sinusitis shows air-fluid levels, mucosal thickening of 6 mm or even more, sinus opacity. The choice of diagnostic test for sinusitis is the coronal CT at a thickness of 3–4 mm. Clinical findings of CT are sinus wall displacement, air-fluid levels, sinus opacification, 4 mm or more mucosal thickening. For the chronic bacterial and fungal sinusitis choice of diagnostic test is culture and biopsy [9].

1.8 Differential diagnosis

Most of the time rhinitis or upper respiratory tract infection are mistakenly diagnose as sinusitis. Maxillary toothache can also be mistaken as pain appeared in maxillary sinusitis. Besides this vascular headache, tension headache, epidural abscesses, brain abscesses, subdural empyema, meningitis and foreign bodies are also madly mistaken as sinusitis [10].

1.9 Malignancy of sinusitis

Sinusitis may spread to the soft tissues of eye orbits, face and bones. Due to the malignancy periorbital cellulitis, facial cellulitis, blindness and orbital abscess may develop. Sinusitis can breach into the brain and cause intra cranial disorders such as meningitis, epidural or subdural empyema and cavernous sinus thrombosis [11].

1.10 Treatment strategies

Treatment for sinusitis include, nasal wash, decongestants, humidification, nasal sprays, corticosteroids, antibiotics and nasal surgery [12].

1.10.1 Saline nasal wash

Saline nasal wash are in the form of nasal sprays or nasal solutions, which are intended to rinse away allergens and irritants and also to reduce drainage [13].

1.10.2 Nasal decongestants

Topical as well as systemic nasal decongestants can be used such as pseudoephedrine. Caution should be taken in using decongestants. Oxymetazoline should not be used for more than 3 days as it causes rebound congestion. Oral decongestants should be used with special care in hypertensive patients [14].

1.10.3 Nasal corticosteroids

Nasal corticosteroids help in reduction and treatment of inflammation. Nasal corticosteroid sprays include beclomethasone, fluticasone, budesonide, mometasone, and triamcinolone. Topical nasal sprays effectively treat mucosal edema but they are more effective in chronic sinusitis [15].

1.10.4 Parenteral or oral corticosteroids

These corticosteroids are used in severe inflammation especially if patient is suffering from nasal polyps. Oral corticosteroids have serious side effects when used for long term so, it should be used only to treat severe symptoms [16].

1.10.5 Antibiotics

Antibiotics are given in case of bacterial sinusitis. In case of bacterial infection amoxicillin or amoxicillin-clavulanate for 10–14 days is the first line treatment. Trimethoprim-sulfamethoxazole is effective for some population but there is high rate of resistance. If symptoms do not resolve in 7 days then broader spectrum agents are used such as augmentin, axetil, cefuroxime, second or third generation cephalosporins, fluoroquinolones and clindamycin. For anaerobic bacterial infection metronidazole can also add in the therapy [17].

1.10.6 Aspirin desensitization treatment

If patient is sensitize to the aspirin and may develop sinusitis then under medical supervision gradually larger doses are given to patient to increase the tolerance of aspirin.

1.10.7 Immunotherapy

Patients who are sensitive to allergens and these allergens may contribute to sinusitis. Immunotherapy is suggested to those individuals. Which help to reduce the body reaction against specific allergens.

1.10.8 Endoscopic sinus surgery

If the medications are not effective in treatment of sinusitis then endoscopic sinus surgery would be an option. In this surgery endoscope is used to explore sinuses. Depending upon the obstruction source different instruments might be used to remove mucous or to scrap polyps [18].

1.11 Use of steroids in atopic patients

Atopy is the development of allergic hypersensitive reactions or IgE-mediated reactions. Atopic patients may develop genetic allergic diseases such as asthma, rhinitis, and atopic dermatitis. Atopy usually associated with the inhaled or food allergens. Topical corticosteroids are the major steroids used for atopy over 40 years. Among steroids hydrocortisone is the first to be used.

1.11.1 Topical steroids

Acute atopic attack is treated by medium to high strength topical steroid for upto 2 weeks. These steroids should not be used for face and neck area because of side effects. Ointment should be apply within 5 min of twice daily bathing. Patients may also suffer from side effects such as atrophy, hypopigmentation, thinning of skin. Generally more potent steroids have more side effects.

1.11.2 Systematic steroids

The use of systematic steroid is under controversy for acute atopy. Most of the prescribers do not prescribe systematic steroids for acute atopy. For severe cases oral prednisone at usual dose of 20 mg/day for 7 days are used. But after discontinuation of the medicine, disease relapses quickly [19].

1.12 Prognosis of sinusitis

Patients with acute sinusitis are treated effectively as outpatient with better prediction of disease. Whereas, severe sinusitis of sphenoid and frontal area associated with air and fluid accumulation require I/V injection of antibiotics and keep under care in hospital. High mortality and morbidity rates are associated with fungal sinusitis. Immunocompromised patients should also get hospitalized [20].

1.13 Progression of acute sinusitis into asthma

Acute sinusitis often begins with the symptoms of common cold. These symptoms may fade away in less than 4 weeks but if symptoms persist for more than 12 weeks despite of proper medical treatment then acute sinusitis is converted into chronic sinusitis. In chronic sinusitis airways get severely inflamed with either bacterial or viral infection, which leads to the development of asthma. Which is known as sinusitis related asthma [21, 22].

2. Sinusitis related asthma

Asthma is a chronic disorder that involves airflow obstruction, an underlying inflammation and bronchial hyper responsiveness. Asthma is complicated disorder that not only involves larger airways but also small airways. Sino nasal disorders are most commonly diagnosed with the asthma. For centuries the continuous existence of these pathological conditions has been known. However the link between upper airways and lower airways has been not clearly understood. Rhinitis and sinusitis are two wide spectrum disorders agonizing the upper airways which are closely related to asthma [23].

2.1 Prevalence, risk factors and causes

Allergic rhinitis and sinusitis are one of the risk factor for asthma. Inherited differences in asthma prevalence, asthma attacks, constructive and appropriate asthma management, thorough education and regular visit to medical health care of patients with asthma associated with sinusitis and rhinitis may lead to effectively control of asthma and also reduce the risk factor for more prevalence.

Clinical trials on the sino nasal pathological conditions has been conducted and it was reported that sinusitis and allergic rhinitis of childhood was severely associated with asthma among them 42% of the patients had asthma with sinusitis whereas 12.9% of the patients only suffered with asthma. Before the age of 7 years if sinusitis is present then it would subsequently lead to asthma. If the sinusitis or allergic rhinitis occurred at the age of seven then the chances of developing asthma increases three fold. The term "The Allergic March" is used to show the progression of the disease from the nose and sinuses to the airways of the lungs [24].

The progression of sino nasal allergic march may proceed before the development of sinusitis. In children and infants atopic eczema may leads to sinusitis and subsequently to asthma. Comparatively in infants with non-atopic eczema, no sinusitis would develop. This confirms that eczema is risk factor for the development of sinusitis and asthma as well. Which further strengthen the concept of an "Allergic March" that sinusitis, allergic rhinitis and asthma are different diseases but still the progressively enhance by allergy [25]. The effect of the first line treatment for eczema on the progression and development of sinusitis is still unknown in patients with sino nasal disorder. Clinical trials have shown that smoking increased three folds the risk of asthma in patients already having sinusitis. Recent publications have shown that obesity is also one of the risk factor for asthma however obesity is not involved in sino nasal disorders as both obesity related asthma and sinusitis related asthma follows different pathway and mechanism [26].

These clinical trials and studies verify that the sinusitis and allergic rhinitis are contributing factors in asthma progression. If sinusitis can be intervene than the development of asthma can be prevented. Another important environmental factor that is smoking elevate asthma can be controlled by quitting tobacco [27] (**Figure 1**).

2.2 Difference between sino nasal disease in asthmatics and non-asthmatics

Sino nasal disease may appear differently in asthmatics then that of general population. Literature survey showed that the patients showing nasal symptoms and undergo to examine the clinical feature of lower airway disease then it is found that most of the patients suffering with the chronic sinusitis and allergic rhinitis along with asthma as compared to non-allergic rhinitis. Asthmatic patients associated with sinusitis progress to nasal polyps and are in much complications of sino nasal disease comparing to non-asthmatics. Sinusitis related asthmatics have more severe and persistent disease and they need multiple of surgeries as well [28].

Studies revealed that sinusitis may develop asthma progressively but there is a difference in between sinusitis related asthma and general population. This is strongly supported by data.

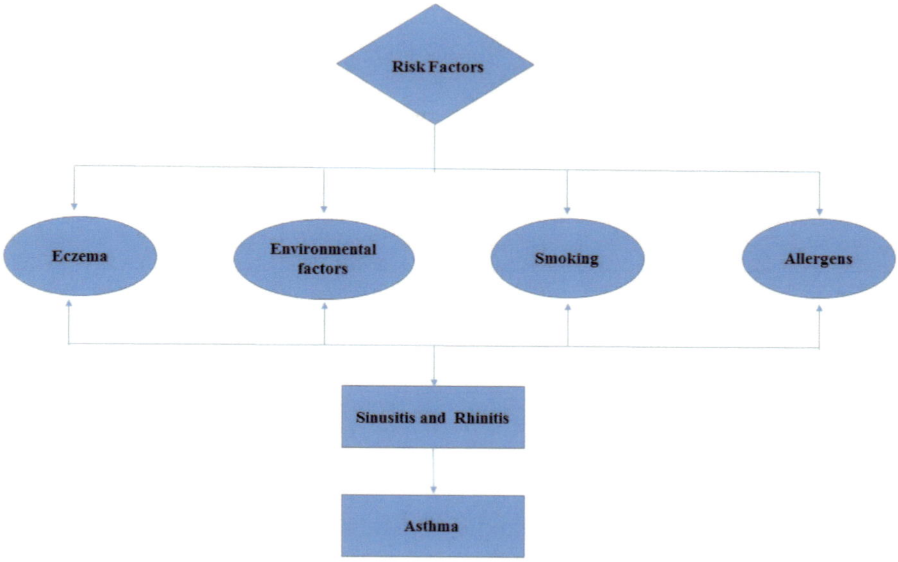

Figure 1.
Risk factors for the development of sinusitis and rhinitis which leads toward asthma.

1. In asthmatics upper air way disease appear differently as compared to general population.

2. Inflammation in upper and lower air ways in both population would be alike.

3. Increasing severity in the upper air ways going parallel to the severity in lower air ways [29, 30].

In asthmatic patients the inflammation in nose and sinuses shows there is disease in the lungs. For instance if patient having nasal polyposis inflammation its clinical identification feature shows antibody IgE production and eosinophilic inflammation. Common inflammatory mediators are release from upper and lower air ways, due to which it is difficult to assess pathways that cause Sino nasal inflammation in asthmatics and non-asthmatics [31]. Further clinical studies have performed in which gene expression of patient with sinus mucosa polyposis and aspirin sensitive asthma was compared with chronic sinusitis and no difference in gene expression was found. Further clinical studies on gene assays that is based on testing of lower air way helps us to understand how sinusitis is different in asthma patient than non-asthmatics [26].

2.3 Upper and lower air way inflammation

From the literature review it is noted that increase in severity of sino nasal disease goes parallel with the lower airways. Recent publication shows that patients having severe sinusitis have severe asthma series. This study suggests that sinusitis, rhinitis and asthma all are common progression of a single systematic disease [32]. Which ids further confirm by more clinical research in which severity in inflammation of lungs is same as in sinuses, nose and systematic inflammation which is measured by circulating eosinophilia, hence the severity in sinusitis or sino nasal disease is parallel to asthma and also same implies that lymphocyte and eosinophil are characteristic feature of upper and lower air way inflammation if upper air way go worse than lower air way also get affected in same way [33] (**Figure 2**).

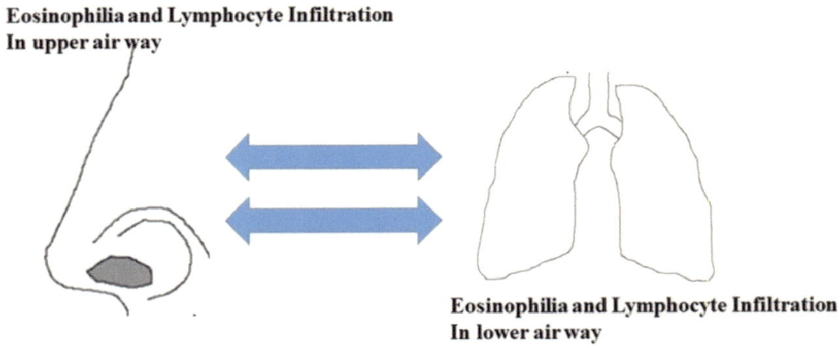

Figure 2.
Physiological relation between upper and lower air way: Inflammation in upper air way (nose, sinuses) develop with parallel to lower air way (lungs) in asthmatic patients.

Sino nasal disorders may increase the risk of lower air way (lungs) diseases which can be seen from the clinical studies. It has been shown that children suffering from allergic asthma and allergic rhinitis due to the dust mites, in that patients there was increased exhalation of nitric oxide was found [34]. Studies have also shown that in patients with allergic asthma allergens can develop the release of eosinophils from bone marrow which shows that sinusitis, rhinitis and asthma could be separate diseases but affected by single systematic disease [35].

2.4 Sino nasal disorder associated with asthma

Sino nasal disorders are linked with asthma is supported by the clinical research studies i.e. non asthmatic patients with allergic rhinitis have inflammation and abnormalities in lower airway. This is further supported by the fact that allergic rhinitis have an increase prevalence for the hyper bronchial activity. Another study showed that sinusitis and allergic rhinitis are associated with impaired lung functions which are significantly related to duration and exposure of sino nasal disorder to the risk factors. These findings suggest that patients with sinusitis and allergic rhinitis may have subclinical abnormalities of their intra thoracic airways and may be at risk of developing the clinical disease of asthma [36, 37] (**Figure 3**).

2.5 Asthma management

Asthma control appears worse in individuals having sino nasal disorder. Recent cross sectional, retrospective and prospective studies between the asthma symptoms and sinusitis symptoms have performed. These studies suggested that severity in sino nasal disorders increase the severity of asthma symptoms [36].

2.6 Treatment outcomes

Important parameters for the treatment outcome include 1. Early treatment of the patient suffering with sino nasal disease to prevent asthma. 2. Treatment regimen should be as effective as to treat asthma symptoms along with sinusitis and rhinitis [38].

Clinical trials are performed on 147 children treated with specific subcutaneous immunotherapy for rhinoconjuctivitis, showed that most of the children do not progress to asthma. Recently study was published in which patients treated

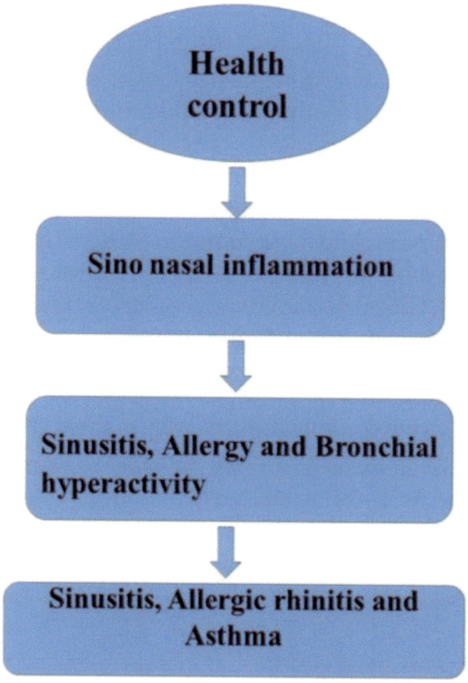

Figure 3.
Progressive gradation of sino nasal disease.

with antihistamine and nasal corticosteroids for the treatment of allergic rhinitis and airflow obstruction investigated by FEF25–75. It was shown that air flow obstruction was treated with in 3 months [39]. Over the decades there has been much interest in finding out and establishing treatment for the sino nasal disorder which may affect the asthma. However studies were performed among which prospective study was disappointing and retrospective study was suggested that by treating sinusitis and rhinitis asthma can be prevented from progression [40, 41]. From the previous trials it was believed that by treating nasal diseases lower air way abnormalities can be controlled which can decrease systemic eosinophilic inflammation. But in the recent trials it was seen that treatment of rhinitis do not affect the lower air way inflammation in any way which was investigated by measuring exhaled (nitric oxide) NO [42]. In these double blinded systemic controlled trials almost 40 children were subjected to treat with nasal steroids along with placebo. The results of the trials suggested that sino nasal inflammation and systemic inflammation was treated, which were investigated by counting eosinophilic cationic protein but unfortunately there was no effect on lower air way inflammation (measured by exhaled by NO). These randomized trials were contraindicated with the previous trials which were carried on the adults. According to previous trials on adults lower air way inflammation was affected by measuring exhaled NO which was decreased by treating with nasal steroids. These results suggested that the effect of nasal treatment to control asthma or lower air way inflammation may vary in different patients sub groups. Not only this but also, studies have suggested that surgical treatment of nasal disease may also help in managing asthma outbreak. Despite of these clinical trials still there is a need to determine how well sino nasal treatment can help in reduction of asthma. Investigation of the patients who may have benefit from the treatment of nasal disease [42, 43].

3. Sinus headache

Headache is a symptom produced by the nervous system in response to disturbance or any threat. Hence it is the physiologically protective symptom of nervous system. About 90% are the life time incidents of the headache [44]. Headache may be primary or secondary as well, depending upon the underlying cause of the pain. When no definite pathological cause is identified then the headache is considered as **primary headache syndrome**. The most common primary headache disorders are migraine, tension type headache, cluster headache and probable migraine. When the cause of headache can be definable under pathological conditions, this type of headache is known as **secondary headache.** Causes of secondary headache include neoplastic, immunologic, metabolic, infectious, traumatic, inflammatory, endocrinologic and sinusitis [45]. Patients visited to the otolaryngologist because of their chronic headache, it is difficult to diagnose depending on the patients' presentation whether the headache is because of sinusitis or may be the other reason. Endoscopic techniques have been well developed for the diagnosis of underlying diseases and their associated symptoms. Sinus headaches are headache in which individual may feel pain and pressure around his eyes, cheeks and forehead. Due to differential diagnosis sometimes migraine and tension headaches may mistakenly consider as sinus headache [46, 47].

3.1 Prevalence, causes and risk factors

Sinus headaches are mostly associated with other chronic secondary headaches. It may cause pain and pressure around facial area and in sinuses and progress the sino nasal disorders. Sinus headaches are not related with the sinus infections therefore they should not be treated with antibiotics. Sinus headaches may affect any individual but they are more prone to those patients who have family history or even previous history of migraine or primary headache disorders. It also affects those patients who have sinusitis and they also suffered with headaches related with hormonal changes [48].

3.2 Symptoms

Symptoms of sinus headache exclusive of causes may include pressure, pain and tension around eyes cheeks and forehead, stuffy filled nose, fatigue, fever, pain may worsen upon bending forward or even lie down and pain sensations in upper jaw and teeth [49].

3.3 Diagnosis

Headache is pathological disorder of nervous system and it is difficult to diagnose the exact cause of headache. After physical examination medical practitioner may perform imaging diagnostic test to find out the real cause of headache. Imaging tests include:

3.3.1 CT-scan

Cross sectional images of brain, spinal cord and sinuses are obtained by X-ray which rotates around the body and displayed on the computer.

3.3.2 Magnetic resonance imaging (MRI)

Cross sectional images of the brain and sinuses are made with magnetic field and radio waves.

These tests are used to diagnose the headache. If sinuses are stuffy filled and inflamed than the sinusitis is the definite cause of headache [50].

3.4 Precaution and prevention

Precautions help in reducing the severity and attacks of headache. Healthy life style changes may prevent from headache other than using medications.

3.4.1 Exercise

Regular aerobic exercise helps in reduction of tension and prevention of headache. Aerobic exercises include swimming, cycling and walking. Before starting intense exercise one should warm up his body because sudden exercise also initiate headache. One of the causes of headache is obesity, in that case obese patients need to exercise daily in order to reduce headache [51].

3.4.2 Avoid trigger factors

If any odor, taste, food and even caffeine, tobacco triggered headache in the past so, one should avoid trigger factors and establish healthy daily routine with regular sleep of at least 8 h, try to reduce stress and take healthy diet.

3.4.3 Reduction of estrogen effects

Women who are taking medications such as birth control pills and hormonal replacement therapy have episodes of headache and estrogen seems to make it worse. Ask your doctor to reduce the dose or to prescribe alternate therapy [52].

3.5 Treatment

Most of the time migraine and chronic headaches are assumed as sinusitis headache. These type of headaches are treated with prescribed medicine on regular basis or to take medicine in order to prevent onset of headache.

3.5.1 OTC analgesics

Chronic headaches can be treated with over the counter pain relievers such as acetaminophen, naproxen and ibuprofen.

3.5.2 Triptans

Triptans are most effective in treating migraine headaches. Triptans include sumatriptan, almotriptan, frovatriptan, naratriptan and eletriptan. They are available in form of nasal sprays, tablets and injections. Triptans effect by constricting blood vessels and block the pain pathways in the brain.

3.5.3 Ergots

Ergots containing active constituent ergotamine. It is available in combination with caffeine. Ergotamine is most effective for the pain which lasts more than 72 h but it is less effective than triptans. Migraine related nausea and vomiting may get worse because of ergotamine. Overuse of ergotamine also leads to headache. Dihydroergotamine is comparatively more effective than ergotamine and have fewer side effects [53].

3.5.4 Anti-emetics

Headaches are mostly associated with nausea and vomiting especially in case of migraine. Anti-emetic medications such as metoclopramide, chlorpromazine and prochlorpromazine are given in combination with other medication to prevent nausea and vomiting.

3.5.5 Steroids (glucocorticoids)

Glucocorticoids such as dexamethasone are used in combination with other headache medication in order to reduce pain severity. Steroids should be used with caution because it causes steroidal toxicity [54, 55].

3.6 Sinusitis or migraine

Sinusitis related headaches and migraine are mostly confused with each other in term of diagnosis because signs and symptoms of both ailments are overlapped each other. In both type of headaches, condition become worse when individual bend forward. However in migraine there are also nasal disorders such nasal congestion, stuffy filled nose with watery discharge and facial pressure. Due to these symptoms migraine is mistakenly taken as sinusitis related headache by 90% of the patients. Whereas in case of sinus headache there is no nausea and vomiting which is usually common in migraine. Duration of sinus related headache is from 7 days or even longer however, migraine may last from hours to 1 or 2 days [56, 57].

4. Conclusion

Sinusitis is a nasal disorder featured by inflammation of mucosal epithelium of sinuses. Clinical studies have published and trials have been conducted which shows that the sinusitis and rhinitis are the two crucial disorders associated with asthmatics. Sinusitis and asthma follows the same inflammatory pathways and temporal sequence of disease which confirms that their progression is manifested by common nasal disorder. Early prevention and treatment of sinusitis is of great interest I order to prevent the progression of sinusitis into asthma. Sinus headache is also one of the symptoms of the sinusitis. Ninety percent life time incidents of headache are reported. Migraine is some time mistakenly taken as sinus headache. Before treating headache it should be diagnosed clearly whether the cause of headache is primary or secondary. After knowing the sinogenic headache, treatment strategies must be followed. Most of the time sinus related headaches are associated with acute or chronic sinusitis.

Acknowledgements

I am thank full to the Faculty of Pharmacy, University of Lahore, for being helpful. My deepest gratitude to Nasir Mahmood Pro Rector Academics, UOL for his great support.

Conflict of interest

No financial support and no other potential conflict of interest.

Author details

Fozia Masood
Faculty of Pharmacy, University of Lahore, Lahore, Pakistan

*Address all correspondence to: fozia.masood@pharm.uol.edu.pk

References

[1] Byeon JY, Choi HJ. Orbital cellulitis following orbital blow-out fracture. Journal of Craniofacial Surgery. 2017;**28**(7):1777-1779

[2] Ali MH, Miller CL. Wolf in sheep's clothing subdural empyema: A rare complication of acute sinusitis. South Dakota Medicine. 2016;**69**(7)

[3] Lloyd CM, Saglani S. T cells in asthma: Influences of genetics, environment, and T-cell plasticity. Journal of Allergy and Clinical Immunology. 2013;**131**(5):1267-1274

[4] Slavin RG, Spector SL, Bernstein IL, Workgroup SU, Kaliner MA, Kennedy DW, et al. The diagnosis and management of sinusitis: A practice parameter update. Journal of Allergy and Clinical Immunology. 2005;**116**(6):S13-S47

[5] Min YG, Kim YK, Choi YS, Shin JS, Juhn SK. Mucociliary activity and histopathology of sinus mucosa in experimental maxillary sinusitis: A comparison of systemic administration of antibiotic and antibiotic delivery by polylactic acid polymer. The Laryngoscope. 1995;**105**(8):835-842

[6] Wald ER. Epidemiology, pathophysiology and etiology of sinusitis. The Pediatric Infectious Disease Journal. 1985;**4**(6):S51-S54

[7] Stewart MG, Johnson RF. Chronic sinusitis: Symptoms versus CT scan findings. Current Opinion in Otolaryngology & Head and Neck Surgery. 2004;**12**(1):27-29

[8] van der Wiel E, ten Hacken NH, Postma DS, van den Berge M. Small-airways dysfunction associates with respiratory symptoms and clinical features of asthma: A systematic review. Journal of Allergy and Clinical Immunology. 2013;**131**(3):646-657

[9] Engels EA, Terrin N, Barza M, Lau J. Meta-analysis of diagnostic tests for acute sinusitis. Journal of Clinical Epidemiology. 2000;**53**(8):852-862

[10] Bushra Mubarak HSFM. Asthma and Lung Biology. London: InTech; 2019

[11] Williams JW, Simel DL, Roberts L, Samsa GP. Clinical evaluation for sinusitis: Making the diagnosis by history and physical examination. Annals of Internal Medicine. 1992;**117**(9):705-710

[12] Hegarty AM, Zakrzewska JM. Differential diagnosis for orofacial pain, including sinusitis, TMD, trigeminal neuralgia. Dental Update. 2011;**38**(6):396-408

[13] Weaver EM. Association between gastroesophageal reflux and sinusitis, otitis media, and laryngeal malignancy: A systematic review of the evidence. The American Journal of Medicine. 2003;**115**(3):81-89

[14] Otten F, Grote J. Treatment of chronic maxillary sinusitis in children. International Journal of Pediatric Otorhinolaryngology. 1988;**15**(3):269-278

[15] Wald ER. Sinusitis in children. New England Journal of Medicine. 1992;**326**(5):319-323

[16] Eisner MD, Zazzali JL, Miller MK, Bradley MS, Schatz M. Longitudinal changes in asthma control with omalizumab: 2-year interim data from the EXCELS study. Journal of Asthma. 2012;**49**(6):642-648

[17] Bruurs ML, van der Giessen LJ, Moed H. The effectiveness of physiotherapy in patients with asthma: A systematic review of the literature. Respiratory Medicine. 2013;**107**(4):483-494

[18] Apter AJ, Wan F, Reisine S, Bender B, Rand C, Bogen DK, et al. The association of health literacy with adherence and outcomes in moderate-severe asthma. Journal of Allergy and Clinical Immunology. 2013;**132**(2):321-327

[19] Williams H. New treatments for atopic dermatitis: Good news, but when and how to use tacrolimus and pimecrolimus is a muddle. 2002:1533-1534

[20] Wald ER, Nash D, Eickhoff J. Effectiveness of amoxicillin/clavulanate potassium in the treatment of acute bacterial sinusitis in children. Pediatrics. 2009;**124**(1):9-15

[21] Jun Kim H, Jung Cho M, Lee J-W, Tae Kim Y, Kahng H, Sung Kim H, et al. The relationship between anatomic variations of paranasal sinuses and chronic sinusitis in children. Acta Oto-laryngologica. 2006;**126**(10):1067-1072

[22] Kupferberg SB, Bent JP III, Kuhn FA. Prognosis for allergic fungal sinusitis. Otolaryngology—Head and Neck Surgery. 1997;**117**(1):35-41

[23] Haselkorn T, Fish JE, Zeiger RS, Szefler SJ, Miller DP, Chipps BE, et al. Consistently very poorly controlled asthma, as defined by the impairment domain of the Expert Panel Report 3 guidelines, increases risk for future severe asthma exacerbations in The Epidemiology and Natural History of Asthma: Outcomes and Treatment Regimens (TENOR) study. Journal of Allergy and Clinical Immunology. 2009;**124**(5):895-902. e4

[24] Pokladnikova J, Selke-Krulichova I. Effectiveness of a comprehensive lifestyle modification program for asthma patients: A randomized controlled pilot trial. Journal of Asthma. 2013;**50**(3):318-326

[25] Oraka E, Iqbal S, Flanders WD, Brinker K, Garbe P. Racial and ethnic disparities in current asthma and emergency department visits: Findings from the National Health Interview Survey, 2001-2010. Journal of Asthma. 2013;**50**(5):488-496

[26] Soler ZM, Mace JC, Litvack JR, Smith TL. Chronic rhinosinusitis, race, and ethnicity. American Journal of Rhinology & Allergy. 2012;**26**(2): 110-116

[27] Hamilos DL. Host-microbial interactions in patients with chronic rhinosinusitis. Journal of Allergy and Clinical Immunology. 2014;**133**(3): 640-653. e4

[28] Hsu J, Peters AT. Pathophysiology of chronic rhinosinusitis with nasal polyp. American Journal of Rhinology & Allergy. 2011;**25**(5):285-290

[29] Wenzel S, Ford L, Pearlman D, Spector S, Sher L, Skobieranda F, et al. Dupilumab in persistent asthma with elevated eosinophil levels. New England Journal of Medicine. 2013;**368**(26):2455-2466

[30] Foreman A, Holtappels G, Psaltis A, Jervis-Bardy J, Field J, Wormald PJ, et al. Adaptive immune responses in *Staphylococcus* aureus biofilm–associated chronic rhinosinusitis. Allergy. 2011;**66**(11):1449-1456

[31] Taillé C, Poulet C, Marchand-Adam S, Borie R, Dombret M-C, Crestani B, et al. Monoclonal anti-TNF-α antibodies for severe steroid-dependent asthma: A case series. The open Respiratory Medicine Journal. 2013;7:21

[32] Ocampo CJ, Peters AT, editors. Medical therapy as the primary modality for the management of chronic rhinosinusitis. In: Allergy & Asthma Proceedings. 2013

[33] Haldar P, Brightling CE, Hargadon B, Gupta S, Monteiro W, Sousa A, et al. Mepolizumab and exacerbations

of refractory eosinophilic asthma. New England Journal of Medicine. 2009;**360**(10):973-984

[34] Madeo J, Frieri M, editors. Bacterial biofilms and chronic rhinosinusitis. In: Allergy & Asthma Proceedings. 2013

[35] Adelson RT, Adappa ND. What is the proper role of oral antibiotics in the treatment of patients with chronic sinusitis? Current Opinion in Otolaryngology & Head and Neck Surgery. 2013;**21**(1):61-68

[36] Kato A, Hulse KE, Tan BK, Schleimer RP. B-lymphocyte lineage cells and the respiratory system. Journal of Allergy and Clinical Immunology. 2013;**131**(4):933-957

[37] Frieri M, editor. Asthma concepts in the new millennium: update in asthma pathophysiology. In: Allergy and Asthma Proceedings. OceanSide Publications; 2005

[38] Smith TL, Kern R, Palmer JN, Schlosser R, Chandra RK, Chiu AG, et al., editors. Medical therapy vs surgery for chronic rhinosinusitis: A prospective, multi-institutional study with 1-year follow-up. In: International Forum of Allergy & Rhinology. Wiley Online Library; 2013

[39] Capetandes A, Haque F, Frieri M. Confluent human pulmonary type II epithelial cells (A549) cells express cytoplasmic VEGF. Journal of Investigative Medicine. 2004;**36**:7

[40] Capetandes A, Horne NS, Frieri M. Dermatophagoides extract-treated confluent type II epithelial cells (cA549) and human lung mesenchymal cell growth. Annals of Allergy, Asthma & Immunology. 2005;**95**(4):381-388

[41] Holgate ST, Arshad HS, Roberts GC, Howarth PH, Thurner P, Davies DE. A new look at the pathogenesis of asthma. Clinical Science. 2010;**118**(7):439-450

[42] Vlastarakos PV, Fetta M, Segas JV, Maragoudakis P, Nikolopoulos TP. Functional endoscopic sinus surgery improves sinus-related symptoms and quality of life in children with chronic rhinosinusitis: A systematic analysis and meta-analysis of published interventional studies. Clinical Pediatrics. 2013;**52**(12):1091-1097

[43] Broide DH. Immunologic and inflammatory mechanisms that drive asthma progression to remodeling. Journal of Allergy and Clinical Immunology. 2008;**121**(3):560-570

[44] Bachert C, Zhang N. Chronic rhinosinusitis and asthma: Novel understanding of the role of IgE 'above atopy'. Journal of Internal Medicine. 2012;**272**(2):133-143

[45] Cady RK, Schreiber CP. Sinus headache: A clinical conundrum. Otolaryngologic Clinics of North America. 2004;**37**(2):267-288

[46] Patel ZM, Setzen M, Poetker DM, DelGaudio JM. Evaluation and management of "sinus headache" in the otolaryngology practice. Otolaryngologic Clinics of North America. 2014;**47**(2):269-287

[47] Seiden AM, Martin VT. Headache and the frontal sinus. Otolaryngologic Clinics of North America. 2001;**34**(1):227-241

[48] Boonchoo R. Functional endoscopic sinus surgery in patients with sinugenic headache. Journal of the Medical Association of Thailand=Chotmaihet thangphaet. 1997;**80**(8):521-526

[49] Headache: Hope through research. March 13, 2018. Available from: https://www.ninds.nih.gov/Disorders/Patient-Caregiver-Education/Hope-Through-Research/Headache-Hope-Through-Research

[50] Sinus headaches. March 13, 2018. Available from: http://www.entnet.org/content/sinus-headaches

[51] Kaur A, Singh A. Clinical study of headache in relation to sinusitis and its management. Journal of Medicine and Life. 2013;**6**(4):389

[52] Parsons DS, Batra PS. Functional endoscopic sinus surgical outcomes for contact point headaches. The Laryngoscope. 1998;**108**(5):696-702

[53] Sinus infection (sinusitis). March 13, 2018. Available from: https://www.cdc.gov/antibiotic-use/community/for-patients/common-illnesses/sinus-infection.html

[54] Allen M, Vincent T. Headache and the frontal sinus. Otolaryngologic Clinics of North America. 2001;**34**:227

[55] Swanson JW. (expert opinion). Mayo Clinic, Rochester, Minn. March 13, 2018

[56] Robertson CE, Black DF, Swanson JW, editors. Management of migraine headache in the emergency department. In: Seminars in Neurology. Thieme Medical Publishers; 2010

[57] Behin F, Behin B, Behin D, Baredes S. Surgical management of contact point headaches. Headache: The Journal of Head and Face Pain. 2005;**45**(3):204-210

Chapter 4

Septoplasty: Endoscopic and Open Techniques

Yi-Tsen Lin

Abstract

Septoplasty is one of the most commonly performed procedures by rhinologists. This article will provide a brief review of the surgical anatomy and the operative techniques of this procedure. Both endoscopic and open septoplasty procedures will be addressed. However, more than 15% of patients undergoing septoplasty fail to achieve symptomatic relief. Incomplete separation of the bony-cartilaginous junction and inadequate correction of the caudal septal deviation are the main reasons for persistent septal deviation after primary septoplasty. In revised septoplasty, correction of the caudal septal deviation can be done by proper correction of the cartilaginous curvature and strengthening of the structure using a batten graft.

Keywords: nasal septum, septoplasty, endoscope, caudal septal deviation

1. Introduction

Septoplasty is one of the most frequently operated procedures by rhinologists and facial plastic surgeons. It is performed mainly for reducing nasal obstruction, but it can also provide a better surgical approach in endoscopic sinus and skull base surgery and an easier access for postoperative treatment. The deviated septum can be cartilaginous, bony, or both. The septum can be curved, tilted, angulated, twisted, present with a formation of spurs, or a combination of these. Therefore, there is no a single "standard" or "routine" operation that can satisfy all variables and complexities of cases. Septoplasty is a reconstructive procedure tailor-made for individual cases. Understanding the anatomy and a thorough preoperative evaluation of all deviated sites will lead to a better surgical outcome.

2. Surgical anatomy

The nasal septum is a vertical midline structure that extends anteriorly to the columella, posteriorly to the sphenoidal rostrum, superiorly to the anterior skull base, and inferiorly to the nasal floor (**Figure 1**). It composed of soft tissue, cartilage, and bone. The most caudal part between the columella and the caudal margin of the septal cartilage is the membranous septum, lying between the medial crura and the caudal septum. The area of the membranous septum may vary between individuals. In people with a large septal cartilage, the membranous septum might be smaller. The cartilaginous part of the nasal septum is quadrangular. It is in conjunction with the upper lateral cartilage and the lower end of the nasal bone anterosuperiorly, the perpendicular plate of the ethmoid bone superiorly, the vomer

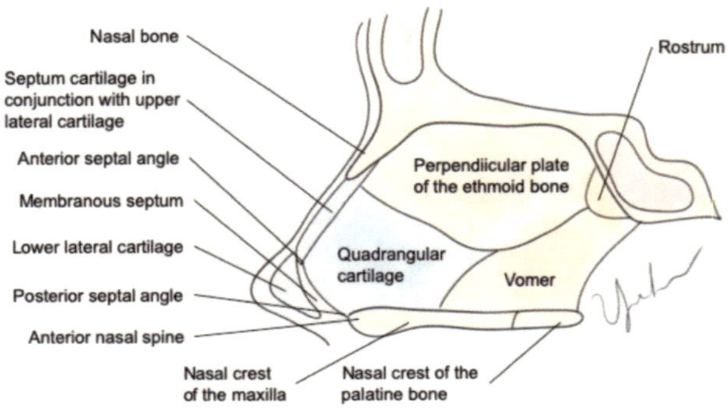

Figure 1.
The anatomy of the nasal septum.

bone posteroinferiorly, and the maxillary crest inferiorly. It usually presents with a tail between the gap of the perpendicular plate and the vomer, and this area is actually considered to be the growth center of the septum. The cartilaginous septum connects to the bony septum by a dense fibrous tissue and usually sits in a groove in the maxillary crest. The bony part of the septum includes the vertical crest of the nasal bone, the perpendicular plate of the ethmoid bone, the vomer, the maxillary crest, and the palatine crest. Because the septum at the bony-cartilaginous junction is the growth center of the nasal septum, we should keep in mind not to manipulate vigorously in this area before 17 and 18 years of age.

Some important landmarks of the nasal septum should be kept in mind when performing septoplasty to avoid unfavorable complications. The keystone area is the confluence of bone and cartilage at the junction of the nasal bone, the septal cartilage, and the upper lateral cartilages. The detachment of the cartilage from the bone and/or damage of the cartilage in the keystone area may cause a complication known as a saddle nose. Another important landmark is the junction of the caudal septum and the anterior part of the maxillary crest. There are three landmarks in the caudal ends of the septal cartilage: the anterior septal angle, middle septal angle, and posterior septal angle. The posterior septal angle contacts the anterior nasal spine, which is the most anterior part of the maxillary crest. Damage to the fibrous connection between the caudal septum and the anterior nasal spine may lead to weakened support of the nasal tip and an increased risk of nasal tip drooping. Usually, the septal cartilage should be preserved at least one 1–1.5 cm in width dorsally and caudally.

Deviation of the nasal septum can be classified as a caudal septal deviation, dislocation of the cartilage out of the maxillary crest, dorsal and high septal deviation, posterior septal deviation, and a bony spur formation. Various techniques have been proposed to deal with the distinct sites of septal deviation.

3. Surgical techniques

Septoplasty can be performed via a traditional headlight approach or by an endoscopic approach. The advantages of using an endoscope are a more accurate diagnosis of septal deviation, better visualization of the contributing factors, prevention of mucosal tears, and visualization of the surgical fields for residents and operating room staff. A systematic review reported that endoscopic septoplasty shortened surgery time and reduced perioperative complications, but the functional result was similar to that with conventional septoplasty [1]. Another systematic review reported that there was a significant improvement in postoperative symptoms (i.e., nasal obstruction and headaches) and fewer complications in patients who underwent endoscopic septoplasty, although these findings should be taken with caution given the poor quality of included studies [2]. Consequently, nowadays, endoscopy has been adopted to perform septoplasty. Many surgical procedures of the nasal septum rely on endoscopes, including septodermoplasty [3, 4], repair of septal perforation [5, 6], and harvesting the nasoseptal flap for skull base reconstruction. The limitation of using endoscopy in septoplasty is correction of the deviated caudal septum. The caudal septal cartilage might be manipulated more easily via a conventional headlight (more details will be described later in this chapter).

3.1 Incision and elevation of the mucoperichondrial flap

Usually, the nose is packed with cotton pledgets soaked with epinephrine 1 mg/ml and 2% lidocaine, followed by a submucoperichondrial injection of 1% lidocaine with 1:100,000 of epinephrine. For better infiltration of the surgical plane and hydrodissection of the subperichondrial and subperiosteal planes, injection into multiple sites of the bilateral septum is performed. For correction of the deviated septum at the junction of the cartilaginous septum and vomer and removal of the bony spur, a Killian incision is made (**Figure 2**). For correction of the caudal septal deviation, a hemitransfixion incision is made to elevate bilateral mucoperichondrial flaps from the caudal septum and to enable straightening of the caudal septum, to add on a batten graft, and to fix the cartilage firmly on the anterior nasal spine (**Figure 2**). A #15 scalpel is used to make the incision, and the subperichondrial plane is identified and dissected. When making the hemitransfixion incision, a sharp instrument can be used first (e.g., a scalpel, Cottle, or iris scissors) to elevate the mucoperichondrial flap. After making the Killian incision, the mucoperichondrial flap can be elevated more easily using a scraping maneuver with a Cottle or Freer elevator. Beginning with a correct plane, the elevation of mucoperichondrial flap can proceed more smoothly. After meticulous separation of the septal mucosal flap from the bony-cartilaginous junction, the subperiosteal plane can be identified by advancing a blunt elevator or even using a suction tip underneath the flap. Usually, the bony-cartilaginous junction is where the septum is most deviated. It would be easier to elevate the flap superiorly and inferiorly to the most deviated and adhesive part and then perform the flap dissection from the most deviated part and/or the spur. Sometimes, as flap tears are unavoidable due to large deviated spurs, we may elevate the concave side of the septal flap first to make sure one side of the septal flap is intact.

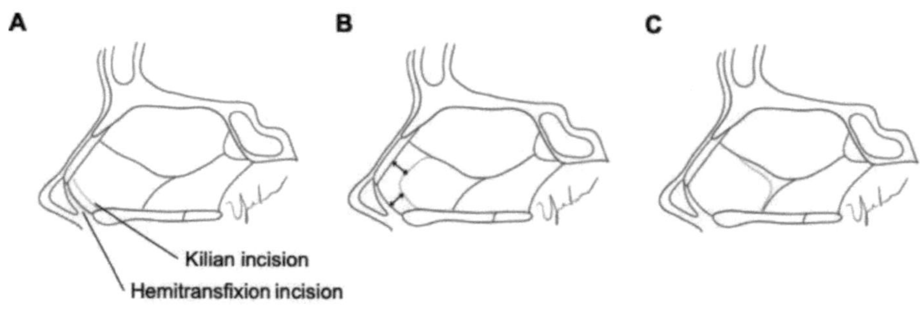

Figure 2.
The incisions in septoplasty. (A) The Kilian incision and the hemitransfixion incision for mucochondrial flap. (B) The septotomy with an adequate preservation of the L-strut. (C) The septotomy made at the bony-cartilaginous junction.

3.2 Septotomy and removal the deviated part

The extent of the incised cartilage depends on the type of septal deviation. For a posterior bony septal deviation or spur formation, the cartilaginous septum may not need to be incised. You can separate the bony-cartilaginous junction during septotomy and enter the contralateral subperiosteal space. Then, the deviated bony septum could be removed precisely using turbinate scissors or through-cutting instruments. For the cartilaginous septal deviation, the septal cartilage may be incised anterior to the deviated part using a Freer septum knife, which can be used to cut the cartilage without injury to the contralateral septal mucosa. If the septal cartilage is to be used as a cartilaginous batten graft for subsequent procedures, it can be harvested using a Freer septum knife as well with an adequate preservation of the L-strut. Then, the contralateral mucoperiosteal flap is elevated, and the deviated bone can be incised using turbinate scissors, through-cutting instruments, or a rongeur.

3.3 Management of the deviation at the maxillary crest

Dislocation of the cartilage from the maxillary crest, widening of the maxillary crest, and a deviated maxillary crest are common causes of airway obstruction at the base of the nose. Sometimes, it could be left untouched if the problem is minor compared to other deviated problems, but at other times, it can be critical and surgical intervention is required. At the junction of the cartilaginous and bony components of the septum, dense decussating fibers are seen at the confluence of the perichondrium and the periosteum. Therefore, when dissecting the subperichondrial plane downward to the maxillary crest, sharp division of the fibrous connection at the cartilaginous-bony junction using a Freer septum knife is helpful. In case of dislocation of the cartilage from the maxillary crest, it is useful to remove a strip of cartilage lateral to the maxillary crest without destabilizing the junction of the caudal septum and the anterior nasal spine. For wide maxillary crests or the deviated crests, we may use a chisel to shave or smooth the bone surface.

3.4 Correction of caudal septal deviation

Aggressive resections of the cartilaginous portion of the septum may lead to loss of nasal tip support. However, inadequate correction of the caudal septal deviation is one of the main reasons for persistent septal deviation after primary septoplasty [7]. The caudal septum is mainly composed of the cartilaginous portion of the septum, and the relationship between the caudal septum and the anterior nasal spine is crucial in the management of caudal septum deviation. In addition, after correcting the curvature of the cartilage and adjusting the relative position of the caudal septum and the anterior nasal spine, the structures need to be strengthened using sutures and/or batten grafts (**Table 1**).

Correction of cartilage is different from correction of bone. Once the bony septum is fractured to be straight, the structure is broken, and it seldom recovers to the original shape. However, the elastic coiling nature of the cartilage renders it with a "memory," which leads to cartilage re-bending even after suture or scoring. To overcome the intrinsic elasticity of the cartilage, Jang et al. proposed a cutting and suture technique [8]. The most convex part of the caudal cartilage is cut while preserving the junction between the cartilaginous septum and the maxillary crest, and then the two segments are sutured side by side with a slight overlap. If the stability of the cut and sutured septum is questionable, a cartilaginous batten graft can be used to provide further support.

To straighten the caudal septum	To strengthen the caudal septum
• Scoring	• Anchoring sutures
• Cut and suture	• Cartilaginous batten graft
• Wedge resection	• Bony batten graft
• Swing door	
• Septum riding on the spine	

Table 1.
Surgical techniques to correct the deviated caudal septum.

The structure of the caudal septum corrected by the cutting and suture technique can also be strengthened with an interpositioned graft [9]. Another way to break the intrinsic elasticity is to make an incomplete incision on the most concave site of the cartilaginous septum (**Figure 3A**). Then, a pair of forceps can be used to reposition the cartilage to the midline, and the excess piece of cartilage can be trimmed (**Figure 3B** and **C**). The septum can be sutured with a 5-0 PDS, and a batten graft can be used.

Dislocation of the lower part of the caudal septum on the side of the maxillary crest can narrow the airway and cause nasal obstruction, and this can be managed in several ways. As mentioned before, the cartilage along the maxillary crest could be shaved as a strip, but the stability of caudal septum may be affected due to loss of the fibrous connections between the cartilage and bone. Therefore, in addition to shaving the base of the cartilaginous septum, anchoring sutures between the cartilage and the soft tissue around the nasal crest can be used to strengthen the stability. Another solution to correct cartilaginous septal deviation is to disarticulate the cartilage from the maxillary crest, and the excessive cartilage can then be resected. Following this, the caudal cartilaginous septum could be replaced in the midline or fixed on the other side, and stabilizing sutures can be used.

While the above techniques are used to correct the curvature of the septal cartilage, additional batten grafts are used to strengthen and stabilize the structure and maintain a longstanding straightened caudal septum. The batten grafts can provide a strong support to overcome the internal coiling strength of the deviated cartilage and also prevent possible nasal tip drooping due to aggressive septation of the bony-cartilaginous junction. The batten grafts can be taken from either the cartilaginous septum [10, 11] or the perpendicular plate of the ethmoid bone [12–14], and it can be performed endonasally. The bony grafts do not cause internal nasal valve obstruction, and the cartilage grafts can be beveled to avoid excessive thickness of the caudal septum.

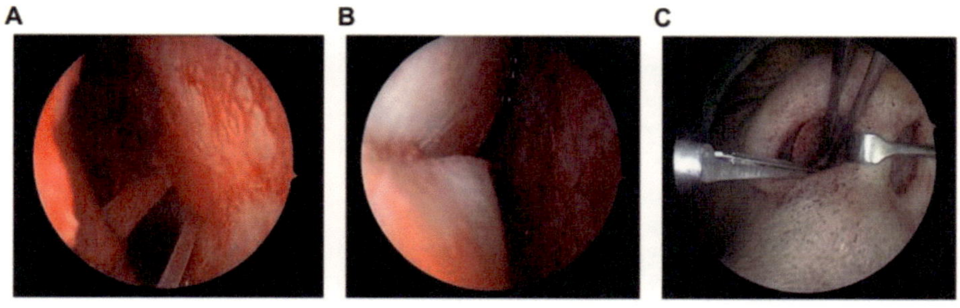

Figure 3.
Correction of the caudal cartilaginous curvature. (A) Making an incomplete incision on the most concave site of the cartilaginous septum. (B) Estimating the overlapping cartilage by repositioning the cartilage to the midline. (C) Trimming of the excess cartilage.

3.5 Wound closure

A reassessment of the nasal airway can be performed after completing the above procedures, and any minor adjustments can be addressed. Then, the septal flap is reapproximated. The hemitransfixion or Kilian incision is closed with simple interrupted 4-0 chromic sutures. The septum can be closed with a through-and-through quilting 4-0 chromic suture, which eliminates dead space and prevents development of septal hematoma. If mucosal tears are present, the silastic splints can be placed at each side of the nasal cavity and removed in 5–7 days.

4. Conclusion

Septoplasty is an individualized procedure, and preoperative evaluation of the deviated site is critical to achieve optimal outcome. Endoscope can provide better visualization of the deviated sites and prevention of mucosal tears, while the deviated caudal septum could be managed via hemitransfixion incision under headlight. Combining the use of headlight and endoscope can deal with most of the deviated sites of the nasal septum, and therefore, septoplasty could be performed endonasally in most of the cases. Open septoplasty may be indicated in cases with deviated or crooked nose, and septoplasty with rhinoplasty can be performed. The surgical intention is to make a straight septum with long-lasting effect.

Conflict of interest

The authors declare no conflict of interest.

Appendices and nomenclature

nasal septum
septoplasty
endoscopic septoplasty
caudal septal deviation
Kilian incision
hemitransfixion incision

Author details

Yi-Tsen Lin
Department of Otolaryngology, National Taiwan University Hospital, Taipei, Taiwan

*Address all correspondence to: yitsenlin@ntu.edu.tw

References

[1] Champagne C, Ballivet de Regloix S, Genestier L, Crambert A, Maurin O, Pons Y. Endoscopic vs. conventional septoplasty: A review of the literature. European Annals of Otorhinolaryngology, Head and Neck Diseases. 2016;**133**(1):43-46

[2] Hong CJ, Monteiro E, Badhiwala J, Lee J, de Almeida JR, Vescan A, et al. Open versus endoscopic septoplasty techniques: A systematic review and meta-analysis. American Journal of Rhinology & Allergy. 2016;**30**(6): 436-442

[3] Rimmer J, Lund VJ. A modified technique for septodermoplasty in hereditary hemorrhagic telangiectasia. The Laryngoscope. 2014;**124**(1):67-69

[4] Bastianelli M, Kilty SJ. Technique modifications for septodermoplasty: An illustrative case. Journal of Otolaryngology—Head & Neck Surgery. 2015;**44**:59

[5] Cassano M. Endoscopic repair of nasal septal perforation with "slide and patch" technique. Otolaryngology—Head and Neck Surgery: Official Journal of American Academy of Otolaryngology-Head and Neck Surgery. 2014;**151**(1):176-178

[6] Cavada MN, Orgain CA, Alvarado R, Sacks R, Harvey RJ. Septal perforation repair utilizing an anterior ethmoidal artery flap and collagen matrix. American Journal of Rhinology & Allergy. 2019;**33**(3):256-262

[7] Jin HR, Kim DW, Jung HJ. Common sites, etiology, and solutions of persistent septal deviation in revision septoplasty. Clinical and Experimental Otorhinolaryngology. 2018;**11**(4):288-292

[8] Jang YJ, Yeo NK, Wang JH. Cutting and suture technique of the caudal septal cartilage for the management of caudal septal deviation. Archives of Otolaryngology—Head & Neck Surgery. 2009;**135**(12):1256-1260

[9] Kim SA, Jang YJ. Caudal septal division and interposition batten graft: A novel technique to correct caudal septal deviation in septoplasty. The Annals of Otology, Rhinology, and Laryngology. 2019;**128**(12):1158-1164

[10] Kim JH, Kim DY, Jang YJ. Outcomes after endonasal septoplasty using caudal septal batten grafting. American Journal of Rhinology & Allergy. 2011;**25**(4):e166-e170

[11] Wee JH, Lee JE, Cho SW, Jin HR. Septal batten graft to correct cartilaginous deformities in endonasal septoplasty. Archives of Otolaryngology—Head & Neck Surgery. 2012;**138**(5):457-461

[12] Lee JW, Baker SR. Correction of caudal septal deviation and deformity using nasal septal bone grafts. JAMA Facial Plastic Surgery. 2013;**15**(2):96-100

[13] Chung YS, Seol JH, Choi JM, Shin DH, Kim YW, Cho JH, et al. How to resolve the caudal septal deviation? Clinical outcomes after septoplasty with bony batten grafting. The Laryngoscope. 2014;**124**(8):1771-1776

[14] Kim DY, Nam SH, Alharethy SE, Jang YJ. Surgical outcomes of bony batten grafting to correct caudal septal deviation in septoplasty. JAMA Facial Plastic Surgery. 2017;**19**(6):470-475

Chapter 5

REAHs and REAH-Like Lesions: Underdiagnosed lesions Often Misconfused with Nasal Polyps

Ph. Eloy, C. Fervaille and M.C. Nollevaux

Abstract

REAH is the eponym for respiratory epithelial adenomatoid hamartoma. The disease is under diagnosed. It is clearly a disease in the olfactory cleft. It is characterized by a polypoid process located in the olfactory cleft which does not evolve in inverted papilloma or malignancy set at 10–15 cm. The lesion can be isolated in one or both olfactory cleft. It can be asymptomatic or can cause nasal obstruction and impairment of smell. More commonly the lesions, often multiple, are associated to the recurrence of the nasal polyposis. They can contribute to the development of loss of smell, nasal obstruction or even the blockage of the frontal recesses. The definitive diagnostic is based upon the histologic examination. Surgery is the treatment. In case of isolated lesion, complete excision without complete ethmoidectomy is the option. In case of lesions embedded in a recurrent massive polyposis, a complete exenteration of the olfactory clefts associated to a revision of full house ethmoidectomy and even a Draf III must be considered.

Keywords: REAHs, REAH-like, nasal polyposis, olfactory cleft

1. Introduction

REAH is the eponysm for Respiratory Epithelial Adenomatoid Hamartoma. It is a relatively new diagnosis, only added to the World Health Organization classification of tumors in 2005 [1].

Wenig and Heffner were the first to describe it in 1995 in a series of 31 cases [2]. They described it as "a proliferation of glands lined by multi-layered ciliated respiratory epithelium, often with admixed mucocytes, arising in direct continuity with the surface epithelium, which invaginated downward into the submucosa."

The lesion is usually diagnosed in middle-aged patients. Clinically it may manifest as a solitary lesion or in association with sinonasal polyposis. The former is far less common than the latter. The lesion takes its origin either in the olfactory cleft, the posterior septum, or the rhinopharynx [1–5] Because the incidence, clinical signs, imaging, modality of treatment, outcomes, and pathogenesis seem to be quiet different between these two clinical patterns, we call the first ones "REAHs" and the second ones "REAH-like." This terminology is proposed by Jankowski [3, 5] and Hawley [4] as well.

The purpose of this paper is to remind the histopathological characteristics and differential diagnosis of REAHs/REAH-like lesions and to report two different cohorts of patients (one with REAHs and the other with REAH like lesions), treated in the ENT department of the CHU UCL Namur.

2. Histopathological characteristics of REAHs and REAH-like lesions

Grossly, REAH looks like a "polypoid fleshy to firm mass with areas of induration." It is yellow or white [6]. It may have varying sizes (**Figures 1–3**).

The histologic picture is dominated by the presence of a glandular proliferation with a polypoid appearance. The proliferation starts from the surface epithelium and tends to be submucosal.

The glands are lined by ciliated respiratory epithelium originating from the surface respiratory epithelium. The glands are typically round to oval in shape and were small to medium in size with prominent dilation. Stromal tissue separates the glands. The epithelium may be cuboidal or flat, and mucinous gland metaplasia is often seen. Occasionally the gland lumina are filled with mucinous or eosinophilic amorphous material. It often demonstrates periglandular stromal hyalinization, and there is often a mixed inflammatory infiltrate within the stroma.

In the literature we can find another type of REAH called **COREAH**. It is characterized by a chondro-osseous differentiation. Flavin [7] and Roffman [8] were the two first authors to publish this entity, respectively, in 2005 and 2006. Since then 11 cases have been reported [9, 10]. It can occur in children or adults.

The histological features are almost exactly the same as REAH, but COREAH has islands of immature hyaline cartilage interspersed throughout the lesion (**Figures 4** and 5).

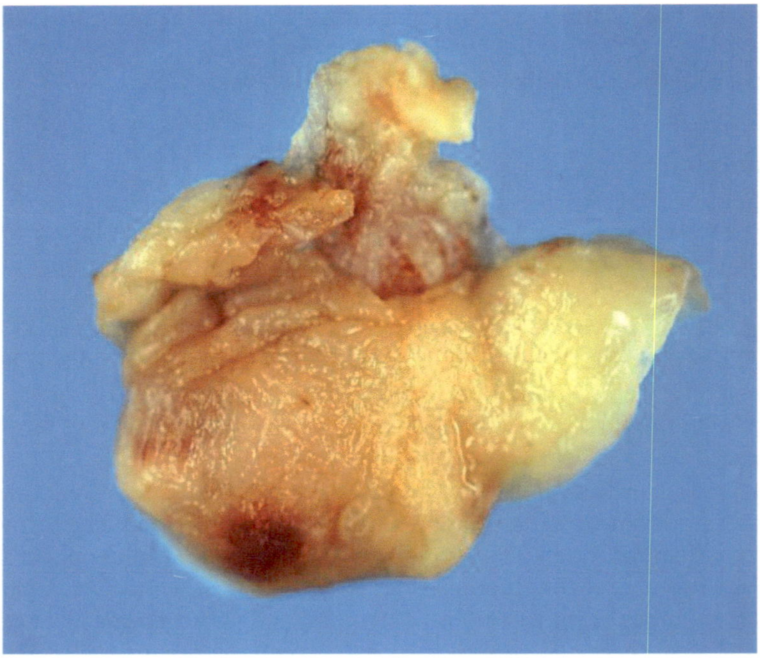

Figure 1.
Gross appearance of a REAH.

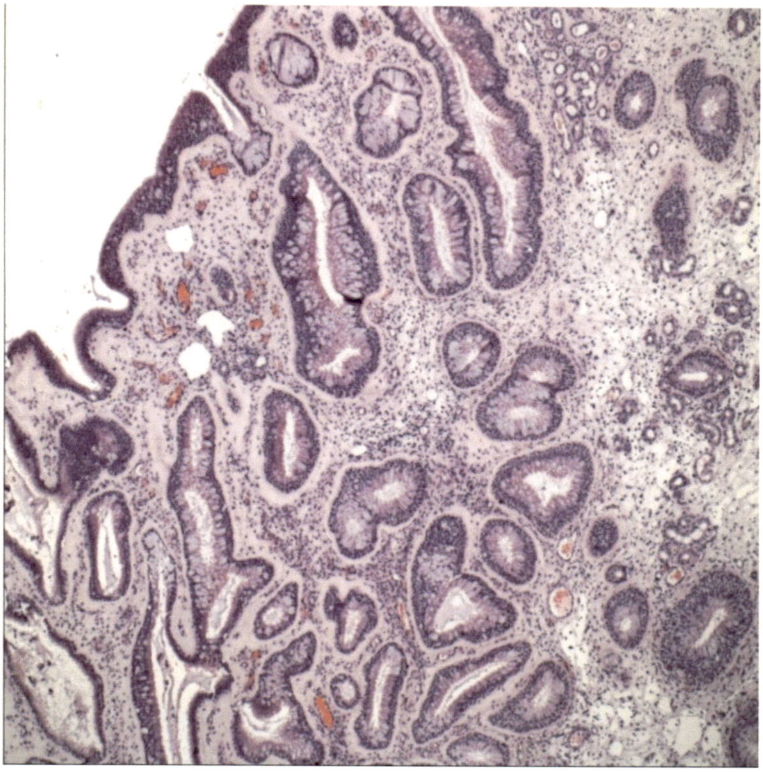

Figure 2.
REAHs: The glandular proliferation arises in direct continuity with the surface epithelium with invagination downward into the submucosa. Clusters of seromucinous glands are seen.

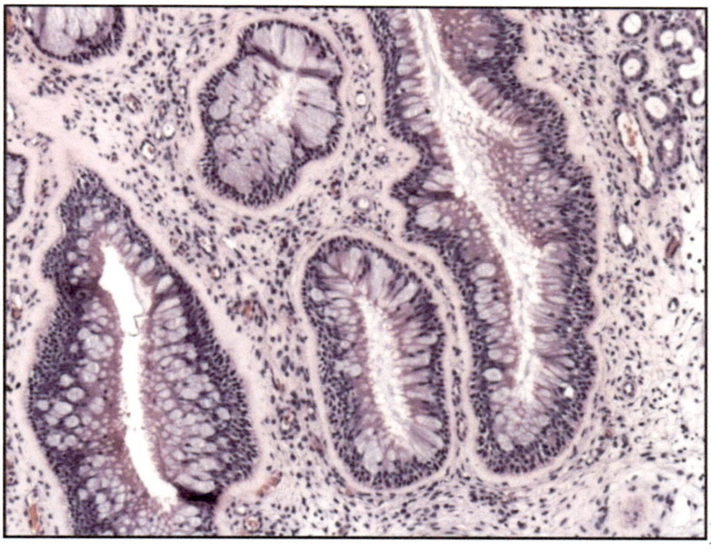

Figure 3.
REAHs: Occasionally the gland lumina are filled with mucinous or eosinophilic amorphous material. It often demonstrates periglandular stromal hyalinization, and there is often a mixed inflammatory infiltrate within the stroma.

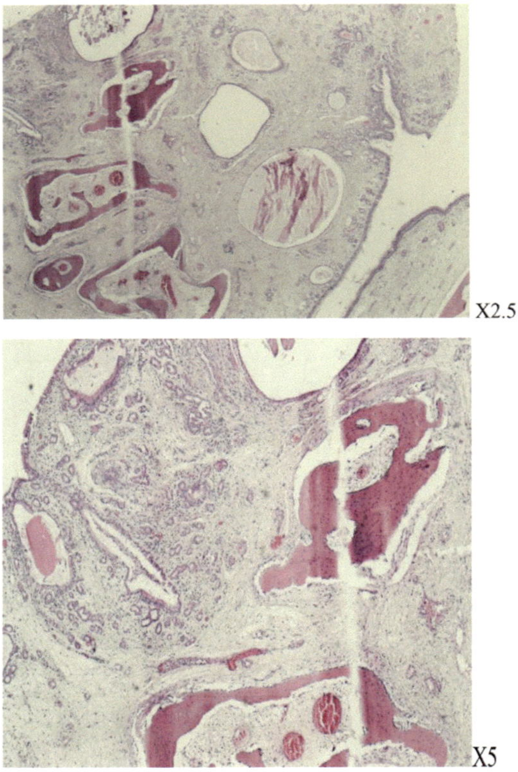

Figure 4.
COREAH: Nasal chondromesenchymal hamartoma. Multiple tumor fragments with a mucosal surface and nodules of cartilage (in red).

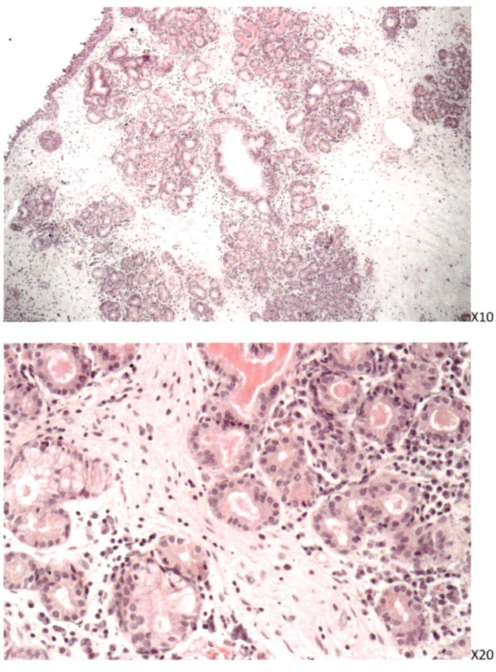

Figure 5.
Seromucinous hamartoma: The mass is covered by respiratory epithelium and is comprised of lobular or haphazard proliferations of small to large glands and ducts which are lined by a single layer of cuboidal or flattened epithelial cells.

3. Immunohistochemistry of REAHs

Immunohistochemistry has not been used to an extensive degree in the diagnosis of REAH, and it is not absolutely necessary to use it to make the definitive diagnosis of it.

However, Ozolek et al. did an immunohistochemical study in which they examined the profile of REAH [11]. REAHs are positive for CK7, negative for CK20 and CDX-2, and positive for MIB1 and Ki67. p63 staining was seen in the basal cells of REAH, which had a low proliferation index. The use of Mindbomb 1 (MIB-1) is useful in distinguishing REAH from other neoplasms, since neoplasms tend to have a high proliferation index.

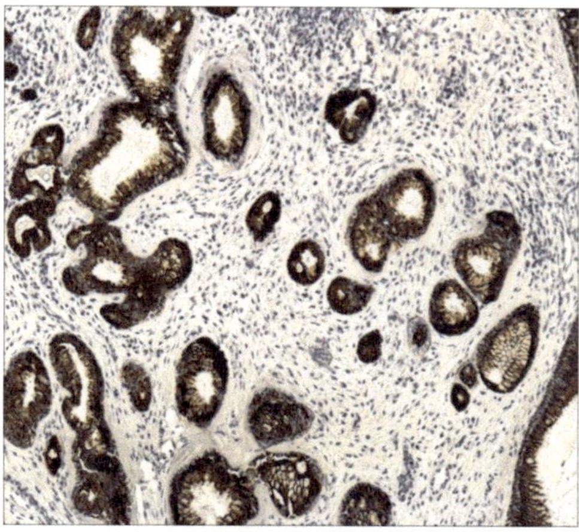

CK7 +

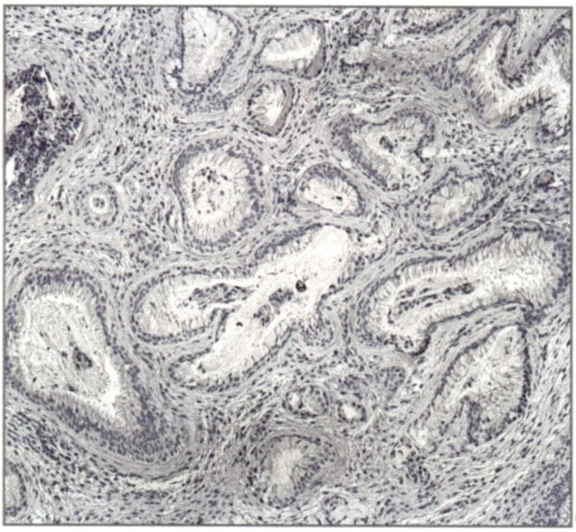

CK20 neg

REAHs: Immunohistochemistry: Positivity for CK7 and negativity for CK20.

4. Differential diagnosis of REAHs

The differential diagnostic of REAHs concerns the inflammatory polyps, Schneiderian papillomas, seromucinous hamartoma, and low-grade non-intestinal adenocarcinoma.

4.1 Inflammatory polyps

Inflammatory polyps are certainly the most common lesions that are confused with REAHs.

The most notable clinical differences between REAHs and inflammatory polyps are the location and their gross appearance.

Inflammatory polyps are typically the clinical manifestation of a sinonasal polyposis. Nasal polyps are rarely isolated. They are multiple and bilateral and usually extrude from the middle and superior meati. They are rarely attached to the posterior septum. REAHs originate specifically from the olfactory cleft.

Nasal polyps are usually edematous and not indurated. On microscopy, both lesions can show fibroblastic and vascular proliferation, stromal edema, a mixed inflammatory cell infiltrate, and seromucinous gland proliferation. However, inflammatory polyps do not have florid adenomatoid proliferation and stromal hyalinization which, when present, favor REAHs (**Figures 6–9**).

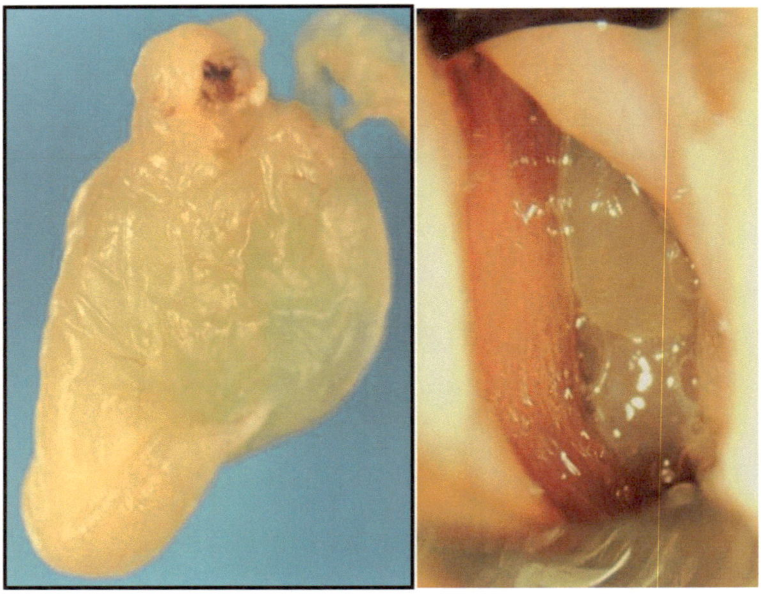

Figure 6.
Macroscopic and endoscopic view of a nasal polyp.

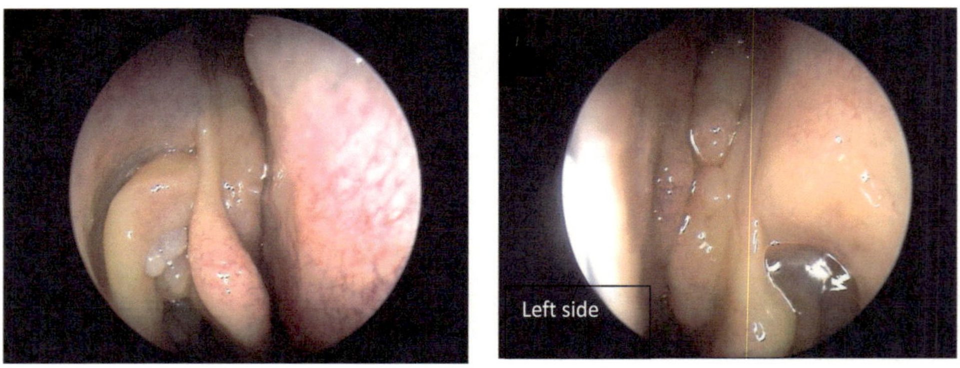

Figure 7.
Endoscopic view: right and left nasal cavity: presence of nasal polyps in the middle and superior meati.

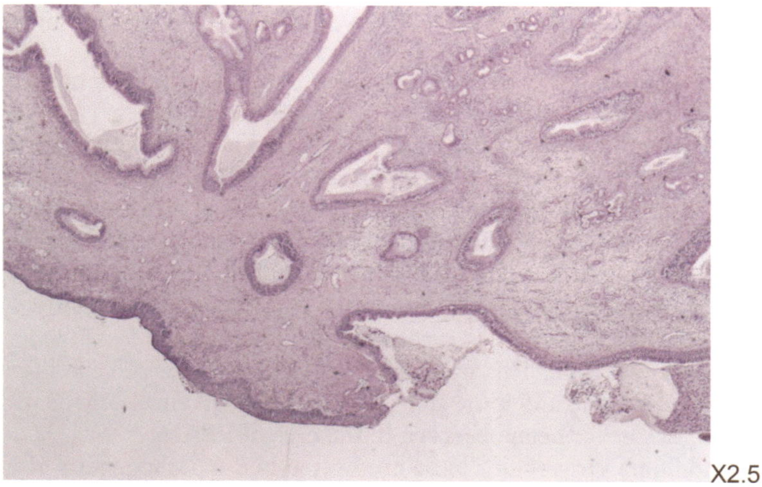

Figure 8.
Inflammatory polyp with edematous inflammatory stroma and single-layered glands.

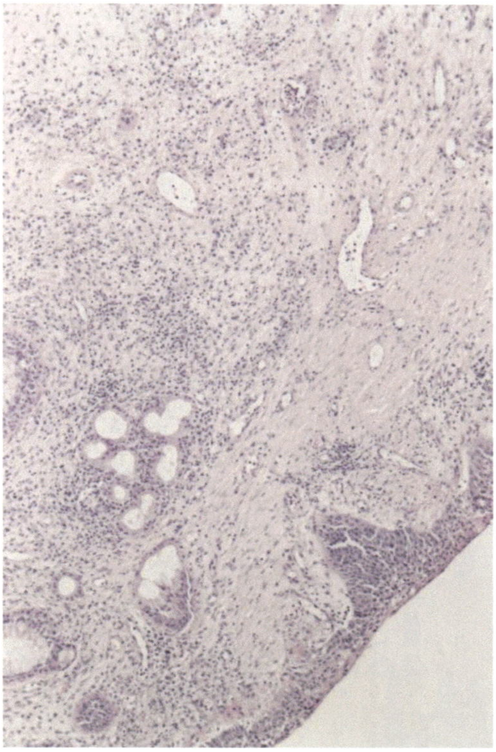

Figure 9.
Inflammatory polyp showing inflammatory stroma without hyalinization.

4.2 Schneiderian papillomas

This is the second important differential diagnosis of REAHs.

Schneiderian papillomas are benign epithelial neoplasms of the sinonasal tract. Their annual incidence ranges between 0.2 and 1.5/100,000 people per year.

They are classified in three types: exophytic/fungiform papilloma, endophytic/inverted papilloma, and oncocytic/cylindrical cell papilloma. The inverted type is the most common, accounting for nearly two thirds of the cases. We limit the description to this type.

It is mostly unilateral. It occurs mainly in adults during the fifth or sixth decade. There is a predilection for men.

Unlike inflammatory polyps and REAHs, inverted papillomas are considered true neoplasms. While REAHs tend to be located medial to the turbinate lamella, inverted papillomas have a predilection for the lateral wall of the nasal cavity or the paranasal cavities. Maxillary and ethmoid sinuses are the most common origins followed by the sphenoid and frontal sinuses. Even if inverted papillomas are benign histologic lesions, clinically they may be aggressive with a relatively strong potential for local destruction, high rate of recurrence (more or less 50%), and a risk of carcinomatous evolution. This transformation in squamous cell carcinoma can be synchrone or metachrone and more likely in case of recurrence. This malignant transformation has never been observed in the case of REAHs.

Human papilloma virus seems to be implicated in the pathogenesis of inverted papillomas. Chronic inflammation seems to be a favorizing factor in REAHs.

The treatment of inverted papilloma requires a more extensive and radical excision with a subperiosteal dissection and a drilling of the base of implantation. Endonasal medial maxillectomy is the golden standard for maxillary sinus origin. Recurrence is more likely in frontal sinus papillomatosis due to the localization and the difficulty to completely eradicate the lesion. The surgical treatment for REAHs is a complete excision without ethmoidectomy.

Grossly, inverted papilloma looks like a reddish-gray lobulated tumor, more firm than an inflammatory polyp, with a fairly characteristic "raspberry" aspect (**Figure 10**).

Histologically inverted papillomas have an endophytic growth pattern. There is an invagination of stratified squamous epithelium with an admixture of mucin containing cells and microcysts. The epithelium may be of squamous, transitional,

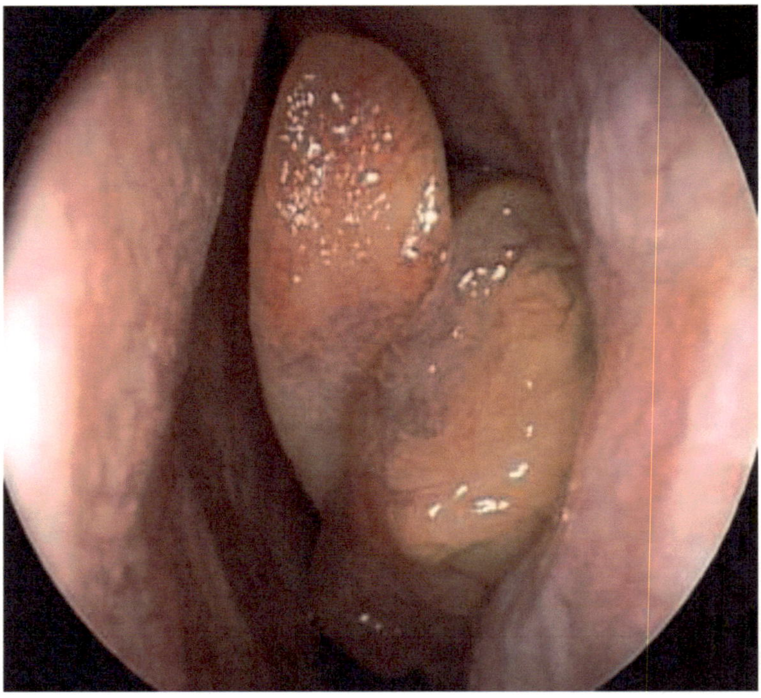

Figure 10.
Endoscopic view of an inverted papilloma originating from the left maxillary sinus.

or respiratory type. The endophytic growth of squamous epithelium is not seen in REAH. Transmigrating neutrophils and neutrophilic microabscesses may be seen. Occasional mitoses may be seen in the basal layer. Mild to moderate atypia may be seen. Edema or chronic inflammatory infiltrate is present in the stroma (**Figures 11–13**).

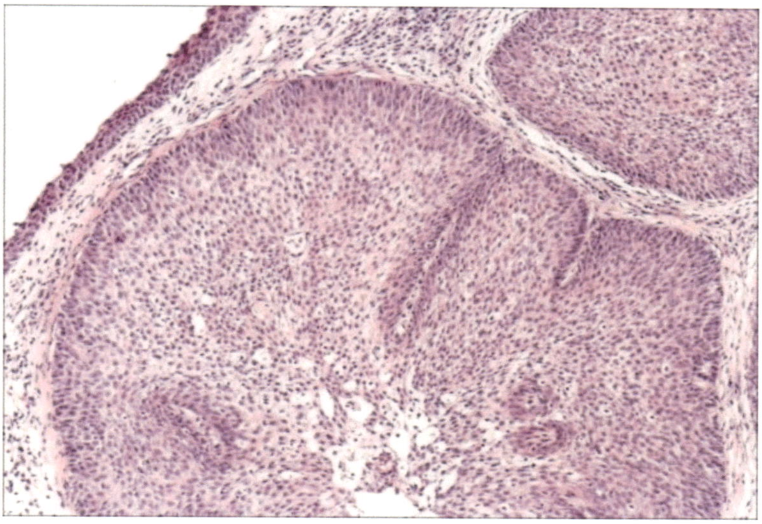

Figure 11.
Low magnification: typical view of an IP: it shows an endophytic growth pattern consisting of markedly thickened squamous epithelial proliferation growing downward into the underlying connective tissue stroma to form large clefts, ribbons, and islands. Note the absence of mucoserous glands. Delicate basement membrane.

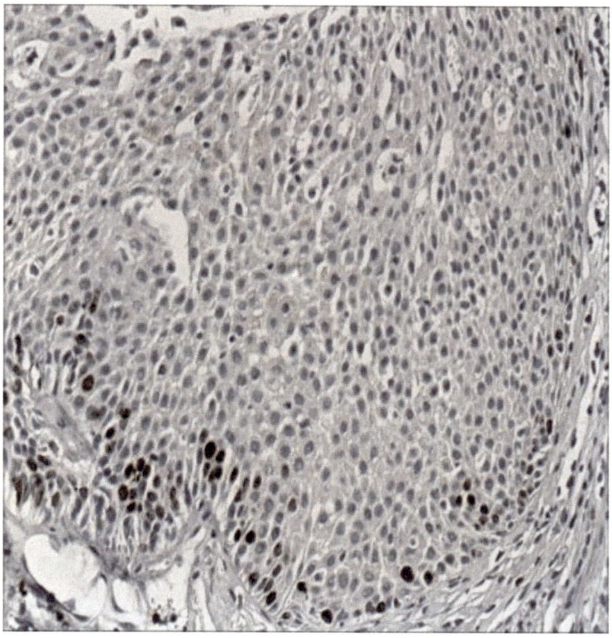

Figure 12.
Immunohistochemistry: high power shows the epithelium to be composed of pseudostratified columnar cells/ positivity of MIB1 in the basal cells.

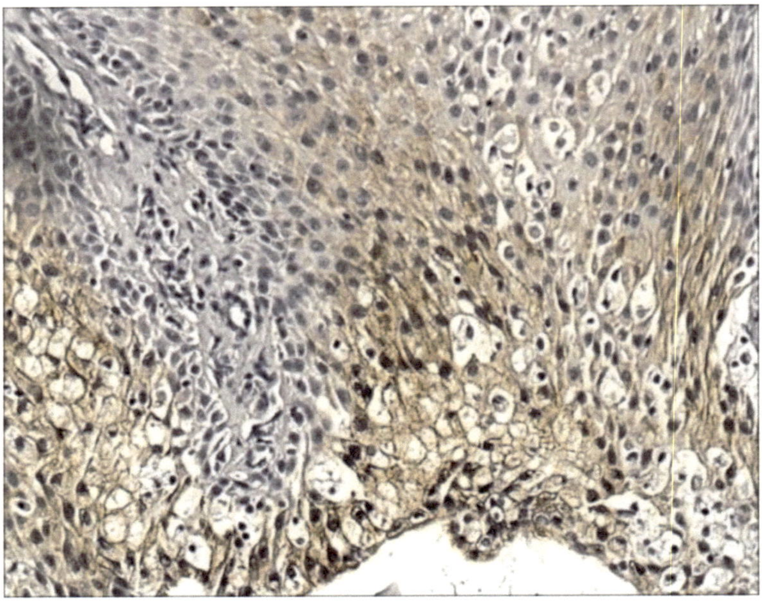

Figure 13.
Immunohistochemistry: high power/positivity of CK7.

4.3 Seromucinous hamartoma

Seromucinous hamartoma is another subtype of hamartoma, recently described. It is a benign lesion of the sinonasal tract as well, located in the posterior nasal cavity or rhinopharynx frequently associated to REAHs. Since its description in 1974 [12], only a small number of additional cases have been reported.

The lesion occurs equally in men and women. Patients are middle-aged to elderly (mean age 50–60) and have complaints with nasal obstruction or nosebleeds. Surgical excision is the treatment of choice. It is included in the differential diagnosis of low grade epithelial proliferations of the sinonasal tract. The differentiation with low-grade non-intestinal adenocarcinoma can be tricky.

Histologically, the mass looks like a benign lesion. Lobular or haphazard proliferations of small to large glands and ducts lined by a single layer of cuboidal or flattened epithelial cells are visualized. Eosinophilic secretions are often present within tubules. The surrounding stroma often contains a lymphoplasmocytic inflammatory infiltrate. Periglandular hyalinization can be observed. There are no features suggesting a malignancy. There are no nuclear atypia.

Seromucinous hamartomas are positive for CK7 and CK19 and negative for CK14 and CK20. The serous glands are usually S100 positive and negative for p63 and muscle-specific antigen.

4.4 Low-grade sinonasal adenocarcinoma (LGSNAC)

Sinonasal adenocarcinoma is the third differential diagnosis for REAH. It accounts for approximately 20% of all sinonasal malignancies and is classified into intestinal and non-intestinal salivary and non-salivary types. Intestinal adenocarcinomas (also called ITAC) take their origin in the olfactory cleftl and then extend into the ethmoid sinus, the orbit, or the anterior cranial fossa. It is an occupational disease; they typically occur in woodworkers. They look like an irregular exophytic pink necrotic and friable mass bulging into the nasal cavity located between the nasal septum and the turbinate lamella.

On microscopy, papillary and colonic types are the most common architectures. Differentiating ITAC from REAH is usually not difficult as the cell types, high-grade features, and increased mitotic index are characteristics for ITAC. ITAC is positive for CK20 and MIB1 and negative for CK7 (**Figure 14**).

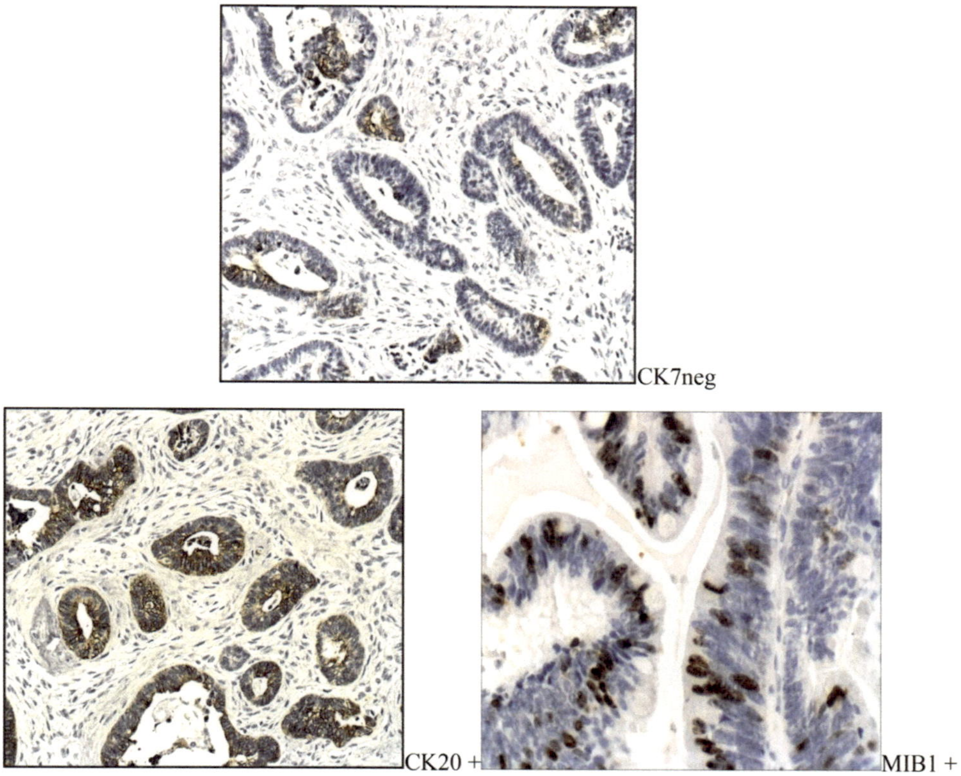

Figure 14.
Intestinal-type adenocarcinoma: Immunohistochemistry—Positivity for CK20, CK7, and MIB1.

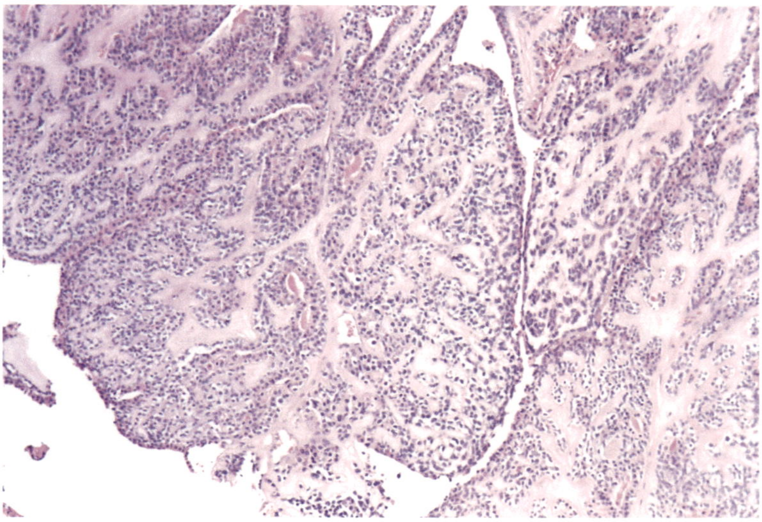

Figure 15.
LGSNAC: Glandular proliferations lined by cuboidal to columnar cells which are usually monomorphic and cytologically bland.

On the other hand, low-grade non-intestinal adenocarcinomas (LGSNAC) are less common and less invasive. There is no sex or racial predilection. There is no association with wood dust exposure. They have no tendency to give systemic metastasis. However, they have a potential for local invasion and destruction of tissue. Extensive surgery is recommended to be associated with radiotherapy in some cases.

Histologically, the mass originates from the surface epithelium and the seromucinous glands of the submucosa. It consists of glandular proliferations lined by cuboidal to columnar cells which are usually monomorphic and cytologically bland. It forms a diverse group of bland tubular and/or papillary tumors. Mitoses are rare. Necrosis, perineural invasion, and lymphovascular invasion are absent. The stroma contains an inflammatory infiltrate as in REAHs.

Immunohistochemistry shows the positivity for CK7 and S100 and negativity for CK20 and CDX2.

The main differential diagnosis is between LGSNAC and seromucinous hamartoma (**Figure 15**).

5. Our experience

5.1 REAHs as a solitary lesion

This clinical presentation of REAHs is actually the less frequent.

Table 1 reports a cohort of eight cases diagnosed and treated in the ENT department of the CHU UCL Namur since 2008.

There were seven women. The mean age was 65 years old. Ranges are 27 and 81.

There was one man: age 53 years old.

The lesions were unilateral in six patients (three left sided; three right sided) and bilateral in two.

Two patients were asymptomatic. REAH was diagnosed by nasal endoscopy and a sinus CT scanner performed for an assessment of epiphora, a case of nasal dysfunction and another one to rule out sinus disease associated to his allergic rhinitis.

The other patients complained with nasal obstruction and rhinorrhea.

Patient	Gender	Side	Symptoms
Br, L.	Female	R/olfactory cleft	Asymptomatic dacryoscan; 2009
Sch, M.	Female	L/septal implantation	Unilateral nasal obstruction 2008
Van rent. M.	Female	X2/olfactory cleft	Bilateral nasal obstruction 2012
W. Jes.	Female Seromucinous hamartoma	R/sphenochoanal recess	Unilateral nasal obstruction 2012
B. Pat.	Female/COREAH	L/sphenochoanal recess	Unilateral nasal obstruction/nasal collapse 2019
H. C.	Female	L/olfactory cleft	Unilateral nasal obstruction 2019
Tr. M.	Female	R/olfactory cleft	Asymptomatic Ct finding 2019
N, A.	Male	X2 R > L	Allergic rhinitis; paucisymptomatic/nasal endoscopy/CT scan 2019

Table 1.
Reports our experience of REAHs.

REAHS originated from the olfactory cleft in six patients and from the anterior wall of the sphenoid sinus in two cases.

On nasal endoscopy the lesion looked fleshy, with no vascular component and no necrosis.

On imaging the lesion was solitary in the olfactory cleft. No chronic rhinosinusitis was present (**Figure 16**).

The MRI performed in three cases was not so helpful. There were no pathognomonic features whatever was the localization. In the literature, REAHs appear as a homogeneous mass with post-contrast enhancement on T1-weighted sequences as well as hyperintensity on T2-weighted images (**Figure 17**) [13].

The diagnosis of REAH was confirmed in all the cases by the pathologist.

In one case it was a COREAH, and in another case it was a seromucinous hamartoma. These two hamartomas were located in the posterior nasal fossa.

A biopsy was performed under local anesthesia in asymptomatic cases to make a formal diagnosis. For the other the diagnosis was made on the surgical specimen.

There was no clear etiologic factor that could have played a role in the development of REAH except in one patient suffering from allergic rhinitis. There was no concomitant chronic sinusitis, asthma, or aspirin intolerance.

Concerning the management, in two patients a wait and see attitude was proposed as the patient was not symptomatic. For the others an endoscopic resection of the lesion was performed under general anesthesia. The dissection was done in a subperiosteal plane. We have never drilled out the site of implantation. There was no need to do a full house ethmoidectomy.

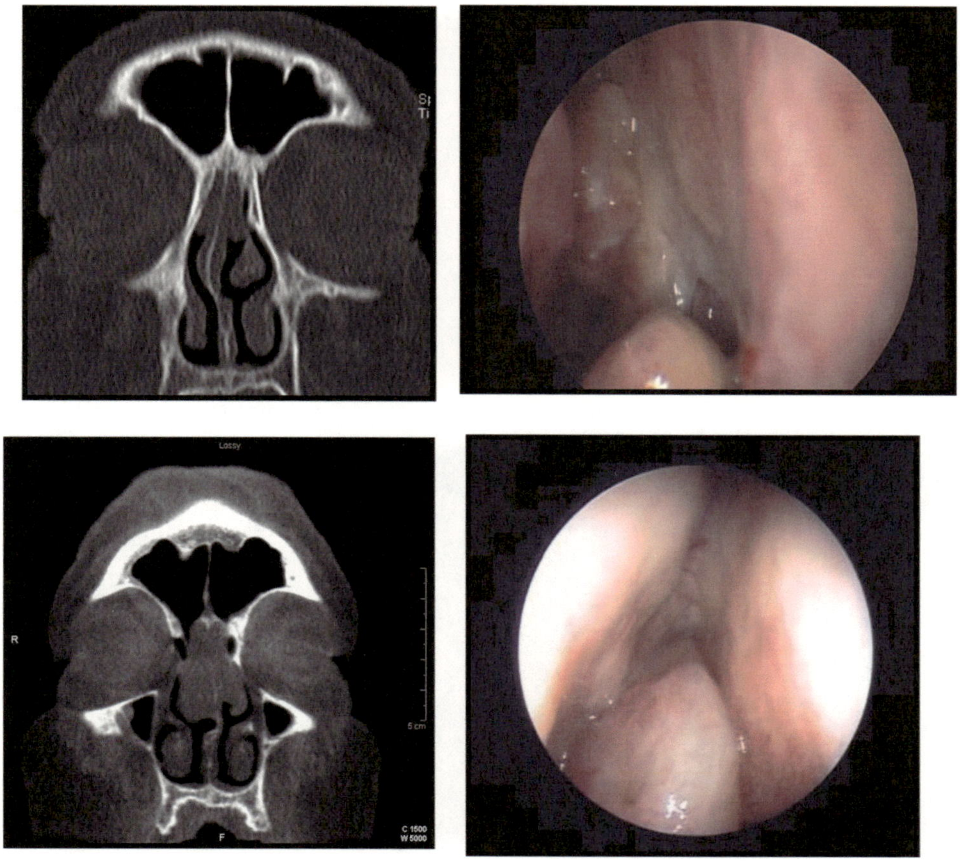

Figure 16.
Comparison between CT scan and nasal endoscopy.

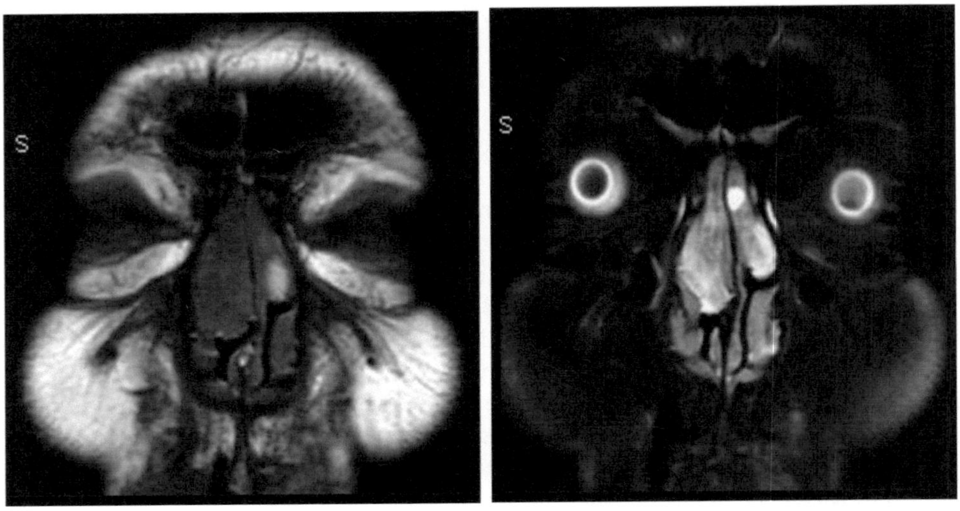

Figure 17.
MRI of a patient with bilateral REAHs: T1- and T2-weighted sequences.

Until now we have had no recurrence (**Figure 18**).

5.2 REAHs associated to a nasal polyposis often previously operated also called REAH-like lesions

This is the second clinical pattern of REAHs, and certainly this is the most common type.

Table 2 reports a cohort of 16 patients diagnosed with such a pattern during the past 18 months.

5.2.1 Epidemiology

The series includes 13 men and 2 women. The mean average is about 63 years old.

The majority of the patients are in the fifth and sixth decades.

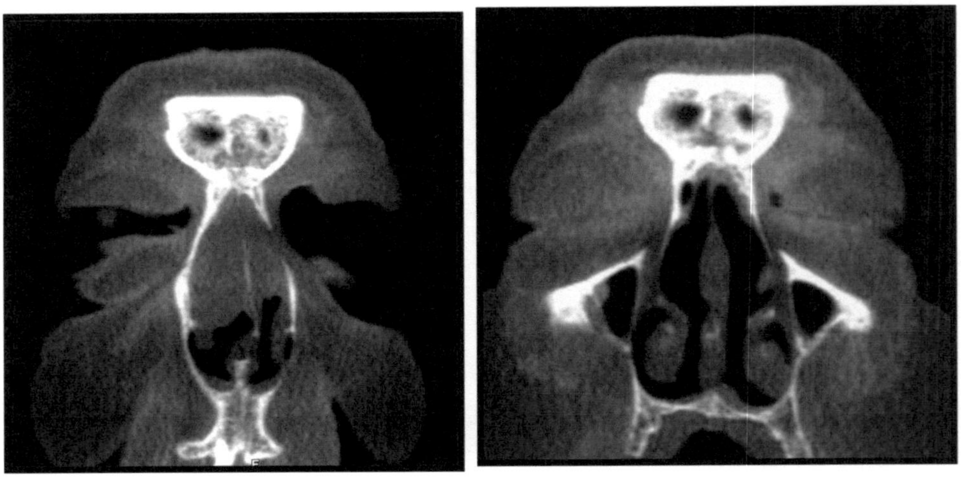

Figure 18.
Illustration of a case with bilateral REAHs: pre- and postop imaging.

Patient	Sex	Disease/surgery
S. Jac.	M	Asthma/rev surgery: REAH-like X2/draf III
Fris. JL	M	Polypose XZ/revision ethmoidectomy/REAH: chronic otitis media
Ros. G	M	Recurrent NP/asthma: REAHs/rev ethmoidectomy
Hub. S.	M	Sever NP/complete ethmoidectomy
L.; Th.	M	Asthma: seromucous otitis media/revision surgery/REAH
Br. Cl.	M	Aspirin intolerance; asthma/recurrence
De Ras.Ge.	M	Nasal polyposis and asthma /previous surgery
Bran. Ar	M	Revison surgery for massive polyposis
De pl. Ph	M	Nasal polyposis operated 3 times/no asthma
Hou. Adr.	M	Recurrentpolyposis/rev ethmoidectomy
Aig; Ph.	M	Recurrentpolyposis/allergic rhinitis/aspirin intolerance/:metabisulfite intolerance
Mas. Cl	F	Revision surgery/asthma/aspirin intolerance
Corl. W.	M	Primary severe nasal polyposis: no asthma: operated in 2013/REAHs
Tri. Fr.	M	Ethmoidectomy 10 y ago/nasal polyposis/ REAHs
V. Mo	F	Nasal polyposis /asthma/previous FESS/REAHs X2

Table 2.
Cohort of patients with REAH-like lesions.

All the patients suffer from a nasal polyposis. In two cases it was a massive primary polyposis. The other patients have a nasal polyposis operated in the past. The REAHs were diagnosed at the revision surgery.

Eight patients have concomitant asthma. Two patients have aspirin intolerance.

Two patients have allergic rhinitis.

Chronic inflammation plays a role in the development of REAHs in this clinical pattern.

5.2.2 Nasal endoscopy

REAHs are located in the olfactory cleft. Their macroscopic aspect is different than usual nasal polyps extruding from the ethmoid sinus. They are more fleshy and firm. There is no necrosis.

As the following pictures show, it is extremely difficult to differentiate with the fibroscopy REAHs and inflammatory polyps in case of recurrent nasal polyposis. The histologic examination of the surgical specimens is mandatory for this differentiation (**Figure 19**).

5.2.3 Imaging

CT imaging findings are described in only a limited number of studies [1, 4, 5, 14]. Lima et al. [5], Hawley et al. [4], and Lee et al. (51 cases) [14] conclude that REAHs cause widening of the olfactory cleft more than 10 mm but generally do not cause bone erosion.

All the paranasal sinus cavities can be opaque as illustrated by the following pictures (**Figures 20–22**):

Some patients have a long-standing disease; REAHs develop after the surgery with time. Some of them are attached to the anterior and superior portion of the

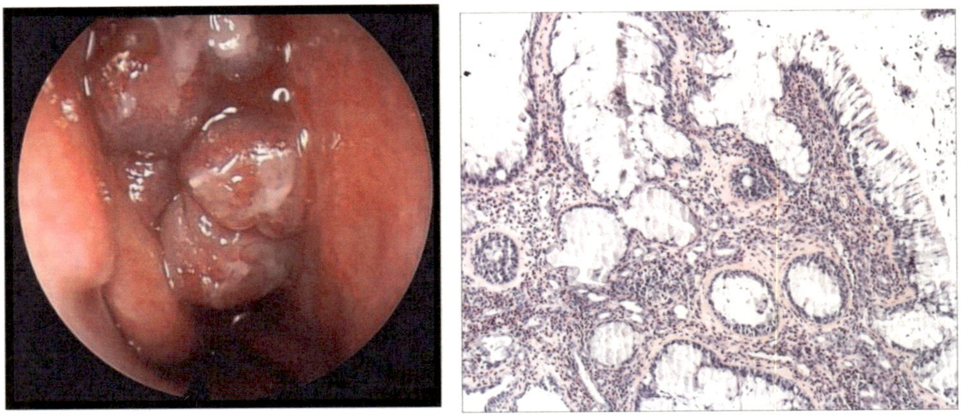

Figure 19.
Comparison of the nasal endoscopy and the histological pattern. The inflammation in the stroma is much more important than in pure REAHs.

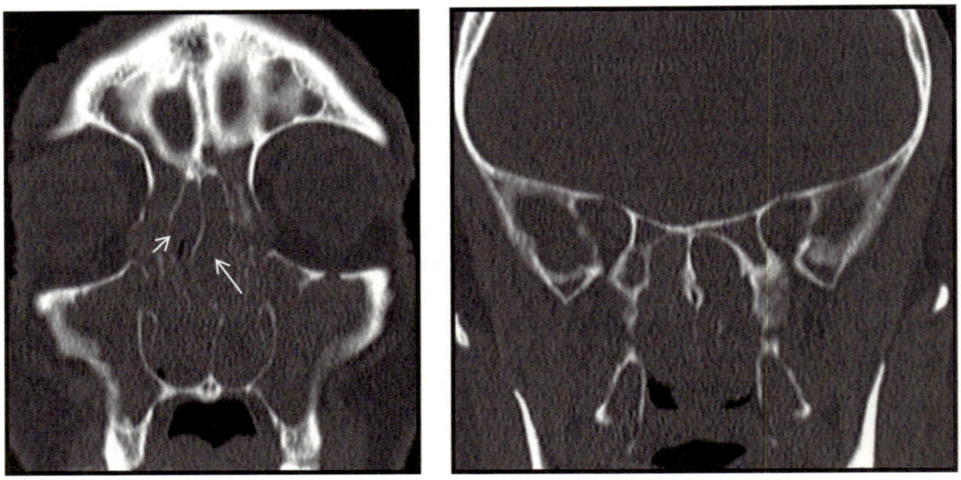

Figure 20.
CT showing a severe nasal polyposis; widening of the olfactory cleft raises suspicion of REAHs.

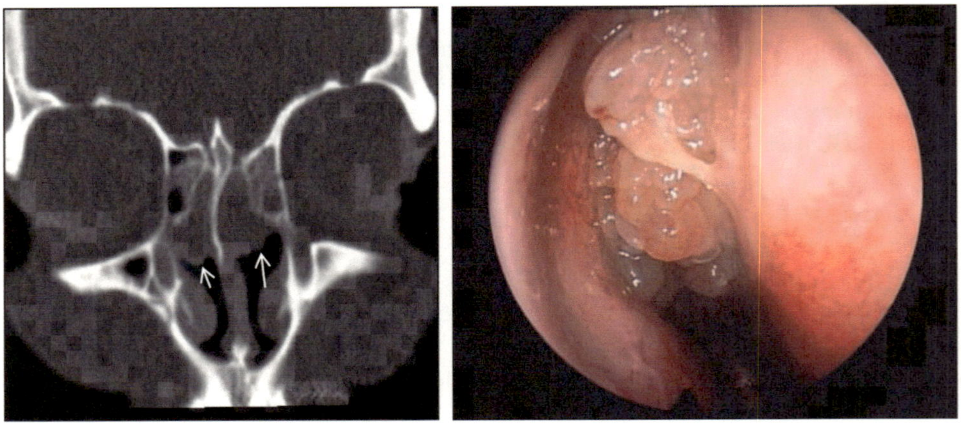

Figure 21.
Patient with REAHs in the olfactory cleft. She had a standard ethmoidectomy for nasal polyposis. We observe REAHs in the olfactory cleft. Correlation between CT scan and nasal endoscopy.

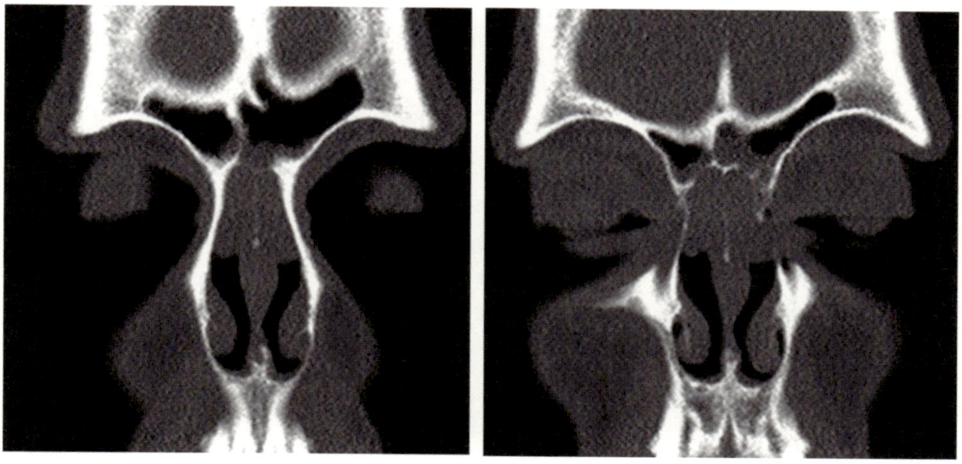

Figure 22.
Typical CT scan showing the opacity of both olfactory clefts caused by REAHs.

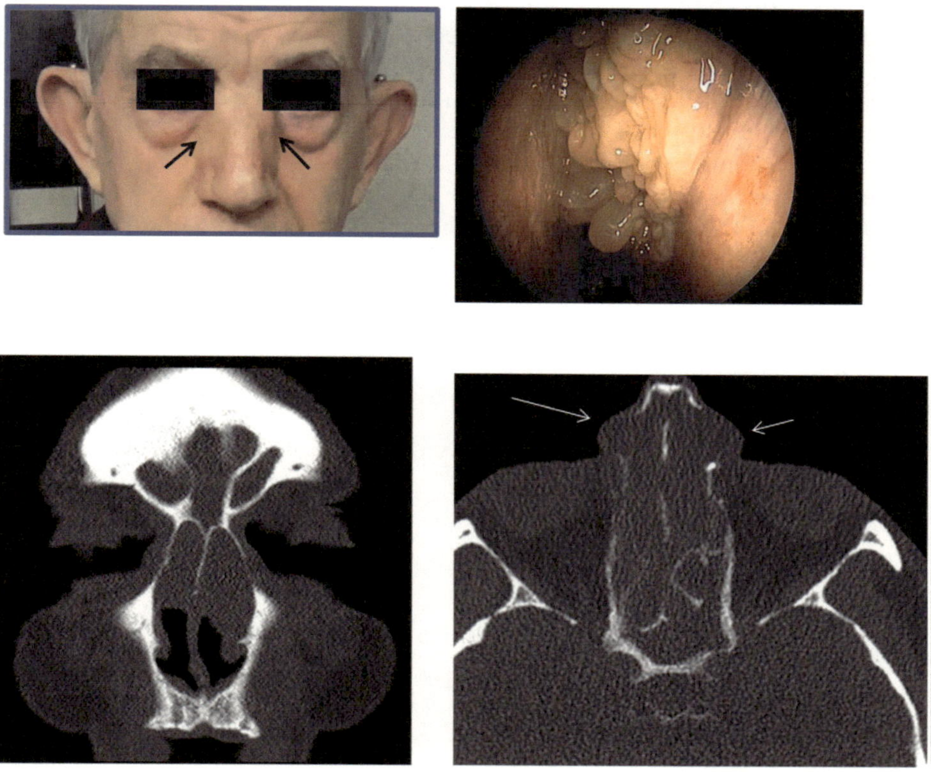

Figure 23.
Same patient with thinning and erosion of the nasal bones (arrows) and opacity of both frontal sinuses.

nasal septum and cause blockage of the frontal sinus pathway or even thinning and erosion of the nasal bones.

Figure 23 show such an exceptional evolution.

MRI can be of some help to rule out other lesions such as encephalocele, olfactory neuroblastoma, or glioma.

The management of REAHs associated with nasal polyposis must be discussed case by case.

A complete sphenoethmoidectomy is usually necessary to manage the recurrent nasal polyposis.

For the REAHs, debulking or better exenteration of the olfactory cleft must be considered. But we know that it can be tricky and risky for the skull base with a risk of CSF leak if the surgery is too aggressive. Resection of the REAHs is usually more bloody than during a polypectomy.

In the case of frontal opacity caused by REAHs attached to the anterior and superior septa, a Draf III procedure must be considered.

After surgery medical treatment of the nasal polyposis and asthma remains absolutely necessary to prevent or delay as much as possible recurrences.

6. Conclusion

REAHs and REAH-like lesions are relatively new clinical entities. Despite numerous publications they are still underdiagnosed. These lesions are located in the olfactory clefts. They can be isolated or in association with nasal polyposis typically in the case of recurrence after FESS.

The clinicians and pathologists must know these lesions. They are usually benign, but in some cases they are associated to frontal sinus blockage and widening of the nasal vault; loss of smell is common. The differential diagnosis includes diseases with more severe morbidities such as inverted papilloma, seromucinous hamartomas, and low-grade non-intestinal adenocarcinoma.

Histological examination of all the surgical specimens is necessary.

The treatment is dictated by the disease.

The extent of the surgery depends on the type and size of the REAHs and the associated disease.

It consists of a limited polypectomy or a complete exenteration of the olfactory cleft associated or not to a full house ethmoidectomy and even a Draf III procedure.

Author details

Ph. Eloy[1*], C. Fervaille[2] and M.C. Nollevaux[2]

1 ENT Department, CHU UCL Namur, Site of Godinne, Yvoir, Belgium

2 Department of Pathology, CHU UCL Namur, Site of Godinne, Yvoir, Belgium

*Address all correspondence to: philippe.eloy@uclouvain.be

References

[1] VandenBossche S, De Vos G, Lemmerling MA. Typical but underdiagnosed nasal cavity Mass. Journal of the Belgian Society of Radiology. 2018;**102**(1):35

[2] Wenig BM, Heffner DK. Respiratory epithelial adenomatoid hamartomas of the sinonasal tract and nasopharynx: A clinicopathologic study of 31 cases. Annals of Otology, Rhinology, and Laryngology. 1995;**104**(8):639-645

[3] Nguyen DT, Gauchotte G, Arous F, Vignaud J-M, Jankowski R. Respiratory epithelial adenomatoid hamartoma of the nose: An updated review. American Journal of Rhinology & Allergy. 2014; **28**(5):187-192

[4] Hawley KA, Ahmed M, Sindwani R. CT findings of sinonasal respiratory epithelial adenomatoid hamartoma: A closer look at the olfactory clefts. American Journal of Neuroradiology. 2013;**34**(5):1086-1090

[5] Lima NB, Jankowski R, Georgel T, Grignon B, Guillemin F, Vignaud J-M. Respiratory adenomatoid hamartoma must be suspected on CT-scan enlargement of the olfactory clefts. Rhinology. 2006;**44**(4):264-269

[6] Bullock MJ. Low-grade epithelial proliferations of the sinonasal tract. Head and Neck Pathology. 2016;**10**(1): 47-59

[7] Flavin R, Russell J, Phelan E, McDermott MB. Chondroosseous respiratory epithelial adenomatoid hamartoma of the nasal cavity: A case report. International Journal of Pediatric Otorhinolaryngology. 2005;**69**:87-91

[8] Roffman E, Baredes S, Mirani N. Respiratory epithelial adenomatoid hamartomas and chondro-osseous respiratory epithelial adenomatoid hamartomas of the sinonasal tract: A case series and literature review. American Journal of Rhinology. 2006; **20**:596-590

[9] Daniel A, Wong E, Ho J, Singh N. Chondro-osseous respiratory epithelial adenomatoid hamartoma (COREAH): Case report and literature review. Case Reports in Otolaryngology. 2019;**2019**. Article ID 5247091. 4p

[10] Ozolek JA, Barnes EL, Hunt JL. Basal/myoepithelial cells in chronic sinusitis, respiratory epithelial adenomatoid hamartoma, inverted papilloma, and intestinal-type and nonintestinal-type sinonasal adenocarcinoma: An immunohistochemical study. Archives of Pathology & Laboratory Medicine. 2007;**131**:530-537

[11] Ozolek JA, Barnes EL, Hunt JL. Basal/myoepithelial cells in chronic sinusitis, respiratory epithelial adenomatoidhamartoma, inverted papilloma, and intestinal-type and nonintestinal-type sinonasal adenocarcinoma: An immunohistochemical study. Archives of Pathology & Laboratory Medicine. 2007;**131**:530-537

[12] Baillie EE, Batsakis JG. Glandular (seromucinous) hamartoma of the nasopharynx. Oral Surgery, Oral Medicine, and Oral Pathology. 1974;**38**: 760-762

[13] Braun J-J, Riehm S, Averous G, Billing A, Veillon F. MRI in respiratory epithelial adenomatoidhamartoma of nasal cavities. Journal of Neuroradiology. 2013;**40**(3):216-219

[14] Lee JT, Garg R, Brunworth J, Keschner DB, Thompson LDR. Sinonasal respiratory epithelial adenomatoid hamartomas: Series of 51 cases and literature review. American Journal of Rhinology & Allergy. 2013; **27**(4):322-328

Section 2

Central Olfactory Function and Disorders

Chapter 6

Neuro-Olfactory Regulation and Salivary Actions: A Coordinated Event for Successful Blood-Feeding Behavior of Mosquitoes

Tanwee Das De and Rajnikant Dixit

Abstract

The synergistic actions of the nongenetic and genetic factors are crucial to shape mosquitoes' feeding behavior. Unlike males, adult female mosquitoes are evolved with unique ability to take blood meals from a vertebrate host for reproductive success which eventually makes them a potential vector. Processing and integration of chemical information in the neuro-olfactory system followed by salivary actions facilitate blood meal uptake process. Thus, deciphering the underlying molecular mechanism of odor sensing through the detection machinery (olfactory system), odor processing and decision-making by decision machinery (brain), and regulation of saliva secretion by the action machinery (salivary gland) is likely to reveal molecular pathways which can be targeted to disrupt mosquitoes' feeding behavior. Here we summarize how smart actions of highly specialized neurosensory systems guide and manage feeding behavior associated complex events of (i) successful navigation to find a suitable host, (ii) making food choice decisions, and (iii) regulation of the salivary gland actions in mosquitoes.

Keywords: mosquito, olfaction, brain, feeding decision, salivary gland, host-seeking, blood feeding

1. Introduction

Mosquitoes that belong to the order Diptera and Culicidae family account for large biomass of insects' community and are one of the most notorious animals on earth which transmit many blood-borne pathogens. It is only the adult female mosquitoes which bite on human and other vertebrate hosts to access the blood and thus have strong impact on epidemiological consequences. So far about 3540 species of mosquitoes have been recognized that are divided into 2 subfamilies and 112 genera [1] which are inhabiting throughout the temperate and tropical regions. *Anopheles* species biodiversity and species richness seem to be one of the dominantly evolved blood-feeding insect species race on earth, impacting millions of lives through transmitting deadliest disease malaria around the globe. In tropical areas, *Anopheles gambiae*, *Aedes aegypti*, and *Culex quinquefasciatus* are the most notorious mosquito vectors of infectious diseases such as malaria, dengue, and filariasis, respectively. The main causative agents of malaria are *Plasmodium falciparum* and *Plasmodium vivax* which infects millions of people each year, posing a major threat to society [2]. Arboviruses, viz. dengue, Zika, chikungunya, and yellow fever viruses, are also significant mosquito-borne pathogens that are mainly vectored by *Aedes* mosquitoes.

The mosquito-borne diseases not only are restricted to underdeveloped countries but also escalate in the developed world. Urbanization, continuous climate change, global warming, and other environmental factors are facilitating mosquitoes' adaptation and survival during adverse situations [3, 4]. Taken together, it is not hard to predict the situation of mosquito and other insect-borne diseases becoming exacerbate in the coming century [5, 6]. Even the diverse ecological and epidemiological settings within Southeast Asia favor the association of diverse Anopheline fauna which makes malaria prevalence and malaria eradication more challenging. In order to save humans from the mosquito's infectious bites, advanced chemical insecticide(s) still play a central role; however, fast emergence of insecticide resistance and increased toxicants to the environment demands the development of new molecular tools. Thus, it is challenging to understand the complex biology of mosquitoes which popularize themselves as the most dangerous animals on earth (https://www.statista.com/chart/2203/the-worlds-deadliest-animals/).

Disease transmission by mosquitoes is restricted to the blood-feeding behavior of adult female mosquitoes which takes blood meal from humans and other vertebrate hosts for the completion of their gonotropic cycle. In order to carry out the successful blood-feeding event, the integration of the "olfactory system," the receiver of the chemical/environmental stimuli; the "central nervous system," the hardware system with high processing efficacy; and the "salivary gland," the output/feedback device are obligatory. Here we provide an overview and update the current knowledge on how the sensory system of mosquito detects essential chemical information which are then processed by the central nervous system for successful navigation and stimulate the salivary gland for salivation to facilitate the feeding event.

2. Mosquito feeding behavior

Feeding is a fundamental need of every animal to achieve their optimal growth, survival, and reproductive requirements. But the strategy of food intake and the feeding preference largely vary depending on the internal metabolic needs, i.e., whether they are starved or satiated; on the internal physiological state, i.e., whether they are virgin or mated and gravid or unfed; and also on the external sensory stimuli. In the case of mosquitoes, plant sugars such as nectar and honeydew are the primary energy source for survival, flight, and foraging activities of both males and females. Only adult female mosquitoes take blood meal as an optional dietary supplement, and this specialization is predicted to evolve for better fitness [7–9]. Genetic architecture and the allelic polymorphism of different mosquito species influence their traits towards selection and preference for feeding hosts. Apart from that other internal factors such as circadian rhythm and physiological status including nutritional and mating status, as well as environmental factors such as temperature and humidity, affect mosquito feeding behavior cumulatively [10, 11] (**Figure 1**).

Each feeding event of mosquitoes is initiated by random navigation from a long distance, which becomes specific when triggered by a certain group of chemicals such as CO_2, lactic acid, 1-Octen-3-Ol, acetone, ammonia, etc. The detection of other additional cues such as visual and thermal factors facilitates the downstream events of host localization, landing over the host and searching for a suitable site for probing by the proboscis to initiate blood-feeding. But, successful navigation does not always corroborate with a successful feeding event, because it involves another level of regulation of the central nervous system by discriminating the

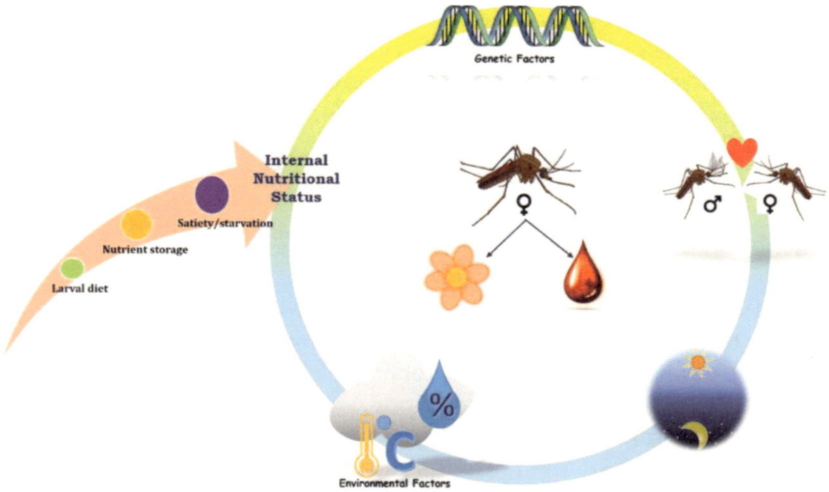

Figure 1.
Factors affecting mosquitoes' feeding behavior. The genetic structure, circadian cycle, mating status, internal nutritional status, and external environmental factors such as temperature and humidity cumulatively work to shape the mosquitoes' feeding preference toward either sugar meal or blood meal. The internal nutritional status is dependent on larval nutrition, the amount of nutrient storage, and the feeding condition of the mosquito, i.e., either starved or satiate.

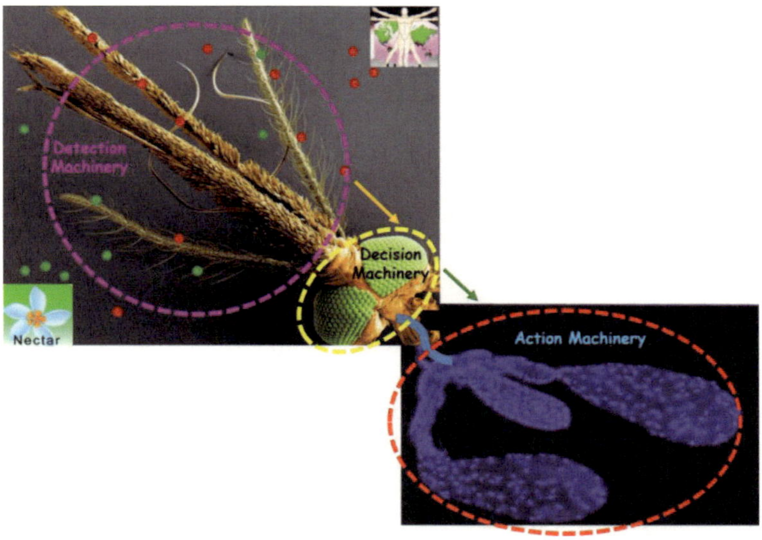

Figure 2.
The path of signal processing for achieving successful mosquito navigation and feeding. The tripartite inter-organ communication among three tissues, viz., olfactory tissue, central nervous system (brain), and the salivary gland, is crucial for the completion of feeding events. The olfactory tissue (highlighted by purple circle) senses and binds to odor molecules emanating from either plant or vertebrate host and sends the respective signal towards the brain system (highlighted as yellow circle). After processing the initial signal of odor in the central nervous system, the decision-making process occurs, and then the brain sends the signal towards the salivary gland (highlighted as red circle), and the process of salivation started to facilitate feeding. Photo credit goes to Zwiebel Lab, Vanderbilt University, for the olfactory system of Anopheles *mosquito. The salivary gland picture was taken from the research article by Ghosh et al. [12].*

odor molecules and making a decision for either to feed or not. Post landing and piercing on a particular site of the vertebrate host, successful uptake of blood meal largely depends on the proper functioning of the salivary gland which acts as the final action machinery by facilitating the feeding process through salivation. Thus, here we provide a detailed integrative description of (1) how mosquitoes detect and discriminate among odorant molecules through olfactory system, (2) how the initial signal of odor is processed in the central nervous system/brain and the molecular factors responsible for feeding decision-making process, and (3) how the brain influences and regulates distant tissue such as salivary gland for salivation and consequently helps in food acquisition (**Figure 2**).

3. Mosquito navigation

A sophisticated olfactory system of mosquitoes enables them to communicate and responds to the diverse array of biological and environmental chemical stimuli throughout their life cycle. They use olfactory cues for locating a food source (nectar sugar), finding a mate partner, locating oviposition site, and most importantly selecting a vertebrate host for blood-feeding. Among these olfactory-guided behaviors, searching and locating the desired plant for nectar-feeding involves both visual and chemical cues emanating from different plant species [13]. Volatiles such as mono- and bicyclic monoterpenes are major floral odors for mosquito attraction, and lighter-colored plant flowers have an additional benefit for successful sugar feeding [14]. But, detection of blood-feeding host requires the integration of olfactory, visual, thermal, and humidity cues [15, 16]. The pattern of host-seeking behavior and selection of a certain host are strictly species-specific. However, the navigation trajectory of all the blood-feeding mosquitoes may have some common events (**Figure 3**).

a. Female mosquitoes are engaged in random, non-oriented navigation until they encounter a plume of host odorants including skin emanates consisting of hundreds of chemicals.

b. Random navigation became oriented when a female mosquito detects fluctuation in the carbon dioxide concentration above the atmospheric measurement, caused by the addition of ~4% CO_2 from human breath. The mosquito then follows the trail of odor plume and initiates to fly upwind in a zigzag pattern which drives mosquitoes to reach the odor source. The concentration gradient of different odorants, initiating from CO_2 from long distance (> 10 m), overlaps with other host odors such as lactic acid and 1-octen-3-ol available at closer vicinity, which acts in a synergistic way to make the navigation successful.

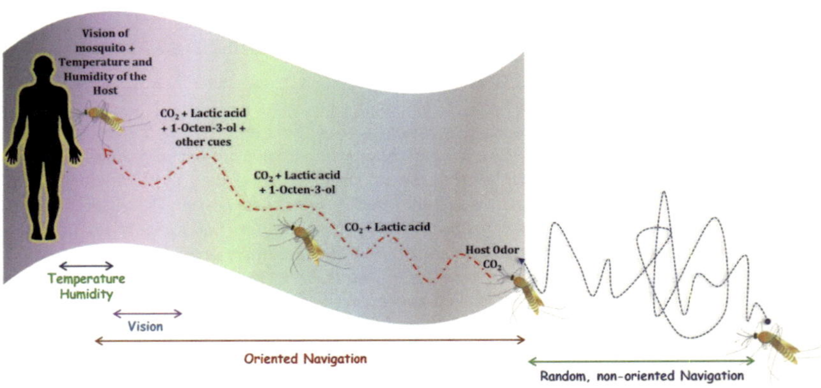

Figure 3.
Mosquito navigation trajectory according to odor plume. The random, non-oriented navigation becomes oriented when mosquitoes sense a gradient of different host odors such as CO_2, lactic acid, 1-octen-3-ol, etc. olfaction along with vision, thermosensation, and hygrosensation facilitates the navigation process and blood meal uptake.

c. When mosquitoes reach in the close vicinity of their potential host through olfactory-guided random to specific navigation, the cumulative role of visual thermosensors enhances. The compound eyes of mosquitoes enable them to visualize a particular host at a distance of 5–10 m by discriminating the light intensity and color of the respective host.

d. After host localization, a mosquito must first land over the host for biting. Temperature and humidity also play a crucial role in short-range host orientation and landing. Then, mosquitoes trace a suitable site for probing through mechanosensory system. The olfactory appendages labellum and stylets along with the peripheral appendages (legs) of mosquitoes finally determine the probing site for successful blood meal uptake.

4. Mosquito sensory system and olfactory signal transduction

It is not difficult to admire that the multimodal sensory system of mosquitoes is the critical regulator of different behavioral processes and thus has a potential impact on disease transmission. In addition, the wide diversity of host preference in mosquitoes is governed by the different genetic makeup of individual species which has strong epidemiological consequences. Therefore, decoding species-specific molecular factors of the mosquitoes' olfactory system may unravel the mechanism of their behavioral plasticity. Two primary components of the chemosensory system are the peripheral system where the chemical information is detected and the central processing unit where the initial signal of odor is processed. The appendages present on the head of the mosquitoes act as the principal detection system, which includes paired antennae, paired maxillary palp, and a labium [8, 17]. These peripheral appendages are equipped with fine hair-like structures called the sensilla, which are distributed nonrandomly across these antennae, maxillary palp, and labium. The type and number of sensilla present on the olfactory organ are highly species-specific [8, 17]. Odorants are thought to penetrate through the numerous pores present on the wall of the sensilla and then traverse through the aqueous sensillar lymph towards the array of molecular receptors present on the dendrites of olfactory receptor neurons (ORNs) [18]. Binding of the diverse odorants with their cognate receptors either activates or inhibits the receptors by changing the ORN action potential. More than two decades of research on insect olfaction uncover several molecular factors that are responsible for odor detection and downstream signal transduction processes. These include odorant-binding proteins (OBPs), odorant-degrading enzymes (ODEs), odorant receptors (ORs), sensory neuron membrane proteins (SNMPs), G proteins, arrestins, and other signaling molecules [8].

4.1 Odorant-binding proteins and odorant-degrading enzymes

Odorant molecules are hydrophobic in nature which require cargo to traverse through the sensillar lymph to reach the receptor molecules, which are present on the dendritic membrane [19–21]. This role is carried out by the odorant-binding proteins (OBPs), which act as a passive carrier of the chemical odorant molecules. OBPs are water-soluble globular proteins containing six α-helical domains with conserved cysteine residues [22]. The number of genes encoding different OBPs varied across different mosquito species and is also dependent on the number of odorant receptors [22]. The availability of this wide and diverse spectrum of OBPs in the insect's tissues facilitates their rapid adaptation in distinct environment. The OBP family broadly includes the pheromone-binding proteins (PBPs) which transport pheromones and different chemosensory proteins (CSPs) which are smaller in size but can bind with a broad spectrum of semiochemicals. In mosquitoes, the OBP genes are classified in three subfamilies: (i) classic OBPs that carry a conserved motif consisting of six cysteine residues; (ii) Plus-C OBPs which contain six additional cysteine residues with novel disulfide connectivity along with three classic OBP motifs; and (iii) atypical OBPs, the longest OBPs that contain a single classic OBP domain in its N-terminal which is extended by a C-terminal extension. Among these three subfamilies, Plus-C OBP class is more divergent in nature and has only been identified from Diptera *Anopheles*, *Culex*, and *Drosophila*; however, Hymenoptera and Lepidoptera did not possess these OBPs. The first OBP of mosquito origin was isolated from the antennae of female *Culex quinquefasciatus* (CquiOBP1) in the early twenty-first century [20, 23]. The availability of genome sequence of several mosquito species in the public domain facilitates the identification and characterization of this large family of OBP genes from different mosquito species, for example, the total number of 69 OBPs from *A. gambiae*, 111 OBPs from *A. aegypti*, 109 OBPs from *C. quinquefasciatus, and* 63 OBPs in *A. culicifacies* [20, 24, 25]. Activation of the chemosensory receptors by odorants also requires timely termination and desensitization of peripheral signaling to maintain sensitivity of ORN-based signaling [26, 27]. In this process, odorant-degrading enzymes (ODEs), particularly several esterases and cytochrome p450s, play a crucial role by terminating the odor-induced signal transduction processes [28–30].

4.2 Odorant receptors

After the OBPs, the principal molecules in odor detection are odorant receptors that convert the chemical signal into electrical outputs and therefore ensure the continuous flow of information from the environment to the insect brain [31–33]. Within the insect phylum, odorant receptors (Ors) were first identified and characterized from the model insect *Drosophila melanogaster*, using an intensive bioinformatics approach [34, 35]. Insects' OR proteins consist of seven transmembrane domains with inverted topology, where N-terminus is intracellular, as compared to mammalian odorant receptors, which are the conventional G protein-coupled receptors (GPCR) [36, 37]. Further experimental evidence suggested that mosquito ORs act as ligand-gated ion channels comprising of heteromeric complexes of two subunits [38, 39]. One subunit is highly conserved and known as olfactory receptor co-receptors (Orco), and the other subunit is largely divergent in terms of number as well as amino acid sequences (Orx) [31, 40–42]. Pilot studies of the OR gene repertoire primarily in *Drosophila melanogaster* [35] and later in mosquitoes [42, 43] suggest that despite having a limited number of ORs, mosquitoes can respond to an array of varied chemicals depending on the specific demand at different life cycle stages [44]. This is possible due to the combinatorial coding mechanism of the insect's olfactory system which increases the perceived odor space of each species. Combinatorial coding increases odor sensitivity to several-fold, where each OR can respond to multiple ligands and a single ligand can activate more than one OR [45]. Moreover, a single odorant can either elicit attractive responses or activate repellent pathway depending on their quality and concentration which subsequently determine insects' behavior [46, 47].

The number of receptors present in each mosquito species is highly variable, e.g., *A. gambiae* genome contains 79 OR genes, *C. quinquefasciatus* has 117, and *A. aegypti* possesses 110 OR genes [47]. Among them the receptor protein Or8 is predominantly studied in mosquitoes because of its conserved nature and specificity towards 1-octen-3-ol, which is a crucial component of human sweat [48, 49]. Deorphanization of other olfactory receptors of mosquitoes was performed using an in vivo heterologous expression system, the "empty neuron" system, originally established in the fruit fly *Drosophila*. The "empty neuron" system is a combination of a GAL4 driver line and a mutant ORN line (UAS—"OR gene") where endogenous odorant receptor is missing and thus gives the opportunity to express and functionally characterize mosquito olfactory receptor gene repertoire. The complexes of both *Drosophila* and mosquitoes using "empty neuron" model indicated that the "odor space" of mosquito and flies is significantly distinct [50, 51]. Furthermore, over the evolutionary time scale, the sensitivity of a particular mosquito OR either increases towards certain predominant hosts or decreases if the host odor profile changes [47]. Thus, it is not difficult to predict that ORs have evolved with highly sensitive and selective property for the detection of diverse odorants which consequently facilitate mosquito adaptation in diverse ecology.

4.3 Other sensory receptors

After detection of a particular odor through synergistic actions of OBPs and ORs, mosquitoes use other sensory modalities such as vision, thermosensation, and hygrosensation to make the differentiation between biting hosts [15, 47, 50]. For visualization, the photoreceptor cells expressing multiple UV-sensitive and long-wavelength sensitive opsin proteins are responsible for detecting and transmitting visual information towards optic lobe (the region of mosquito brain where optic information is processed) [52]. But how mosquitoes integrate visual information with other cues to differentiate hosts remains unclear. Following visual selection, the temperature and humidity are intricately linked to make biting decision [47, 50]. The thermosensory transient receptor potential (TRP) channel protein present on the tips of the antennae of mosquitoes can sense the variation of temperature associated with vertebrate skin [53]. For hygrosensory information processing, the ionotropic receptors (IRs) are reported to play a crucial role in *Drosophila* [47]. Although the role of IRs in humidity sensing in mosquitoes remains elusive, few recent studies highlight their sensitivities against narrow range of odorants such as amines and carboxylic acids and thus have potential function in host-seeking [54].

Once the host is located by the harmonious actions of all the sensory modalities, the mosquito first lands over the host and engages in a mission of locating a proper site for probing by repeated contacting of the skin with the labellum [50]. The gustatory receptors (taste receptors) (GRs), expressing on the labellum and the tarsae (the last segment of their legs through which mosquitoes make contact with the host), may play a pivotal role in biting behavior of mosquitoes [47, 55]. While the functional characterization of mosquito OR genes are of prime focus, a significant number of studies reported that the putative gustatory receptors (Gr1, Gr3 in *A. aegypti* and *C. quinquefasciatus*; Gr22, Gr24 in *A. gambiae*) of mosquitoes are sensitive to CO_2 and thus influence host-seeking behavioral activities [47, 50].

4.4 Olfactory signal transduction

The information, i.e., hidden within the odor molecules, are amplified by activating the sensory neurons. The activation of a different subset of sensory neurons to a different degree is the basis for neuronal coding. When compared with the vertebrate OR, the insect's ORs show a high degree of variation with different topologies, which strongly suggest a different signal transduction mechanism [8]. Some previous studies highlight that olfactory signal transduction in insects involving a ligand-gated ion channel that is formed by the hetero-dimerization of diverse odorant receptor and its co-receptors [27]. This fast ionotropic response does not postulate the involvement of any G proteins and any intracellular second messengers. In contrast, another study indicated the entanglement of G protein and the synthesis of cAMP, IP3, and other secondary messengers that consequently induce the downstream effector enzymes and also affect the membrane potential through activating the co-receptor protein [27, 56]. The resultant change in the membrane potential/permeability by either process causes the generation and propagation of action potentials along the ORN axon membrane towards the antennal lobes. In contrast to the rapid ionotropic pathway, the G protein-mediated metabotropic pathway is slower. However, it plays an important role when the odor cues are present in lower concentration, whereas high concentration directly involves the ionotropic pathway [8, 27, 57].

5. The decision-making unit: the brain

The discrimination and integration among the odor molecules and the exchange of electrochemical information consequently influence the neuronal decision-making abilities of the brain system [58]. When an animal is given preference for food, several decisions can be made such as whether to eat or not, what to eat, and when to eat, which not only depends on the internal physiological condition but also relies on the biological clock of the respective animal. In the case of mosquito species, making a choice among the different available foods requires a fine-tuning of the nasal system and strong integration of the decision-making machinery. The availability of diverse nature of blood-feeding hosts not only makes the decision-making process more complex but also has an impact on mosquito survival, fitness, and fecundity [59].

5.1 Structural basis of signal processing

The knowledge about insect olfactory coding is strongly rooted in the fruit fly *Drosophila melanogaster*. Over the last two decades, the cellular and molecular bases of *Drosophila* olfaction have been studied well with the assistance of varied genetic tools. The three milestones of olfaction have been documented comprehensively in the fruit fly on how odor information is received, concatenated, and processed by the peripheral and central nervous systems, respectively [60, 61]. Apart from that, "the parallel olfactory processing" and "feature detection" mechanism has also been unlocked in honey bee brain and sphinx moth, respectively [62–64]. Several studies on *Drosophila* and other insects (*Manduca sexta and Bombyx mori*) suggested that the primary brain structures responsible for receiving initial information of odor are the antennal lobes (ALs) [62, 63, 65, 66]. These antennal lobes consist of a specific number of spherical condensed neuropil structures, which are known as glomeruli. Depending on the nature and sex of the insect species, the number of glomeruli varied between 50 and 200, whereas each respective species possess the same number of glomeruli having identical features (shape, size, location) [67, 68]. Olfactory receptor neurons that express a particular type of receptor on their dendrites project their axons into the same glomerulus [8, 45, 67, 69]. Furthermore, each glomerulus is housed with the arms of the local interneurons (LNs) and the dendrites of the projection neurons (PNs) [69]. Thus, within the antennal lobe, a synaptic connection is formed between olfactory receptor neurons and antennal lobe interneurons. From the antennal lobe, the olfactory information is transmitted to a higher brain center by the projection neurons [8, 69, 70] (**Figure 4**). Horizontal innervation of the local interneurons within the glomerulus facilitates interglomerular communication. The primary neurotransmitter found to communicate between local interneurons is the gamma-aminobutyric acid (GABA) which facilitates the generation of Na^{+}-mediated action potential in response to olfactory stimulation [8].

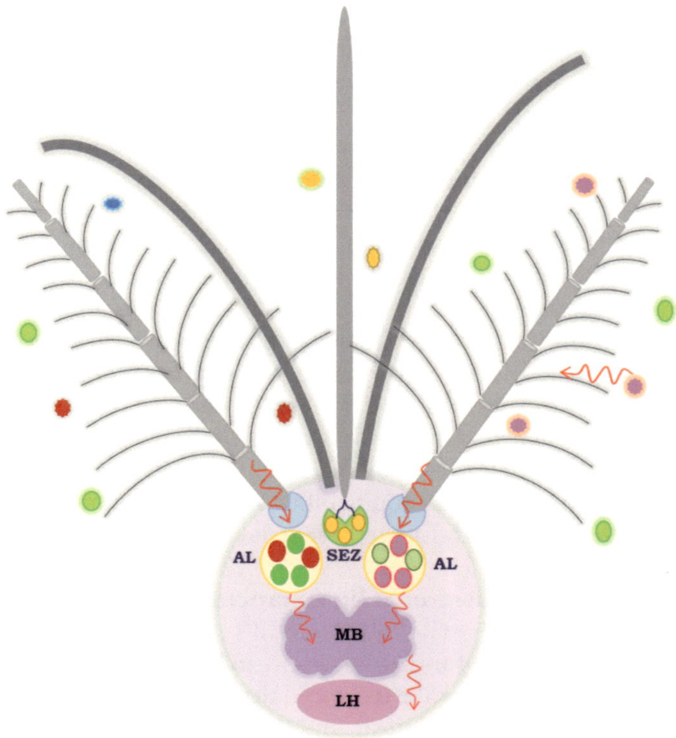

Figure 4.
Schematic presentation of flow of odor signals from the environment to the central nervous system. Odor molecules of diverse nature (highlighted as multicolored small circle) bind to their respective receptors present on the olfactory receptor neurons of antennae of mosquitoes. Then the initial signal of odor is transmitted to the antennal lobe (AL), and from the AL the signal is transmitted to higher brain centers, i.e., mushroom body (MB) and lateral horn (LH) for signal processing and decision-making. The red arrow indicates the path of signal flow.

Vertically arranged distinct fiber tract of the projection neurons connects the ALs to the higher brain centers such as calyces of the mushroom body and the lateral horn of the protocerebrum [8], where olfactory information is integrated with other sensory cues. The cell bodies of the PNs are located at the periphery of the antennal lobe glomeruli and their axons spread in the higher brain center. The branching pattern of PNs is either uniglomerular or multiglomerular [69]. The functional characterization of odor coding properties of individual ORN targeting each glomerulus revealed the existence of strong sexual dimorphism between male and female AL glomeruli which lead to a highly specialized odorant response towards general odorants and sex pheromones. PN odor response is not identical to the ORN odor response. The majority of the PNs are broadly tuned with respect to the general odors and send their dendritic arbor into the ordinary glomeruli (OG) (both uniglomerular and multiglomerular) which respond vigorously during the odor onset [69, 70]. This results from the high convergence of ORNs expressing the same odorant receptor into a single glomerulus. Generally, ORNs project its axon into a particular glomerulus, and PNs receive input from all of the ORN axons entering into that cognate glomerulus. As a result, the signal gets amplified many folds which makes the PNs very sensitive to small changes in the presynaptic ORN input. But the PNs associated with sex pheromone target different regions of the lateral horn in a sexually dimorphic manner, and thus the same pheromone elicits distinct behavior in males and females [32, 68, 71]. Most of the ORNs to PN synapses are cholinergic, and PNs respond more strongly to the fluctuating amount of odors in the odor plume [8, 32, 68]. Next, the PNs form synaptic connections with Kenyon cells, neurons of the protocerebrum, and mushroom bodies. Odor information from multiple glomeruli finally merges into narrowly tuned Kenyon cells which affect memory formation [65].

Despite the knowledge about the neuronal firing path during odor transmission, a pilot question arises in mosquito neurobiology on how discrete sensory inputs integrate and translate into varied behavior. An in-depth understanding of the neuronal circuitry involved in olfactory signaling and decision-making in mosquitoes is limited due to the absence of established neurogenetic methods. A recent study by Olena Riabinina et al. suggested that an integration of the olfactory and gustatory signals commenced within the antennal lobe and subesophageal zone of the brain, respectively [72]. Furthermore, Clement Vinauger et al. reported that despite having a synergistic effect during mosquito navigation, the visual and odor modulation is asymmetric and processed by distinct loci of the brain, where olfaction always works preceding to visual selection. But detailed understanding of the molecular and neurophysiological bases of mosquito olfactory behaviors and crucial decision-making events in the brain needs further research.

5.2 Molecular physiology of neuronal signal processing

Mosquitoes are well known for their plasticity in host preference. The selection of host species for blood meal uptake is skewed depending on the availability of the preferred host, the quality of blood meal, and the defensive behavior of the host. Apart from the neuronal firing and neurotransmitter-mediated signal transmission, the molecular factors of the brain are shown to play a crucial role in olfactory learning, neuronal decision-making, and memory formation in insects [73, 74]. The diverse neuromodulators that include neurotransmitters, neuropeptides, neurohormones, and biogenic amines facilitate the nervous system to transduce varied signals and thus enable the insects to manage the complex behavioral events with amazing accuracy [8, 11]. Neurotransmitters are the primary and potent neurochemicals that make synaptic connections between neurons and thus relay information from presynaptic cells to postsynaptic cells. The crucial neurotransmitters in the insect chemosensory system are acetylcholine, gamma-aminobutyric acid (GABA), and nitrous oxide (NO) [17, 75, 76]. Our ongoing study has shown that blood meal intake causes dynamic changes in the neurotransmitter abundance within the brain, suggesting their possible contribution in cognition and food-associated memory formation in adult female mosquitoes [77]. Furthermore, we also showed that the gut of the mosquitoes also can synthesize neurotransmitters and play a crucial role in gut-brain-axis communication during metabolic switch (sugar-fed condition to blood-fed condition) and thus modulate neuronal decision-making process [77].

Neuromodulators include the neuropeptide and biogenic amines, which have an intense effect on mosquito chemosensation, feeding, social behavior, circadian rhythm, and also maintenance of general physiological homeostasis [11, 17, 78–81]. Usually, these neuromodulators are produced by the specialized neurosecretory cells and released into the local vicinity of the brain circuits and in the hemolymph. Both neuropeptides and biogenic amines modulate the response through G protein-coupled receptor signaling pathway [11, 79]. Two important amine neuromodulators are dopamine and serotonin which are found to modulate mosquitoes' learning and memory response. The immunoreactive neurons of serotonin and dopamine innervate all the glomeruli of AL and higher brain regions such as lateral horn and mushroom body, indicating their role in memory formation [73]. Apart from the biogenic amines, 28 neuropeptides have been predicted from the genome

Sl. no.	Peptide hormone name	Function
1.	Adipokinetic hormone	Mobilizes stored carbohydrate
2.	Allatostatin A and C	Regulate juvenile hormone biosynthesis and gut motility
3.	Allatotropin	Stimulates juvenile hormone biosynthesis
4.	CCHamide 1	A nutrient-responsive hormone in *Drosophila* but function not known in mosquitoes
5.	Corazonin	Cardioactive peptide
6.	Diuretic hormone	Myotropic activity, regulation of Malpighian tubule for fluid secretion, osmoregulation, and diuresis
7.	Ecdysis triggering hormone	Trigger ecdysis during larval and pupal molting
8.	Eclosion hormone	Function not known in mosquitoes
9.	FMRFamide	Heart contraction
10.	Insulin-like peptide	Elevate carbohydrate and lipid storage, female reproduction, vitellogenesis, hemocyte differentiation, blood meal digestion
11.	Leukokinin	Diuresis
12.	Neuropeptide F	Inhibition of anterior midgut peristalsis in larval stage
13.	Ovary ecdysteroidogenic hormone	Induces ecdysone production and egg development
14.	Prothoracicotropic hormone	Regulates metamorphosis
15.	Pyrokinin	Regulation of diuresis
16.	Short neuropeptide F	Regulation of host-seeking behavior
17.	Sulfakinin	Function not known in mosquitoes
18.	Tachykinin	Function not known in mosquitoes

Table 1.
List of peptide hormones and their possible functions.

database of *Aedes aegypti* through the bioinformatics approach [82]. Among them, short neuropeptide F (sNPF) was found to play a crucial role in mosquito feeding and inhibition of host-seeking behavior following blood feeding [83, 84]. Recent studies provide contrasting evidence that either sNPF is synthesized from male accessory gland and transferred to the female during mating or female's own sNPF titer is increased in the hemolymph after consumption of blood meal significantly and reduces host-seeking behavior in adult females. While the functions of different neurohormones have been studied in many insects, functional studies in mosquitoes are limited. The wide distribution of peptide hormones throughout the mosquito body from the neurosecretory cells of the brain (corpora allata, corpus cardiacum) to the endocrine cells of the gut enable them to perform diverse function in mosquito physiology such as (1) regulation of metabolism, (2) maintenance of physiological homeostasis, (3) metamorphosis and eclosion, (4) osmoregulation, and (5) regulation of vitellogenesis and gonotropic cycle [11]. **Table 1** summarizes the name of peptide hormones in mosquitoes and their possible functions.

6. The action machinery: salivary gland

A successful feeding event of mosquitoes is regulated by the synchronized action of mosquito navigation and food choice decision which finally tuned with the salivary gland action for successful food uptake. The endocrine system of the salivary gland induces saliva secretion that gets mixed with foods and facilitates the food intake [85]. Mosquitoes have paired salivary glands in their thorax which is flanking in the esophagus. During sugar feeding saliva is mixed with the sugar, and the mixture enters into the crop where digestion commenced. During blood meal ingestion, salivary gland secretions serve in blood vessel localization [86]. The hemostatic and immune factor of the vertebrate host makes the blood meal uptake process challenging for mosquitoes [86]. Thus, salivary glands of mosquitoes are evolved and adapted with a unique ability to serve the leading function during blood meal ingestion by providing secretory salivary factors such as vasodilators, anticoagulant, antihistamines, etc. [86, 87]. Furthermore, salivary gland components not only support mosquitoes to overcome host homeostasis and defense response but also serve as the primary route for parasite transmission and maintenance of disease cycle [86, 88]. Due to the involvement of salivary gland in malaria transmission, most of the previous studies are restricted to the role of salivary gland in blood feeding and pathogen survival [89]. A recent study by Sharma et al. showed that salivary gland has a distinguished ability of gene expression switching to manage the meal-specific (sugar vs. blood meal) molecular responses [90]. But, our understanding of the regulatory mechanism of the neuro-olfactory system modulating salivary gland cocktail composition depending on the type of food is still in infancy.

6.1 Mosquito sialome leads to feeding success

To feed on a vertebrate host, the arthropods are required to overcome a series of obstacles [86]. The saliva produced by the hematophagous insects contains bioactive molecules that counteract host defense [91]. Mosquitoes are reported to feed on arterioles and venules rather than capillaries, and they often probe multiple times at different sites to find a suitable site for feeding [86]. Initiation of feeding induces hemostatic cascade within the host including the platelet aggregation followed by collagen interaction with ADP which supports the blood coagulation pathway [87, 92]. The presence of secretory apyrase enzyme in the salivary gland of blood-feeding arthropods inhibits platelet aggregation by hydrolyzing ATP and ADP into AMP and inorganic phosphate [93]. Vasoconstriction is a common phenomenon following laceration of blood vessels due to insect bite to minimize blood flow and hence loss of blood [87]. The hematophagous insects, including *Aedes aegypti* mosquito saliva, contain sialokinins which act as a vasodilatory molecule by stimulating nitric oxide (NO) production by the endothelial cells via cGMP induction [87, 94, 95]. Except apyrase and sialokinin, salivary specific D7 family proteins have been implicated to function as a scavenger molecule of serotonin, histamine, and norepinephrine and antagonize their vasoconstrictor, platelet-aggregating, and pain-inducing properties [94, 96]. Salivary peroxidases are well known for their potent function as a vasodilator, as it might act as a hydrogen peroxide-dependent destructor of serotonin and noradrenaline [97]. Furthermore, the secretory anophelin protein is reported to inhibit thrombin activity and collagen sequestration and hence delay platelet aggregation [98]. An additional challenge arises from the immune components of the blood meal itself which have been generated during previous exposure of mosquito bites [86]. Thus, successful blood feeding is dependent on the evolution of salivary composition possessing anti-immune molecules to suppress the action of host immune factors. Antitumor necrosis factor in female salivary glands is one of the crucial molecule that may play anti-immune function in hematophagous insects [86].

6.2 Neurological control over salivation

The experimental evidence about the classical conditioning of salivation in dogs was demonstrated by Pavlov in the early nineteenth century [99, 100]. By definition, classical conditioning refers to the learning procedure where a conditioned stimulus (CS), for example, the sound of a bell, is paired with an unconditioned stimulus (US), such as food which eventually triggers salivation [100], although secretion of saliva is obligatory to facilitate feeding for majority of animals from invertebrates to vertebrates. However, the knowledge of classical conditioning of salivation is restricted to mammals and invertebrate cockroaches [99]. The salivary gland and the saliva make the bridge that joins the mosquito vectors, parasite, and the host together by facilitating blood meal uptake and parasite transmission [86]. But, the cellular and molecular mechanisms underlying the classical conditioning of salivation in mosquitoes remain unknown. Considering the finicky host-seeking behavior of mosquitoes and their preference towards a certain host [47], it can be hypothesized that mosquitoes can learn during the repeated exposure of conditioned stimulus such as host odor and unconditioned stimulus, which is a reward of blood meal [47]. Reward may be appetitive when mosquitoes get benefited from the blood meal or aversive if mosquitoes experience any kind of host defensive behavior [47]. Thus, it can be speculated that mosquitoes should exhibit classical conditioning of salivation, i.e., increase saliva secretion which is tightly regulated by the neuro-olfactory system (**Figure 5**).

Our knowledge about control of insects' salivary secretion is limited to cockroaches, locusts, and blowflies, where neuronal innervation of the salivary gland or neuro-hormonal regulation was reported to play a significant role in salivation [101, 102]. Insects' salivary glands are innervated with nerves that are originated from different sources of the central nervous system [102]. Stomatogastric nervous system projects its nerves in the salivary gland of *Manduca sexta* [103]. The salivary gland of cockroaches (*Periplaneta americana*) is innervated with nerves that are projected from both the stomatogastric system and the subesophageal ganglion [102, 104, 105]. An exception to that is that the blowfly salivary glands are not innervated, but the salivary secretion is regulated by the secretion of the biogenic amine serotonin [102, 106]. Gustatory stimulation leads to the release of

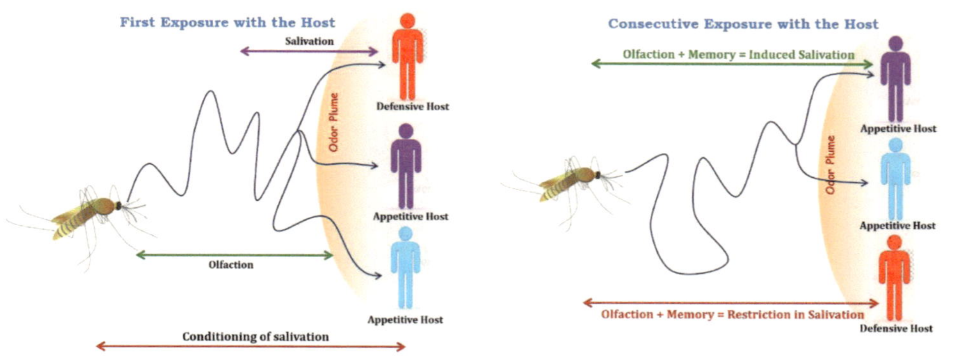

Figure 5.
Graphical illustration of conditioning of salivation in mosquitoes. Mosquitoes navigate towards vertebrate host through olfaction when they sense the odor plume emanating from the host (both appetitive and defensive). Olfaction also induces the salivary secretion (conditioning of salivation) with the aim to facilitate blood meal uptake. But the host's defensive behavior interrupts successful encountering of the mosquito with the host (red-colored human), which mosquitoes can memorize, and during consecutive exposure they probably restrict the salivation process to avoid the respective host, whereas mosquitoes get a reward from the appetitive host through successful blood-feeding without any interference. This positive memory along with olfaction further empowers the navigation process by induction of salivation.

serotonin from the neurons into the hemolymph which acts as a neurohormone and alters the cytosolic calcium (Ca^{2+}) and adenosine cyclic monophosphate (cAMP) concentration within the secretory cells of the salivary gland [107]. The increased calcium level consequently facilitates the movement of chloride (Cl^-) ions from the hemolymph side into the lumen of the gland. On the contrary, cAMP was found to stimulate potassium (K^+) transport towards the luminal side of the salivary gland. The simultaneous induction of two different pathways leads to the activation of either phospholipase C (PLC)/inositol 1,4,5-trisphosphate (IP3)/diacylglycerol/Ca^{2+} signaling pathway or cyclic AMP/adenylyl cyclase signaling cascade which

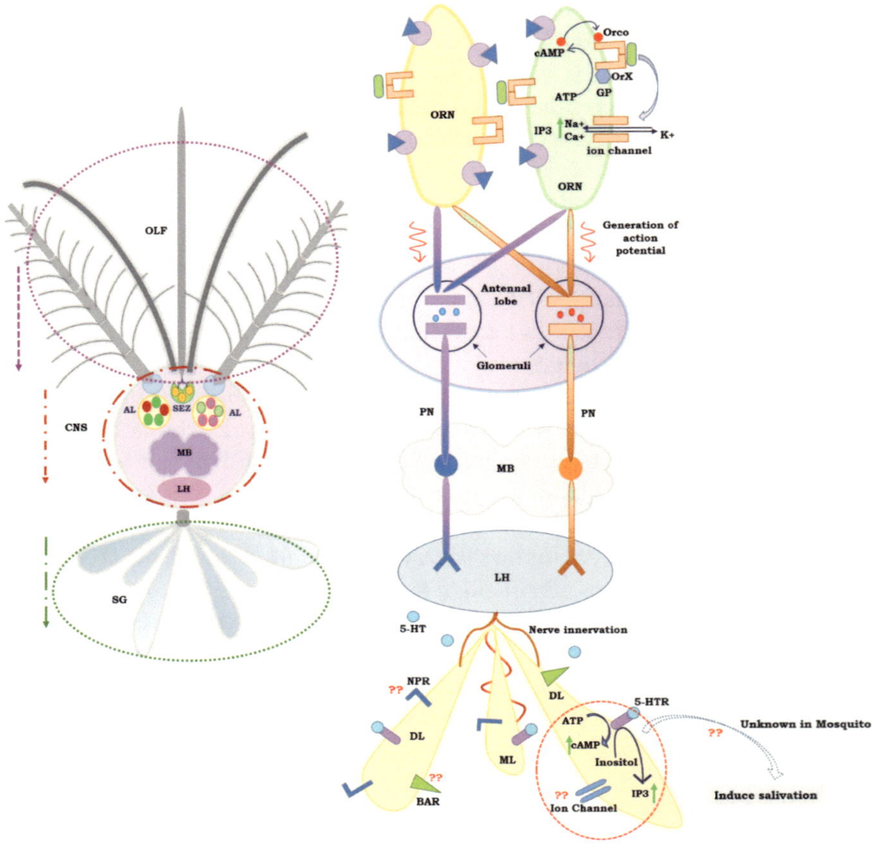

Figure 6.
The tripartite communication of three tissues [olfactory tissue (OLF), central nervous system (CNS)/brain, and salivary gland (SG)] for successful feeding. The left picture showed the flow of signal from odor response to salivary action, which is indicated by the downward arrows. The right picture is the detailed representation of the left one. Primarily, odorants bind with their cognate receptors, present on the dendritic membrane of the olfactory receptor neurons (ORNs). Odor binding initiates the downstream signal transduction procedure, which includes the synthesis of either the second messengers (cAMP, IP3) or change in the membrane ion channel conformation which then allows the flow of ions (Na^+, Ca^+, and K^+) and facilitates the change in membrane potential and consequently generates the action potential. This action potential rapidly moves through the axons towards the CNS (indicated as red arrow). The antennal lobe (AL) is the primary site for odor perception in mosquitoes. The axons of the ORNs expressing the same receptors which bind to a particular odor molecule merge in a single AL (indicated by orange and blue rods). From the AL, the odor signal then transmitted to higher brain centers [mushroom body (MB), and lateral horn (LH)] through projection neurons (PNs). Along with the neuromodulator-mediated regulation, nerve innervation (originating from the higher brain region) also regulates salivation of the salivary gland in insects (indicated by red zigzag lines over the salivary gland). One of the biogenic amines, the 5-hydroxy tryptamine (5-HT), and its cognate receptor (highlighted in sky blue circle and purple rods) facilitate salivation. But this receptor-mediated downstream signal transduction events and the resultant change in salivary gland membrane potential is not known in the case of mosquitoes (highlighted in red circle). The involvement of other biogenic amine receptors (BAR) and neuropeptide receptors (NPR) in saliva regulation is also yet to be explored. DL, distant lobe; ML, medial lobe of the salivary gland.

are the potent secondary messengers found to play a significant role in insect salivation [107, 108]. Studies in blood-feeding insects are limited to *Aedes aegypti* mosquito and on tsetse flies *Glossina pallidipes*, depicting the presence of serotonergic innervation in their salivary glands [109, 110]. Together it can be stated that both the biogenic amines and neuropeptides play a crucial role in insect salivation by modulating the salivary glands' ability to alter second messenger level and ion channel conformation. Furthermore, olfactory conditioning of salivation is directly linked to long-term memory formation which is accomplished by the active involvement of NO signaling for the induction of protein synthesis required for memory signature [111]. Salivary conditioning is also suitable to monitor the activity pattern of salivary neurons located in specific regions of the brain; thus this conditioning system will be suitable for the study of molecular mechanisms of learning and memory formation in mosquitoes' brains (**Figure 6**).

7. Conclusion and future direction

Evolution and adaptation to blood-feeding behavior in adult female mosquitoes provided a natural mechanism for their reproductive success. Here, we propose a system biology approach which defines the harmonious actions of the olfactory, the brain, and salivary glands, regulating the complex feeding behavior of mosquitoes. However, deciphering the molecular basis on how mosquitoes meet and manage the conflicting demands of sugar feeding vs. blood-feeding and how olfactory conditioning of salivation commenced may lead to the identification of crucial molecular targets including different neurohormones, biogenic amines, neuropeptides, and their receptors for genetic manipulation. Functional genomics and the advancement of electrophysiological techniques illuminate our understanding of mosquitoes' sensory systems. Although it is challenging to identify the species-specific potential olfactory factors that play a pivotal role in mosquitoes' host-seeking and blood-feeding behavior, it will be very effective for the development of novel approaches to control different mosquito populations. The efficacy of emerging genetic tools such as CRISPR/Cas9, a gene drive technology in mosquitoes, can facilitate the molecular understanding of neuronal mechanism of olfactory selection and differential learning and memory formation across different mosquito species which can be manipulated for more effective disruption of host-seeking behavior. Furthermore, unraveling the microbiome-gut-brain-axis communication mechanism during metabolic switch in mosquitoes may enlighten the innovative idea of microbiome-mediated alteration of mosquitoes' olfactory perception.

Acknowledgements

We are thankful to the Indian Council of Medical Research (ICMR), Government of India (No. 3/1/3/ICRMR-VFS/HRD/2/2016), and Tata Education and Development Trust (Health-NIMR-2017-2101-03/AP/db) for financial and infrastructural support to conduct the research at NIMR. Tanwee Das De is the recipient of the ICMR postdoctoral fellowship scheme (3/1/3/PDF(18)/2018-HRD).

Author details

Tanwee Das De and Rajnikant Dixit*
Laboratory of Host-Parasite Interaction Studies, National Institute of Malaria Research, Dwarka, Delhi, India

*Address all correspondence to: dixit2k@yahoo.com

References

[1] Harbach RE, Garros C, Manh ND, Manguin S. Formal taxonomy of species C of the *Anopheles minimus* sibling species complex (Diptera: Culicidae). Zootaxa. 2007:41-54

[2] Petersen E, Severini C, Picot S. Plasmodium vivax malaria: A re-emerging threat for temperate climate zones? Travel Medicine and Infectious Disease. 2013:51-59

[3] Ramasamy R, Surendran SN. Global climate change and its potential impact on disease transmission by salinity-tolerant mosquito vectors in coastal zones. Frontiers in Physiology. 2012;**3**:1-14

[4] Ogden NH, Lindsay LR. Effects of climate and climate change on vectors and vector-borne diseases: Ticks are different. Trends in Parasitology. 2016:646-656

[5] Medlock JM, Leach SA. Effect of climate change on vector-borne disease risk in the UK. The Lancet Infectious Diseases. 2015:721-730

[6] Wu X, Lu Y, Zhou S, Chen L, Xu B. Impact of climate change on human infectious diseases: Empirical evidence and human adaptation. Environment International. 2016:14-23

[7] Attardo GM, Hansen IA, Raikhel AS. Nutritional regulation of vitellogenesis in mosquitoes: Implications for anautogeny. Insect Biochemistry and Molecular Biology. 2005:661-675

[8] Takken W, Knols BGJ. Olfaction in vector-host interactions. Olfaction Vector-Host Interact. 2010. DOI: 10.3920/978-90-8686-698-4

[9] Gulia-Nuss M, Eum J-H, Strand MR, Brown MR. Ovary ecdysteroidogenic hormone activates egg maturation in the mosquito *Georgecraigius atropalpus* after adult eclosion or a blood meal. The Journal of Experimental Biology. 2012;**215**:3758-3767

[10] Takken W, Verhulst NO. Host preferences of blood-feeding mosquitoes. Annual Review of Entomology. 2013:433-453

[11] Stay B, Tobe SS, Bendena WG. Allatostatins: Identification, primary structures, functions and distribution. Advances in Insect Physiology. 1995;**25**:267-337. Available from: http://www.sciencedirect.com/science/article/pii/S0065280608600661

[12] Ghosh a K, Ribolla PE, Jacobs-Lorena M. Targeting *Plasmodium* ligands on mosquito salivary glands and midgut with a phage display peptide library. Proceedings of the National Academy of Sciences of the United States of America. 2001;**98**:13278-13281

[13] Foster WA, Hancock RG. Nectar-related olfactory and visual attractants for mosquitoes. Journal of the American Mosquito Control Association. 1994;**10**: 288-296

[14] W a F. Mosquito sugar feeding and reproductive energetics. Annual Review of Entomology. 1995;**40**:443-474

[15] Van Breugel F, Riffell J, Fairhall A, Dickinson MH. Mosquitoes use vision to associate odor plumes with thermal targets. Current Biology. 2015;**25**: 2123-2129

[16] Cardé RT. Multi-cue integration: How female mosquitoes locate a human host. Current Biology. 2015;**25**:R793-R795

[17] Siju KP. Neuromodulation in the chemosensory system of mosquitoes—Neuroanatomy and physiology. 2009. Available from: http://pub.epsilon.slu.se/1956/%5Cnhttp://pub.epsilon.slu.se/1956/1/Thesis_K.P..Siju.pdf

[18] Pelosi P, Iovinella I, Felicioli A, Dani FR. Soluble proteins of chemical communication: An overview across arthropods. Frontiers in Physiology. 2014;**5**:1-13

[19] Fan J, Francis F, Liu Y, Chen JL, Cheng DF. An overview of odorant-binding protein functions in insect peripheral olfactory reception. Genetics and Molecular Research. 2011:3056-3069

[20] Manoharan M, Chong MNF, Vaïtinadapoulé A, Frumence E, Sowdhamini R, Offmann B. Comparative genomics of odorant binding proteins in *Anopheles gambiae*, *Aedes aegypti*, and *Culex quinquefasciatus*. Genome Biology and Evolution. 2013;**5**:163-180

[21] Brito NF, Moreira MF, Melo ACA. A look inside odorant-binding proteins in insect chemoreception. Journal of Insect Physiology. 2016:51-65

[22] Yin J, Choo YM, Duan H, Leal WS. Selectivity of odorant-binding proteins from the southern house mosquito tested against physiologically relevant ligands. Frontiers in Physiology. 2015;**6**

[23] Zhou J-J, Huang W, Zhang G-A, J a P, Field LM. "Plus-C" odorant-binding protein genes in two Drosophila species and the malaria mosquito *Anopheles gambiae*. Gene. 2004;**327**:117-129

[24] Das De T, Thomas T, Verma S, Singla D, Rawal C, Srivastava V. A synergistic transcriptional regulation of olfactory genes derives complex behavioral responses in the mosquito *Anopheles culicifacies*. Frontiers in Physiology. 2017;**9**:1-15

[25] Das DT, Thomas T, Verma S, Singla D, Chauhan C, Srivastava V, et al. A synergistic transcriptional regulation of olfactory genes drives blood-feeding associated complex behavioral responses in the mosquito *Anopheles culicifacies*. Frontiers in Physiology. 2018

[26] Suh E, Bohbot JD, Zwiebel LJ. Peripheral olfactory signaling in insects. Current Opinion in Insect Science. 2014;**6**:86-92

[27] Kaupp UB. Olfactory signalling in vertebrates and insects: Differences and commonalities. Nature Reviews. Neuroscience. 2010;**11**:188-200. DOI: 10.1038/nrn2789

[28] Younus F, Chertemps T, Pearce SL, Pandey G, Bozzolan F, Coppin CW, et al. Identification of candidate odorant degrading gene/enzyme systems in the antennal transcriptome of *Drosophila melanogaster*. Insect Biochemistry and Molecular Biology. 2014;**53**:30-43

[29] Younus F, Fraser NJ, Coppin CW, Liu J-W, Correy GJ, Chertemps T, et al. Molecular basis for the behavioral effects of the odorant degrading enzyme esterase 6 in Drosophila. Scientific Reports. 2017;**7**:46188 Available from: http://www.nature.com/articles/srep46188

[30] Leal WS. Odorant reception in insects : Roles of receptors, binding proteins, and degrading enzymes. Annual Review of Entomology. 2013;**58**:373-391

[31] Bohbot JD, Pitts RJ. The narrowing olfactory landscape of insect odorant receptors. Frontiers in Ecology and Evolution. 2015;**3**:1-10 Available from: http://journal.frontiersin.org/article/10.3389/fevo.2015.00039/abstract

[32] Su CY, Menuz K, Carlson JR. Olfactory perception: Receptors, cells, and circuits. Cell. 2009:45-59

[33] Chesler A, Firestein S. Neuroscience: Current views on odour receptors. Nature. 2008;**452**:944. DOI: 10.1038/452944a

[34] Gao Q, Chess A. Identification of candidate Drosophila olfactory receptors from genomic DNA sequence. Genomics. 1999;**60**:31-39. Available from: http://www.ncbi.nlm.nih.gov/pubmed/10458908

[35] Clyne PJ, Warr CG, Freeman MR, Lessing D, Kim J, Carlson JR. A novel family of divergent seven-transmembrane proteins: candidate odorant receptors in Drosophila. Neuron. 1999;**22**:327-338. Available from: http://www.ncbi.nlm.nih.gov/pubmed/10069338

[36] Lundin C, Käll L, Kreher SA, Kapp K, Sonnhammer EL, Carlson JR, et al. Membrane topology of the Drosophila OR83b odorant receptor. FEBS Letters. 2007;**581**:5601-5604

[37] Tsitoura P, Andronopoulou E, Tsikou D, Agalou A, Papakonstantinou MP, Kotzia GA, et al. Expression and membrane topology of *Anopheles gambiae* odorant receptors in lepidopteran insect cells. PLoS One. 2010;**5**:1-11

[38] Sato K, Pellegrino M, Nakagawa T, Nakagawa T, Vosshall LB, Touhara K. Insect olfactory receptors are heteromeric ligand-gated ion channels. Nature. 2008;**452**:1002-1006

[39] Wicher D, Schafer R, Bauernfeind R, Stensmyr MC, Heller R, Heinemann SH, et al. Drosophila odorant receptors are both ligand-gated and cyclic-nucleotide-activated cation channels. Nature. 2008;**452**:1007-1011

[40] Nichols AS, Chen S, Luetje CW. Subunit contributions to insect olfactory receptor function: Channel block and odorant recognition. Chemical Senses. 2011;**36**:781-790

[41] Larsson MC, Domingos AI, Jones WD, Chiappe ME, Amrein H, Vosshall LB. Or83b encodes a broadly expressed odorant receptor essential for Drosophila olfaction. Neuron. 2004;**43**:703-714

[42] Liu H, Liu T, Xie L, Wang X, Deng Y, Chen C-H, et al. Functional analysis of Orco and odorant receptors in odor recognition in *Aedes albopictus*. Parasites & Vectors. 2016;**9**:363 Available from: http://parasitesandvectors.biomedcentral.com/articles/10.1186/s13071-016-1644-9

[43] Xia Y, Zwiebel LJ. Identification and characterization of an odorant receptor from the West Nile virus mosquito, *Culex quinquefasciatus*. Insect Biochemistry and Molecular Biology. 2006;**36**:169-176

[44] Bohbot JD, Dickens JC. Selectivity of odorant receptors in insects. Frontiers in Cellular Neuroscience. 2012;**6**:2010-2013

[45] Andersson MN, Löfstedt C, Newcomb RD. Insect olfaction and the evolution of receptor tuning. Frontiers in Ecology and Evolution. 2015;**3**:1-14. Available from: http://journal.frontiersin.org/article/10.3389/fevo.2015.00053/abstract

[46] Clark JT, Ray A. Olfactory mechanisms for discovery of odorants to reduce insect-host contact. Journal of Chemical Ecology. 2016;**42**:919-930

[47] Wolff GH, Riffell JA. Olfaction, experience and neural mechanisms underlying mosquito host preference. The Journal of Experimental Biology. 2018;**221**:1-13

[48] Wang G, Carey AF, Carlson JR, Zwiebel LJ. Molecular basis of odor coding in the malaria vector mosquito *Anopheles gambiae*. Proceedings of the National Academy of Sciences of the United States of America. 2010;**107**:4418-4423. Available from: http://www.pubmedcentral.nih.gov/articlerender.fcgi?artid=2840125&tool=pmcentrez&rendertype=abstract

[49] Bohbot JD, Durand NF, Vinyard BT, Dickens JC. Functional development of the octenol response in *Aedes aegypti*. Frontiers in Physiology. 2013;**4**:1-8

[50] Montell C, Zwiebel LJ. Mosquito sensory systems. Advances in Insect Physiology. 2016;**51**:293-328

[51] Carey AF, Wang G, Su C-Y, Zwiebel LJ, Carlson JR. Odorant reception in the malaria mosquito *Anopheles gambiae*. Nature. 2010;**464**:66-71 Available from: http://www.nature.com/doifinder/10.1038/nature08834

[52] Vinauger C, Van Breugel F, Locke LT, Tobin KKS, Dickinson MH, Fairhall AL, et al. Visual-olfactory integration in the human disease vector mosquito *Aedes aegypti*. Current Biology. 2019;**29**:2509-2516

[53] Wang G, Qiu YT, Lu T, Kwon HW, Jason Pitts R, Van Loon JJA, et al. *Anopheles gambiae* TRPA1 is a heat-activated channel expressed in thermosensitive sensilla of female antennae. The European Journal of Neuroscience. 2009;**30**:967-974

[54] Pitts RJ, Derryberry SL, Zhang Z, Zwiebel LJ. Variant ionotropic receptors in the malaria vector mosquito *Anopheles gambiae* tuned to amines and carboxylic acids. Scientific Reports. 2017;**7**:40297 Available from: http://www.nature.com/articles/srep40297

[55] Dennis EJ, Goldman OV, Vosshall LB. *Aedes aegypti* mosquitoes use their legs to sense DEET on contact. Current Biology. 2019;**29**:1551-1556

[56] Nakagawa T, Vosshall LB. Controversy and consensus: Noncanonical signaling mechanisms in the insect olfactory system. Current Opinion in Neurobiology. 2009:284-292

[57] Sparks JT, Botsko G, Swale DR, Boland LM, Patel SS, Dickens JC. Membrane proteins mediating reception and transduction in chemosensory neurons in mosquitoes. Frontiers in Physiology. 2018

[58] Lin HH, Lin CY, Chiang AS. Internal representations of smell in the Drosophila brain. Journal of Biomedical Science. 2007:453-459

[59] Olayemi IK, Ande AT, Danlami G, Abdullahi U. Influence of blood meal type on reproductive performance of the malaria vector, *A. gambiae* ss. (Diptera: Culicidae). Journal of Entomology. 2011;**8**:459-467. Available from: http://scialert.net/abstract/?doi=je.2011.459.467

[60] Ruebenbauer A. Olfactory coding—From molecule to the brain. Introductory Paper 181. 2006;**41**. Available from: www4.lu.se/upload/biologi/pheromone/introaga.pdf

[61] Masse NY, Turner GC, Jefferis GSXE. Olfactory information processing in Drosophila. Current Biology. 2009;**19**:R700-R713

[62] Carcaud J, Giuria M, Sandoz JC. Parallel olfactory processing in the honey bee brain: Odor learning and generalization under selective lesion of a projection neuron tract. Frontiers in Integrative Neuroscience. 2016;**9**:1-13

[63] Heinbockel T, Shields VDC, Reisenman CE. Glomerular interactions in olfactory processing channels of the antennal lobes. Journal of Comparative Physiology A: Neuroethology, Sensory, Neural, and Behavioral Physiology. 2013;**199**:929-946

[64] Christensen TA, Hildebrand JG. Frequency coding by central olfactory neurons in the sphinx moth *Manduca sexta*. Chemical Senses. 1988;**13**:123-130

[65] Silbering AF, Okada R, Ito K, Galizia CG. Olfactory information processing in the Drosophila antennal

lobe: Anything goes? The Journal of Neuroscience. 2008;**28**:13075-13087

[66] Martin JP, Beyerlein A, Dacks AM, Reisenman CE, Riffell JA, Lei H, et al. The neurobiology of insect olfaction: Sensory processing in a comparative context. Progress in Neurobiology. 2011:427-447

[67] Hansson BS, Stensmyr MC. Evolution of insect olfaction. Neuron. 2011:698-711

[68] Mucignat-Caretta C. Neurobiology of chemical communication. Neurobiology of Chemical Communication. 2014

[69] Wilson RI. Early olfactory processing in Drosophila: Mechanisms and principles. Annu Rev Neurosci. 2013;**36**:217-241 Available from: http://www.pubmedcentral.nih.gov/articlerender.fcgi?artid=3933953&tool=pmcentrez&rendertype=abstract

[70] Kim AJ, Lazar AA, Slutskiy YB. Projection neurons in Drosophila antennal lobes signal the acceleration of odor concentrations. eLife. 2015;**4**:1-16

[71] Schlief ML, Wilson RI. Olfactory processing and behavior downstream from highly selective receptor neurons. Nature Neuroscience. 2007;**10**:623-630

[72] Riabinina O, Task D, Marr E, Lin C-C, Alford R, O'Brochta DA, et al. Organization of olfactory centres in the malaria mosquito *Anopheles gambiae*. Nature Communications. 2016;7:13010. DOI: 10.1038/ncomms13010

[73] Lutz EK, Lahondère C, Vinauger C, Riffell JA. Olfactory learning and chemical ecology of olfaction in disease vector mosquitoes: a life history perspective. Curr. Opin. Insect Sci. 2017:75-83

[74] Dubnau J, Chiang AS, Grady L, Barditch J, Gossweiler S, McNeil J, et al. The staufen/pumilio pathway is involved in drosophila long-term memory. Current Biology. 2003;**13**:286-296

[75] Osborne RH. Insect neurotransmission: Neurotransmitters and their receptors. Pharmacology & Therapeutics. 1996:117-142

[76] Martin CA, Krantz DE. Drosophila melanogaster as a genetic model system to study neurotransmitter transporters. Neurochemistry International. 2014;**73**:71-88

[77] Das De T, Tevatiya S, Chauhan C, Kumari S, Srivastava V, Rani J, et al. Microbiome-gut-brain-axis communication regulates metabolic switch in the mosquito *Anopheles culicifacies*. bioRxiv. 2019. DOI: https://doi.org/10.1101/774430

[78] Jacklet J. Nitric oxide signaling in invertebrates. Invertebrate Neuroscience. 1997:1-14 Available from: http://www.ncbi.nlm.nih.gov/entrez/query.fcgi?db=pubmed&cmd=Retrieve&dopt=AbstractPlus&list_uids=4023606943429281325related:LcblcjK51jcJ

[79] Blenau W, Baumann A. Molecular and pharmacological properties of insect biogenic amine receptors: Lessons from *Drosophila melanogaster* and *Apis mellifera*. Archives of Insect Biochemistry and Physiology. 2001;**48**:13-38

[80] Fuchs S, Rende E, Crisanti A, Nolan T. Disruption of aminergic signalling reveals novel compounds with distinct inhibitory effects on mosquito reproduction, locomotor function and survival. Scientific Reports. 2014;**4**:5526. Available from: http://www.pubmedcentral.nih.gov/articlerender.fcgi?artid=4078307&tool=pmcentrez&rendertype=abstract

[81] Fukumitsu Y, Irie K, Satho T, Aonuma H, Dieng H, Ahmad A, et al. Elevation of dopamine level reduces host-seeking activity in the adult

female mosquito *Aedes albopictus*. Parasites & Vectors [Internet]. 2012;**5**:92 Available from: http://parasitesandvectors.biomedcentral.com/articles/10.1186/1756-3305-5-92

[82] Predel R, Neupert S, Garczynski SF, Crim JW, Brown MR, Russell WK, et al. Neuropeptidomics of the mosquito Aedes aegypti. Journal of Proteome Research. 2010;**9**:2006-2015

[83] Riehle MA, Garczynski SF, Crim JW, Hill CA, Brown MR. Neuropeptides and peptide hormones in *Anopheles gambiae*. Science (80-). 2002;**298**:172-175. Available from: http://www.ncbi.nlm.nih.gov/pubmed/12364794%5Cnhttp://www.sciencemag.org/content/298/5591/172%5Cnhttp://www.sciencemag.org/content/298/5591/172.full.pdf

[84] Liesch J, Bellani LL, Vosshall LB. Functional and genetic characterization of neuropeptide Y-like receptors in *Aedes aegypti*. PLoS Neglected Tropical Diseases. 2013;**7**:1-16

[85] Dhar R, Kumar N. Role of mosquito salivary glands. Current Science. 2003:1308-1313

[86] James AA, Rossignol PA. Mosquito salivary glands: Parasitological and molecular aspects. Parasitology Today. 1991:267-271

[87] Xu XQ, Lai R. Antihemostatic molecules from saliva of blood-feeding arthropods. Progress in Biochemistry and Biophysics. 2008

[88] Brennan JD, Kent M, Dhar R, Fujioka H, Kumar N. Anopheles gambiae salivary gland proteins as putative targets for blocking transmission of malaria parasites. Proceedings of the National Academy of Sciences of the United States of America. 2000;**97**:13859-13864 Available from: http://www.pnas.org/cgi/content/long/97/25/13859

[89] Arthropod saliva and its role in pathogen transmission: Insect saliva. In: Ski Arthropod Vectors. 2018

[90] Sharma P, Sharma S, Mishra AK, Thomas T, Das De T, Rohilla SL, et al. Unraveling dual feeding associated molecular complexity of salivary glands in the mosquito *Anopheles culicifacies*. Biology Open. 2015;**4**:1002-1015. Available from: http://www.pubmedcentral.nih.gov/articlerender.fcgi?artid=4542284&tool=pmcentrez&rendertype=abstract

[91] Andrade BB, Teixeira CR, Barral A, Barral-Netto M. Haematophagous arthropod saliva and host defense system: A tale of tear and blood. Anais da Academia Brasileira de Ciências. 2005;**77**:665-693

[92] Francischetti IMB, Mather TN, Ribeiro JMC. Cloning of a salivary gland metalloprotease and characterization of gelatinase and fibrin(ogen)lytic activities in the saliva of the Lyme disease tick vector *Ixodes scapularis*. Biochemical and Biophysical Research Communications. 2003;**305**:869-875

[93] Champagne DE, Smartt CT, Ribeiro JMC, James AA. The salivary gland-specific apyrase of the mosquito *Aedes aegypti* is a member of the 5′-nucleotidase family. Proceedings of the National Academy of Sciences of the United States of America. 1995;**92**:694-698

[94] Ribeiro JMC, Arcà B, Lombardo F, Calvo E, Phan VM, Chandra PK, et al. An annotated catalogue of salivary gland transcripts in the adult female mosquito, *Aedes aegypti*. BMC Genomics. 2007;**8**:1-27

[95] Champagne DE, Ribeiro JMC. Sialokinin I and II: Vasodilatory tachykinins from the yellow fever mosquito *Aedes aegypti*. Proceedings of the National Academy of Sciences of the United States of America. 1994;**91**:138-142

[96] Calvo E, Mans BJ, Andersen JF, Ribeiro JMC. Function and evolution of a mosquito salivary protein family. The Journal of Biological Chemistry. 2006;**281**:1935-1942

[97] Anderson JM, Valenzuela JG. Tick saliva: From pharmacology and biochemistry to transcriptome analysis and functional genomics. Ticks: Biology, Disease and Control. 2008

[98] Francischetti IMB, Valenzuela JG, Ribeiro JMC. Anophelin: Kinetics and mechanism of thrombin inhibition. Biochemistry. 1999;**38**:16678-16685

[99] Watanabe H, Mizunami M. Classical conditioning of activities of salivary neurones in the cockroach. The Journal of Experimental Biology. 2006;**209**:766-779

[100] Fearing F, Pavlov IP, Anrep GV. Conditioned reflexes. An investigation of the physiological activity of the cerebral cortex. Journal of the American Institute of Criminal Law and Criminology. 1929

[101] Ekstrom J, Khosravani N, Castagnola M, Messana I. Saliva and the control of its secretion. Rinshō Shinkeigaku. 1999;**39**:102-103

[102] Ali DW. The aminergic and peptidergic innervation of insect salivary glands. The Journal of Experimental Biology. 1997;**200**:1941-1949

[103] Robertson HA. The innervation of the salivary gland of the moth, Manduca sexta: Evidence that dopamine is the transmitter. The Journal of Experimental Biology. 1975;**63**:413-419 Available from: http://ovidsp.ovid.com/ovidweb.cgi?T=JS&PAGE=reference&D=med1&NEWS=N&AN=448

[104] Walz B, Baumann O, Krach C, Baumann A, Blenau W. The aminergic control of cockroach salivary glands. Archives of Insect Biochemistry and Physiology. 2006;**62**:141-152

[105] Just F, Walz B. The effects of serotonin and dopamine on salivary secretion by isolated cockroach salivary glands. The Journal of Experimental Biology. 1996;**199**:407-413

[106] Trimmer BA. Serotonin and the control of salivation in the blowfly *Calliphora*. The Journal of Experimental Biology. 1985;**114**:307-328

[107] Röser C, Jordan N, Balfanz S, Baumann A, Walz B, Baumann O, et al. Molecular and pharmacological characterization of serotonin 5-HT2α and 5-HT7 receptors in the salivary glands of the blowfly *Calliphora vicina*. PLoS One. 2012;**7**:1-13

[108] Voss M, Fechner L, Walz B, Baumann O. Calcineurin activity augments cAMP/PKA-dependent activation of V-ATPase in blowfly salivary glands. American Journal of Physiology. Cell Physiology [Internet]. 2010;**298**:C1047-C1056 Available from: http://www.ncbi.nlm.nih.gov/pubmed/20164380

[109] Novak MG, Ribeiro JM, Hildebrand JG. 5-Hydroxytryptamine in the salivary glands of adult female *Aedes aegypti* and its role in regulation of salivation. The Journal of Experimental Biology. 1995;**198**:167-174

[110] Guerra L, Stoffolano JG, Belardinelli MC, Fausto AM. Serotonergic innervation of the salivary glands and central nervous system of adult *Glossina pallidipes* Austen (Diptera: Glossinidae), and the impact of the salivary gland hypertrophy virus (GpSGHV) on the host. Journal of Insect Science. 2016;**16**:1-7

[111] Matsumoto CS, Kuramochi T, Matsumoto Y, Watanabe H, Nishino H, Mizunami M. Participation of NO signaling in formation of long-term memory in salivary conditioning of the cockroach. Neuroscience Letters. 2013;**541**:4-8

Chapter 7

Neurological and Neuropsychiatric Disorders in Relation to Olfactory Dysfunction

Naina Bhatia-Dey and Thomas Heinbockel

Abstract

Olfaction is an underestimated sensory modality in terms of its predictive value as an indicator of disorders. It is a well-known phenomenon that a significant percentage of people afflicted with certain prevalent disorders causing degenerative neuropathology, progressive loss of memory and communication function, normal age-based decline of physiological functions, intellectual challenges, depressive and anxiety disorders as well as post-traumatic stress disorders, present with a range of olfactory deficits. Here, we review our understanding of these deficits and their relation to various clinical manifestations such as neurological and neuropsychiatric diseases and disorders. At the outset, we will briefly describe the olfactory pathway from olfactory sensory neurons in the nasal epithelium to the olfactory bulb and on to olfactory cortical and subcortical structures involved in olfaction such as the amygdala.

Keywords: aging, Alzheimer's disease, amygdala, dementia, hippocampus, limbic system, mood disorders, olfactory bulb, olfactory cortex, olfactory sensory neuron, Parkinson's disease

1. Introduction

This chapter provides a cursory description of a well-known phenomenon, namely that a significant percentage of people afflicted with certain prevalent disorders causing degenerative neuropathology, depressive and anxiety disorders, progressive loss of memory and communication function such as Autism Spectrum Disorder (ASD), intellectual challenges, as well as post-traumatic stress disorders present with a range of olfactory deficits. Here, we review our understanding of these deficits and their relation to various clinical manifestations such as neurological and neuropsychiatric diseases and disorders, disorders affecting mood, cognition, communication and memory and finally, olfactory deficits as secondary outcome of therapeutic drugs. At the outset, we will briefly describe the olfactory pathway from olfactory sensory neurons in the nasal epithelium to the olfactory bulb and on to olfactory cortical structures and subcortical structures involved in olfaction such as the amygdala. Then, we shall discuss olfaction in the context of normal age-based decline of physiological functions relating olfactory deficits to the onset of neurodegenerative pathology, decline in cognition, memory, ability to communicate as well as with episodes of depression and anxiety.

2. The olfactory system

The main role of the olfactory system is the detection of odors. This function is critical for food selection by detecting olfactory and gustatory signals. Moreover, our sense of smell plays a role in reproductive and neuroendocrine regulation and is relevant for memory, aggression, emotion, social organization, and recognition of prey and predators [1]. Social chemical stimuli or semiochemical signals are processed by the olfactory system in most mammals. These chemicals differ from general odorants and mediate physiological aspects of mating and aggression. These chemical signals are processed in the accessory olfactory bulb in the brain which is part of the vomeronasal system [1].

The olfactory pathway starts deep in the nasal cavity with an olfactory epithelium that sits on the superior conchae (**Figure 1**). This pseudostratified ciliated columnar epithelium houses olfactory sensory neurons, supporting cells (sustentacular cells), and basal stem cells. In addition, Bowman's glands located in the connective tissue under the epithelium (lamina propria) send ducts to the surface of the epithelium and secrete a serous fluid that immerses the cilia of olfactory receptor neurons in a mucous layer to trap odorant molecules. Odorant molecules bind to olfactory receptor proteins in the cilia of olfactory sensory neuron dendrites. The number of cilia that emerges from the dendrite of an olfactory sensory neuron is relatively small, 20 to 30, compared to the ciliated cells that are found in the respiratory epithelium (~300 cilia). Air-borne odorant molecules in the air that we breathe in activate the olfactory receptor proteins in the olfactory cilia. Odorant molecules can find their way to the olfactory sensory neurons either through the

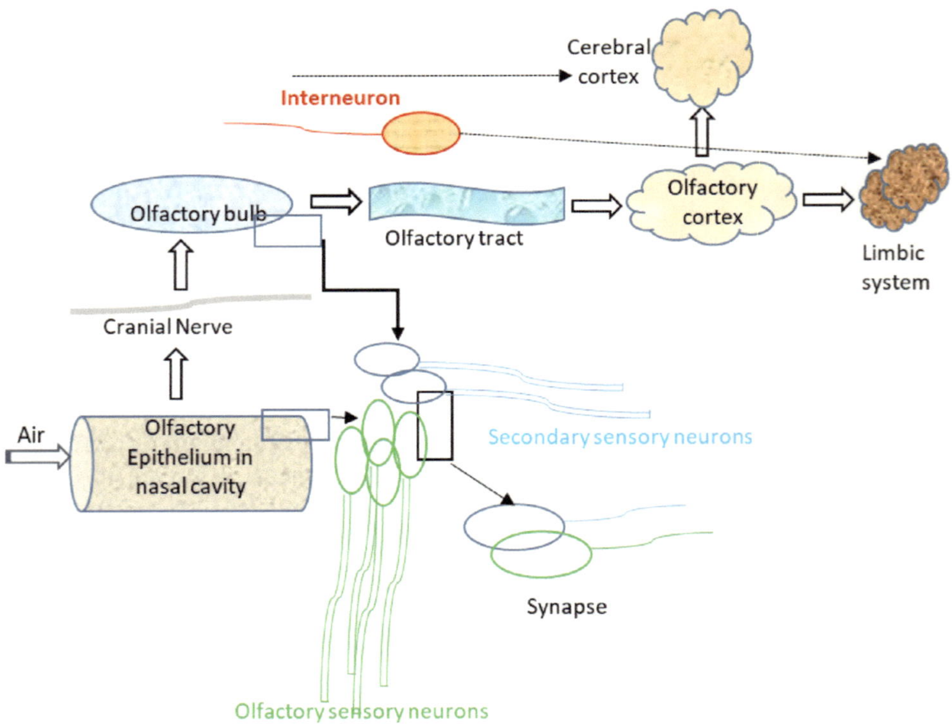

Figure 1.
Schematic representation of olfactory pathways. Olfactory sensory neurons in the olfactory epithelium of the nasal cavity send their axons to form synapses with secondary sensory neurons in the olfactory bulb. A small number of neurons from the olfactory bulb participate in olfactory processing as they exchange information with both limbic system components and cortical structures.

nose (orthonasal stimulation) or from the mouth to the nose (retronasal stimulation) [2]. Often this retronasal olfactory stimulation is confused with taste, which takes place in taste buds in the tongue and soft palate of the oral cavity. However, food odors and the consistency of the food ('crunchiness') together with tastants contribute to the flavor or aroma of food. The membrane of olfactory sensory neuron cilia houses odorant receptor proteins and thereby activates these neurons in the nasal epithelium. The olfactory receptor proteins form a large gene family (1000 genes in rodents, 350 in humans, [3, 4]). Each olfactory sensory neuron sends an axon through the cribriform plate of the ethmoid bone to the ipsilateral main olfactory bulb in the brain (**Figure 1**). The axons of olfactory sensory neurons coalesce to form the olfactory nerve (cranial nerve I) and olfactory nerve layer of the main olfactory bulb.

The main olfactory bulb is a cortical structure of the cerebrum. However, the main olfactory bulb is not part of the neocortex but part of the allocortex as shown by its fetal development and cytoarchitecture. Neocortical structures undergo a prenatal phase that results in six layers, whereas allocortical structures have three or four layers in the mature brain [5]. While the main olfactory bulb presents itself as a small extension of the brain in humans, in rodents, the main olfactory bulb is a large structure that fills roughly a quarter of the length of the cranial cavity [6] and is dedicated to the processing of odorant information [1, 2, 7].

Several million sensory neurons are present in the olfactory epithelium. A given olfactory receptor protein is expressed by several thousand of them. The olfactory sensory neurons that express the same olfactory receptor protein send their axon to the same one or two glomeruli in the main olfactory bulb to form synaptic contacts (**Figure 1**). The dendrites of interneurons (juxtaglomerular cells) and output neurons (mitral and tufted neurons) in the olfactory bulb synapse with olfactory sensory neurons. Compared to the large number of olfactory sensory neurons, only relatively few output neurons innervate each glomerulus. These output neurons send their axons to higher order brain centers for brain processing of olfactory signals [8]. The precise sending of olfactory sensory neuron axons to specific glomeruli is critical for the discrimination of odorants [2]. The axons of output neurons leave the main olfactory bulb through the lateral olfactory tract and terminate in various higher order olfactory centers such as the anterior olfactory nucleus (AON), piriform cortex, the anterior parahippocampal cortex (entorhinal cortex), and the cortico-medial amygdala, all of which belong to limbic system (**Figure 1**) and are on the ipsilateral brain side. In contrast to other sensory modalities, the olfactory pathway routes sensory information directly from the olfactory bulb to cortical centers and bypasses the thalamus [1, 2].

The amygdala is a collection of nuclei in the limbic system [9]. The basolateral nucleus is the largest one and receives input from sensory cortices (vision, hearing) as well as direct auditory signals through a subcortical structure, the medial geniculate nucleus which is part of the thalamus. The olfactory bulb and piriform cortex send sensory information to the cortical and medial nuclei of the amygdala, the cortico-medial nucleus [10, 11]. In addition, the amygdala receives input from other cortical and subcortical brain systems, such as the prefrontal cortex with the anterior cingulate and orbitofrontal cortices. In turn, both piriform cortex and amygdala project to the orbitofrontal cortex to regulate emotion and associative learning. The amygdala is also connected with the entorhinal and hippocampal system for long-term memory [12]. Furthermore, the amygdala is a target for fibers from the hippocampus and rhinal (olfactory) cortices [10, 11]. Functionally, it has been established that odors have the ability to evoke strong emotions and trigger the recall of emotional memories and modulate cognition [11].

Not only does the olfactory bulb send axons to higher order olfactory centers (afferent fibers), an even larger number of centrifugal axons originating in higher olfactory centers innervate the olfactory bulb glomeruli (efferent fibers) [6, 13, 14]. These centrifugal neurons have been shown to provide modulatory feedback to neurons in the different layers of the main olfactory bulb which is important for experience-dependent modulation [13]. The origin of the centrifugal fibers is in the locus coeruleus (noradrenergic), the horizontal limb of the diagonal band of Broca (cholinergic), and the raphe nucleus (serotonergic) [15–18]. The centrifugal fibers travel mainly through the anterior olfactory nucleus and the anterior commissure, and very little through the lateral olfactory tract [13].

3. Aging effects in the olfactory system

Age-associated impairment in the sense of olfaction has been well documented [19–23]. Akin to neurodegenerative pathology, a decline in olfactory acuity and olfactory dysfunction are common features of the normal aging process [24–27] detectable in over 50% individuals ranging in age from 65 to 80 years and almost in 75% of those above 80 years [24, 28–30]. This decline in olfactory function is detected using different kinds of tests such as psychophysical, psychophysiological and electrophysiological tests that determine odor detection, identification and discrimination, odor related physiological changes in cardiac and respiratory system as well as odor-event related potentials [29]. However, studies analyzing the mechanism of non-pathological, normal chronological age-related decline of olfactory acuity and impaired olfactory function are limited, despite the fact that deficits in the olfactory sense are considered as important symptom for early and differential diagnosis of neurodegenerative disorders [28]. At the anatomical level, the sense of olfaction is affected by age-associated ossification and closure of foramina of the cribriform plate [29, 31]. There is evidence of a quantitative reduction in the olfactory epithelium and its replacement by respiratory epithelium in normal subjects of the aging population which is evident in biopsies of the upper nasal septum [32]. It is now clearly evident that in the course of normal aging, suboptimal olfaction and olfactory dysfunction are associated with a number of anatomical and physiological features such as age-associated thinning of the olfactory neuroepithelium, altered cellular patterns and regional distribution of nuclei of olfactory sensory and sustentacular cells [29], reduction of mucosal metabolizing enzymes and sensory loss of olfactory sensory cells to various odorants along with a cumulative effect of environmental exposure to the olfactory epithelium [30]. An additional causative factor is the parallel loss of olfactory function in direct correlation with a clear age-associated decline in the volume of the olfactory bulb in adults of both genders [33–35]. Other than the olfactory bulb, a reduction in volume of AON, amygdala, hippocampus and piriform cortex in the limbic system contribute to a loss of olfaction due to their pivotal role in olfactory processing [36]. Testing the sensitivity and response of isolated sensory neurons to odorant mixtures indicates a loss of olfactory sensitivity and specificity in neurons derived from older subjects [37]. In older individuals, there is evidence of decreased beta-event related synchronization in response to certain pleasant odorants and, therefore, these individuals rated such odorants as less pleasant, thereby, denoting a decline in olfactory processing [38]. A change in olfactory perception represents subtle olfactory dysfunction that appears to precede a number neurodegenerative disorders and is presumed due to loss of synaptic function [39, 40]. Subsequent studies have shown that loss in olfactory sensitivity and perception is heterogeneous and appears to be more specific to heavier molecules [41]. Inherent allelic variations of brain derived neurotrophic factor (BDNF) also affect and add to age-dependent olfactory decline [29, 42]. A comparative research study quantifying heritability of odor identification and cognition detected a role of common genes in both olfaction and cognition. However, heritability of odor identification was lower in contrast to that of cognition [43]. Quantitative analysis of olfaction using odor identification (OI) scale in community dwelling subjects of age group 70–79 years reveals association of higher risk of dementia with poor OI score [44] and reduction in OI has been linked to advanced physiological brain aging as well as with a number of neurodegenerative diseases [45]. An aging cortical synapse in limbic structures has been considered as a hallmark of age-associated decline in cognition [46]. However, such studies are still preliminary for the olfactory bulb, despite evidence of growth factor dependent induction of synaptic strength in olfactory bulb cell layers during odor-dependent social transmission of food preference [47]. Chronological age adds to the impact of environmental exposure through living and working conditions on all physiological systems and their functions [48]. Experimental analysis indicates age-dependent accumulation of somatic mutations using both proliferative and non-proliferative cell types from human brain tissue [49]. It further indicates the probability of mutation accumulation in neurons. Genome-wide single somatic nucleotide variant analysis on DNA of 159 single neurons of 15 normal individuals with a wide age range (4 months to 82 years) and 9 individuals diagnosed with early onset of neurodegeneration revealed linear increase in both sets, indicating age-dependent accumulation of somatic mutations as significant factor affecting neurodegeneration [50]. Research studies of classical neurodegenerative disorders have proposed that the observed variability of olfactory dysfunction in diverse neurological and neuropsychiatric diseases could aid in early differential diagnosis of Alzheimer's disease (AD), Parkinson's disease (PD), mild cognitive impairment (MCI), progressive supranuclear palsy (PSP) and frontotemporal lobar degeneration known as FTLD-TDP43 [51–54]. A cell biology oriented experimental approach to detect the presence of neurodegeneration-associated proteins used nasal brushing to collect olfactory neurons from olfactory mucosa of normal subjects and detected four different characteristic proteins involved in neurodegenerative pathology: α-synuclein, transactive response DNA-binding protein 43 (TDP-43), hyperphosphorylated tau and β-amyloid proteins [55]. These findings have prompted an analysis of the parallel progression of loss of olfaction with onset of neurodegenerative pathology and/or decline in cognitive abilities as initial symptoms of neurological and neuropsychiatric disorders.

4. Alzheimer's disease, dementia and olfactory deficits

Olfactory deficiencies are evident in a number of neurodegenerative disorders such as AD, dementia with Lewy bodies (DLB), frontotemporal dementia (FTD), MCI, PD and Huntington disease [40, 51, 56–59]. In an extensive two year study with six-monthly follow up, all MCI patients with lower range of olfaction score but no subjective smelling loss detected by standard UPSIT (University of Pennsylvania Smell Identification Test) developed AD. In contrast, in a control group of higher olfaction score, AD occurrence was nil [60]. A similar association of lower olfaction score with development of AD pathology was evident in a multiethnic community cohort with UPSIT test [61]. In a comparative OI analysis of FTD and AD patients with normal age matched control individuals, OI score of FTD patients differed significantly with control group, however, there was a close resemblance in OI pattern of FTD patients with OI in AD patients [62]. An analysis using Pocket Small Test as indicator of OI performance in AD patients and healthy young and age matched control group of individuals detected reduced OI in an older control group than in a younger control group, and AD patients had even reduced OI compared to their age matched control group [27]. At the cellular level, a characteristic neuropathological feature of AD is the appearance of neurofibrillary tangles consisting of hyperphosphorylated tau protein [63]. In relation to olfactory dysfunction, the two key hallmarks of AD neuropathology are the detection of amyloid-beta (Aβ) and hyperphosphorylated tau protein in the olfactory system; both have been detected together with impaired olfaction much before a clinical presentation of the disease [57]. An analysis assessing OI as indicator of presymptomatic AD pathogenesis in cognitively normal aged individuals shows an association of reduced OI with lower cognitive score and older age as well as increased ratio of total tau protein to phosphorylated tau protein in cerebrospinal fluid [64]. Therefore, at the behavioral level, diminished OI has emerged as a practical and affordable biomarker of AD pathology [64] as well as prodromal symptom of AD [65].

5. Parkinson's disease and olfactory impairment

A major factor leading to neurodegenerative PD pathology is the loss of dopaminergic neurons from the substantia nigra, resulting in slow but substantial loss of dopamine that eventually leads to many clinical motor symptoms such as bradykinesia, rigidity, tremor, instability of posture and decline of cognitive function [66]. The olfactory system is a severely affected non-motor system in PD patients with early appearance of olfactory dysfunction that remains independent of progressive PD symptoms, their duration and treatment [67]. Additional research studies have indicated association of olfactory dysfunction with PD for over three decades [25, 68]. Olfactory dysfunction, including hyposmia and decline in olfactory acuity, has been established as one of the earliest features of PD. These are detectable in approximately 90% of early stage PD patients, where they may precede the onset of the motor symptoms by a margin of years [69–73]. Hyposmia and progressive olfactory decline in PD patients have been attributed to central olfactory processing, since the olfactory epithelium biopsy samples of PD patients were normal [74]. Subsequent MRI studies indicate a varying degree of reduction in olfactory bulb volume and depth of olfactory sulcus in PD patients than in normal control individuals. These studies indicate an association of anatomical changes with altered olfaction in PD patients [75]. Lewy bodies and Lewy neurites comprised of α-synuclein are histological hallmarks of neurodegenerative pathology in PD [76]. The olfactory bulb and lower brainstem have been considered as the induction site for the onset of histopathological features comprising of both Lew bodies and Lewy neurites [73, 77]. Along with the peripheral nervous system, such histological aberrations also begin to appear in gut nerve plexa and the olfactory bulb, thereby indicating participation of olfactory bulb cell layers in the progression of neurodegenerative pathology of PD [78].

Dementia associated with PD, known as Parkinson's disease dementia (PDD), is one of the most debilitating symptoms of PD and is difficult to predict during early stages of the disease. A research study using OSIT-J (odor stick identification test for Japanese) shows over 18 fold increase in risk of dementia for PD patients with severe hyposmia [79]. Indeed OI has emerged as a reliable tool for providing excellent diagnostic accuracy for PD distinguishing it from PD mimics [80].

6. Mood and communication disorders

In addition to aging, neurodegenerative and psychiatric conditions, olfactory deficits including low OI appear as characteristic feature of mild to severe major depressive disorders [81, 82]. As there is overlap in brain regions involved in AD, depression and olfactory processing, olfactory dysfunction could be the potential early biomarker of both AD and depressive disorders [83]. Similar to research studies using animal models that indicate a strong link between loss of olfaction and depressive behavior, a comparative analysis of age matched control individuals and patients diagnosed with depression showed loss of normal olfaction as marker of depression in humans [84]. Literature reviews of multiple research findings using specific parameters indicate a clear and consistent relation between depression and poor life quality in individuals from both clinical and community setting in age dependent manner [85]. Encoded olfactory stimuli activate emotional memory [86]; olfactory system and brain circuits participating in memory and cognition show a close anatomical link as well as frequent functional alteration in patients with depression [87–89]. Additional analysis clearly denotes a reciprocal relationship between olfaction and depression; patients with olfactory dysfunction show worsening depressive symptoms while olfactory performance is clearly reduced in depression patients in comparison to normal controls [90]. Moreover,

Declined olfactory acuity and olfactory dysfunction are also evident in individuals suffering with post-traumatic stress disorder (PTSD) and in patients diagnosed with major depressive disorder (MDD). PTSD leads to decreased olfactory bulb volume, thereby leading to decreased olfactory acuity, additional olfactory deficits and dysfunction [35]. MDD indicates decline in both primary and secondary olfactory processing [84, 91]. MDD patients denote lower score for olfactory threshold, odor discrimination in 40-point smell identification test in comparison to normal controls At the same time, patients with olfactory dysfunction show clear symptoms of depression that become acute in comparative analysis of hyposmic to anosmic subjects [90].

ASD adult patients show decline in odor identification ability [92]. Experimental evidence in two different mouse models of ASD indicates weaker and fewer synapses between olfactory sensory nerve terminals and olfactory bulb tufted cell layer; and weaker synapses between olfactory sensory nerve terminals and inhibitory periglomerular cells of the olfactory bulb [93]. Duplication of GABA receptor genes and deletion of TOP3B, topoisomerase involved in relaxation of supercoiled DNA contribute to autism susceptibility and have been assigned to gene families with specific contribution to neurodevelopmental disorders [94]. Out of 102 identified genes that contribute to ASD, most genes are expressed and enriched early in excitatory and inhibitory neuronal lineages and affect synapses [95].

7. Drugs

The regenerative ability of olfactory epithelium has made it an attractive target for exploring and evaluating therapeutic strategies to distinguish and treat drug induced olfactory disorders [96]. More than 86% of cancer patients of wide age range display smell and taste disorders that persist even after completion of chemotherapy for cancer [97]. However, not every therapeutic chemotherapy drugs has negative impact on olfactory acuity (personal communication). *Bacopa monnieri* extracts administration reverses bulbectomy induced neurochemical and histological alterations in mouse model of depression; cognition dysfunction is reversed through a mechanism that enhances synaptic plasticity related signaling, BDNF transcription and protection of cholinergic systems [98].

The flavonoid Naringenin functions as antidepressant by restoring serotonin and noradrenaline levels in brain tissue [99]. In bulbectomized mice, two weeks of Naringenin treatment ameliorated depression like behavioral alterations, decreased elevated pro-inflammatory cytokines and increased levels of BDNF and serotonin in hippocampus and cortex [100].

Depression with psychomotor agitation (PMA) is a putative psychiatric disorder associated with substance dependence, specifically, opioids. It remains unaffected by drug induced major depressive episodes indicating complex interplay of therapeutic drugs in treating depression [101].

The AON, a key area of the olfactory system, shows accumulation of characteristic neuropathological markers such as hyperphosphorylated tau, α-synuclein and β-amyloid proteins at the earliest stages of AD in a Somatostatin (SST) expressing subpopulation of interneurons. In the limbic system, the same accumulation is evident in same subpopulation of interneurons [102]. However, SST is unequally involved in two predominant neurodegenerative disorders with a very strong involvement in AD pathology but quite weaker participation in PD. In early stages of AD, SST is reduced in olfactory areas whereas it is preserved in non-demented PD cases [102]. Further analysis of SST related olfactory deficiencies will pave the way of SST based therapeutic approaches.

Olfactory dysfunctions unrelated to blocked nasal passages are present in a significant percentage of Covid-19 patients [103–105]. Altered expression of SARS-CoV-2 entry genes in supporting cells of the olfactory epithelium has been proposed as a mechanism underlying COVID-19-associated anosmia [106, 107].

8. Discussion and conclusions

The mammalian olfactory bulb has been termed the "brain inside the brain", due to the presence of sensory inputs, neuronal lamination and contribution of new neural elements throughout the lifetime [108]. It plays a pivotal role in olfactory processing [8, 109]. In addition to AD, PD, MCI and depressive disorders, inadequate and/or improper olfactory function together with impaired olfactory processing exist in many other neurodegenerative and neuropsychiatric disorders. For instance, in the case of multiple sclerosis (MS), prevalence of olfactory dysfunction ranges from 20 to 45% of the MS population. However, the mechanism of loss of olfaction remains unknown, except for decreased olfactory bulb and brain volume [110, 111]. In patients with a diagnosis of a behavioral FTD variant, OI and odor discrimination did not show any difference from control cases, but there was a significant difference in the odor association test. It has been attributed to impaired olfactory processing [112]. Within the healthy population, impulsive tendencies exhibit some link to olfactory defects [113]. Narcolepsy is associated with hypocretin deficiency of the limbic system. Despite genetic predisposition, it has been postulated to increase by environmental substances that may access the olfactory bulb, triggering neuroinflammation and induce neurodegeneration [114].

Single cell transcriptome analysis during mouse olfactory neurogenesis in early development reveals that expression of olfactory receptor (OR) genes becomes progressively restricted to one gene per neuron in each mature neuron instead of several receptor genes that express in immature neurons [115, 116]. Expression of a single OR allele in olfactory sensory neurons is the outcome of coalescence of multiple intergenic enhancers to a multi-chromosomal hub that allows the expression of a single OR allele while the remaining OR genes converge into few heterochromatic compartments leading to effective transcriptional silencing [117]. Age associated chromosomal breakage and DNA damage lead to an increase in markers of genome instability [118] and requires many layers of regulatory functions such as inducing senescence [48], reducing accumulation of DNA damage and enhancing DNA repair pathways [119]. Genome protection from DNA damage to minimize aging effects is also an effective strategy to minimize risk factor for neurodegeneration [119]. This is likely to retain olfactory acuity and ability based on the model proposed by Bashkirova and Lomvardas [117].

Single cell RNA sequencing reveals differentially regulated and expressed genes as neuronal markers specific to adult born interneurons that may serve as molecular markers for synapse formation, synapse maintenance, and neural plasticity of adult brain circuits [120]. Research studies analyzing functional mechanisms of these markers and their regulation are likely to facilitate the understanding of decreased OI, olfactory dysfunction and onset of neurodegenerative pathology.

Olfactory ensheathing glial cells help olfactory bulb neurons to connect with both the peripheral and central nervous system, and, therefore, they have been widely used as therapeutic tools for neural repair and olfactory/neural regeneration for injuries and neurodegenerative pathological conditions [121]. Indeed, the olfactory bulb has emerged as an attractive target for many novel therapeutic approaches [122].

Another fast growing research topic addresses the role of microRNAs in regulating genes that participate in cognition and neurodegeneration [123–125] and olfactory acuity. Such findings would also add to a better understanding of the relationship between olfactory dysfunction and neurodegenerative pathologies.

Targeting synaptic deficits in AD patients and aging individuals by improving synaptic plasticity though alteration of structural deficits in dendritic spines through microRNA mediated regulatory pathways could be an effective and novel therapeutic strategy for AD as well as other neurodegenerative disorders [126].

Acknowledgements

This work was supported in part by grants from the National Science Foundation (NSF IOS-1355034) and the **Charles and Mary** Latham Trust Fund.

Conflict of interest

The authors declare that there is no conflict of interests regarding the publication of this chapter.

Author details

Naina Bhatia-Dey and Thomas Heinbockel*
Department of Anatomy, Howard University College of Medicine, Washington, DC, USA

*Address all correspondence to: theinbockel@howard.edu

References

[1] Shipley, MT; Ennis, M. Functional organization of olfactory system. J. Neurobiol. 1996; 30: 123-176.

[2] Ennis M, Hamilton KA, Hayar A. Neurochemistry of the main olfactory system. In Handbook of Neurochemistry and Molecular Neurobiology: Sensory Neurochemistry; Springer: New York, NY, USA, 2007; 137-204.

[3] Buck L, Axel R. A novel multigene family may encode odorant receptors: a molecular basis for odor recognition. Cell. 1991; 65:175-187.

[4] Young JM, Friedman C, Williams EM, Ross JA, Tonnes-Priddy L, Trask BJ. Different evolutionary processes shaped the mouse and human olfactory receptor gene families. Hum Mol Genet. 2002; 11:535-546. Doi. org/10.1093/hmg/11.5.535

[5] Schiebler TH, Schmidt W, Zilles K. Anatomie, 8 ed.; Springer Verlag, Berlin, Germany, 1999.

[6] Swanson LW. Brain Maps: Structure of the Rat Brain. A Laboratory Guide with Printed and Electronic Templates for Data, Models and Schematics, 3rd ed.; Elsevier: Amsterdam, the Netherland. 2004.

[7] Heinbockel T, Heyward PM. Glutamate synapses in olfactory neural circuits. In Amino Acid Receptor Research; Paley, B.F., Warfield, T.E., Eds.; Nova Science Publishers: New York, NY, USA, 2009; 16: 379-414

[8] Shepherd, G.M.; Chen, W.R.; Greer, C.A. Olfactory Bulb. In Synaptic Organization of the Brain, 5th ed.; Shepherd, G.M., Ed.; Oxford University Press: New York, NY, USA, 2004a; 165-216.

[9] Pape HC, Driesang RB, Heinbockel T, Laxmi TR, Meis S, Seidenbecher T, Szinyei C, Frey U, Stork O. Cellular processes in the amygdala: gates to emotional memory? Zoology, 2001; 104: 232-240. Doi. org/10.1078/0944-2006-00029

[10] Bernardi S, Salzman CD. The contribution of nonhuman primate research to the understanding of emotion and cognition and its clinical relevance. Proc Natl Acad Sci USA. 2019; 116: 26305-26312. Doi: 10.1073/pnas.1902293116.

[11] Kadohisa M. Effects of odor on emotion, with implications. Front Syst Neurosci. 2013; 7:66. Doi: 10.3389/fnsys.2013.00066.

[12] Seidenbecher T, Laxmi TR, Stork O, Pape HC. Amygdalar and hippocampal theta rhythm synchronization during fear memory retrieval. Science. 2003; 301:846-50. Doi: 10.1126/science.1085818

[13] Kiselycznyk C, Zhang S, Linster C. Role of Centrifugal Projections to the Olfactory Bulb in Olfactory Processing. Learn. Mem. 2006, 13, 575-579. Doi:10.1101/lm.285706

[14] Laaris N, Puche, A, Ennis, M. Complementary postsynaptic activity patterns elicited in olfactory bulb by stimulation of mitral/tufted and centrifugal fiber inputs to granule cells. J. Neurophysiol. 2007; 97:296-306. Doi. org/10.1152/jn.00823.2006

[15] Macrides F, Davis BJ, Youngs WM, Nadi NS, Margolis, FL. Cholinergic and catecholaminergic afferents to the olfactory bulb in the hamster: A neuroanatomical, biochemical, and histochemical investigation. J. Comp. Neurol. 1981:203: 495-514.

[16] Halasz N. The Vertebrate Olfactory System; Akademia Kiado: Budapest, Hungary, 1990.

[17] Shipley MT. Olfactory System. In: The Rat Nervous System; Academic Press: Sydney, Australia, 1995; 899-928.

[18] Cleland TA, Linster C. Central Olfactory Structures. In Handbook of Olfaction and Gustation; Marcel Dekker: New York, NY, USA, 2003; 165-181.

[19] Murphy C, Schubert CR, Cruickshanks KJ, Klein BE, Klein R, Nondahl DM. Prevalence of olfactory impairment in older adults. JAMA. 2002; 288:2307-2312.Doi:10.1001/jama.288.18.2307

[20] Brämerson A, Johansson L, Ek L, Nordin S, Bende M. Prevalence of olfactory dysfunction: The Skövde population-based study. Laryngoscope 2004; 114: 733-737. Doi.org/10.1097/00005537-200404000-00026

[21] Vennemann MM, Hummel T, Berger K. The association between smoking and smell and taste impairment in the general population. J Neurol 2008; 255: 1121-6. Doi.org/10.1007/s00415-008-0807-9

[22] Schubert CR, Cruickshanks KJ, Fischer ME, Huang G-H, Klein BEK, Klein R. et al. Olfactory impairment in an adult population: the beaver dam offspring study. Chem. Senses. 2012; 37:325-334. Doi:10.1093/chemse/bjr102

[23] Masurkar AV, and Devanand DP. Olfactory dysfunction in the elderly: basic circuitry and alterations with normal aging and Alzheimer's disease. Curr. Geriatr. Rep. 2014; 3, 91-100. Doi.org/10.1007/s13670-014-0080-y

[24] Doty RL. The olfactory system and its disorders. Semin.Neurol. 2009; 29: 74-81. Doi 10.1055/s-0028-1124025. ISSN 0271-8235.

[25] Masaoka Y, Yoshimura N, Inoue M, Kawamura M, Homma I. Impairment of odor recognition in Parkinson's disease caused by weak activations of the orbitofrontal cortex. Neuroscience Letters. 2007; 412:45-50. Doi:10.1016/j.neulet.2006.10.055

[26] Huttenbrink KB, Hummel T, Berg D, Gasser T, Hähner A. Olfactory dysfunction: common in later life and early warning of neurodegenerative disease. Dtsch Arztebl Int. 2013; 110: 1-7. Doi: 10.3238/arztebl.2013.0001

[27] Makowska I, Kloszewska I, Grabowska A, Szatkowska I, Rymarczyk K. Olfactory deficits in normal aging and Alzheimer's disease in the polish elderly population. Arch Clin Neuropsychol 2011; 26:270-279. Doi:10.1093/arclin/acr011

[28] Mobley AS, Rodriguez-Gil DJ, Imamura F, Greer CA. Aging in the olfactory system. Trends Neurosci. 2013; 37:77-84. Doi.org/10.1016/j.tins.2013.11.004

[29] Doty RL, Kamath V. The influences of age on olfaction: a review. Front Psychol 2014; 5:20. Doi: 10.3389/fpsyg.2014.0020

[30] Attems J, Walker L, Jellinger KA. Olfaction and aging: a mini-review. Gerontology. 2015; 61:485-490. Doi: 10.1159/000381619

[31] Kalmey JK, Thewissen JG, Dluzen DE. Age-related size reduction of foramina in the cribriform plate. Anat Rec 1998;251:326-329

[32] Paik SI, Lehman MN, Seiden AM, Duncan HJ, Smith DV. Human Olfactory Biopsy: The Influence of Age and Receptor Distribution. *Arch Otolaryngol Head Neck Surg.* 1992; 118:731-738. Doi:10.1001/archotol.1992.01880070061012

[33] Buschhuter D, Smitka M, Puschmann S, Gerber JC, Witt M, Abolmaali ND, Hummel T. Correlation

between olfactory bulb volume and olfactory function. Neuroimage. 2008; 42:498-502. Doi 10.1016/j.neuroimage.2008.05.004

[34] Yousem DM, Geckle RJ, Bilker WB, McKeown DA, Doty RL. Posttraumatic olfactory dysfunction: MR and clinical evaluation. AJNR. 1996; 17:1171-1179. Doi 0195-6108/96/1706-117

[35] Yousem DM, Geckle RJ, Bilker WB, Kroger H, Doty RL. Posttraumatic smell loss: Relationship of psychophysical tests and volumes of the olfactory bulbs and tracts and the temporal lobes. Acad Radiol. 1999; 6:264-272. Doi: 10.1016/S1076-6332(99)80449-8

[36] Segura B, Baggio HC, Solana E, Palacios EM, Vendrell P, Bargallo N, Junque C. Neuroanatomical correlates of olfactory loss in normal aged subjects. Behav Brain Res. 2013; 246: 148-153. Doi.org/10.1016/j.bbr.2013.02.025

[37] Rawson NE, Gomez G, Cowart BJ, Kriete A, Pribitkin E, Restrepo D. Age-associated loss of selectivity in human olfactory sensory neurons. Neurobiol Aging. 2012; 33:1913-1919. Doi.org/10.1016/j.neurobiolaging.2011.09.036

[38] Joussain P, Thevenet M, Rouby C, Bensafi M. Effect of Aging on Hedonic Appreciation of Pleasant and Unpleasant Odors. PLoS ONE 2013; 8: e61376. Doi:10.1371/journal.pone.0061376

[39] Acebes A, Martín-Peña A, Chevalier V, Ferrús A. Synapse loss in olfactory local interneurons modifies perception. J Neurosci 2011; 31:2734-45. Doi.org/10.1523/JNEUROSCI.5046-10.2011

[40] Barresi M, Ciurleo R, Giacoppo S, Foti CV, Celi D, Bramanti P et al. Evaluation of olfactory dysfunction in neurodegenerative diseases. J. Neurol. Sci. 2012; 323, 16-24. Doi.org/10.1016/j.jns.2012.08.028

[41] Sinding C, Puschmann L, Hummel T: Is the age-related loss in olfactory sensitivity similar for light and heavy molecules? Chem Senses 2014; 39: 383-390. Doi:10.1093/chemse/bju004

[42] Hedner M, Nilsson LG, Olofsson JK, Bergman O, Eriksson E, Nyberg L et al. Age-related olfactory decline is associated with the BDNF Val66met polymorphism: evidence from a population-based study. Front. Aging Neurosci. 2010; 2:24. Doi.org/10.1080/13803391003683070.

[43] Doty RL, Petersen I, Mensah N, & Christensen, K (2011). Genetic and environmental influences on odor identification ability in the very old. Psychology and Aging, 26(4), 864-871. Doi.org/10.1037/a0023263

[44] Yaffe K, Freimer D, Chen H, et al. Olfaction and risk of dementia in a biracial cohort of older adults. Neurology 2017; 88: 456-462. Doi.org/10.1212/WNL.0000000000003558

[45] Van Regemorter V, Hummel T, Rosenzweig F, Mouraux A, Rombaux P and Huart C (2020) Mechanisms Linking Olfactory Impairment and Risk of Mortality. Front. Neurosci. 14:140. Doi: 10.3389/fnins.2020.00140

[46] Morrison JH and Baxter MG. The ageing cortical synapse: hallmarks and implications for cognitive decline. Nat. Rev. Neurosci. 2012; 13:240-250. Doi.org/10.1038/nrn3200

[47] Liu Z, Chen Z, Shang C, Yan F, Shi Y, Zhang J, Qu B, Han, H, Wang Y, Li D, Südhof TC, Cao P. IGF1-dependent synaptic plasticity of mitral cells in olfactory memory during social learning. Neuron. 2017; 95: 106-122. Doi.org/10.1016/j.neuron.2017.06.015

[48] Bhatia-Dey N, Kanherkar RR, Stair SE, Makarev EO and Csoka AB (2016) Cellular Senescence as the Causal

Nexus of Aging. Front. Genet. 7:13. doi: 10.3389/fgene.2016.00013

[49] Hoang ML, Kinde I, Tomasetti C, McMahon KW, Rosenquist TA, Grollman AP, et al. Genome-wide quantification of rare somatic mutations in normal human tissues using massively parallel sequencing. Proc Natl Acad Sci U S A. 2016; 113:9846-51. Doi:10.1073/pnas.1607794113/

[50] Lodato MA, Rodin RE, Bohrson CL, Coulter ME, Barton AR., Kwon M, ... Walsh, C. A. (2018). Aging and neurodegeneration are associated with increased mutations in single human neurons. Science, 359, 555-559. Doi.org/10.1126/science.aao4426

[51] Djordjevic J, Jones-Gotman M, De Sousa K, Chertkow H. Olfaction in patients with mild cognitive impairment and Alzheimer's disease. Neurobiol Aging 2008; 29:693-706. Doi.org/10.1016/j.neurobiolaging.2006.11.014.

[52] Doty, RL Olfactory dysfunction in neurodegenerative diseases: is there a common pathological substrate? Lancet. Neurol. 2017, 16, 478-488. Doi.org/10.1016/S1474-4422(17)30123-0

[53] Marin C, Vilas D, Langdon C, Alobid I, López-Chacón M, Haehner A, Hummel T, Mullol J Olfactory dysfunction in neurodegenerative diseases. Curr Allergy Asthma Rep 2018; 18, 42. Doi.org/10.1007/s11882-018-0796-4

[54] Doty RL and Hawkes CH. Chemosensory dysfunction in neurodegenerative diseases. Smell and Taste. 2019; 325-360. Doi:10.1016/B978-0-444-63855-7.00020-4,

[55] Brozzetti L, Sacchetto L, Cecchini MP, Avesani A, Perra D, Bongianni M, Portioli C, Scupoli M, Ghetti B, Monaco S, Buffelli M and ZanussoGNeurodegeneration-Associated Proteins in Human Olfactory Neurons Collected by Nasal Brushing. Front. Neurosci. 2020; 14:145.Doi: 10.3389/fnins.2020.00145

[56] Heyanka DJ, Golden CJ, McCue RB II, Scarisbrick DM, Linck JF, Zlatkin NI (2014). Olfactory deficits in frontotemporal dementia as measured by the Alberta smell test. Appl. Neuropsychol. Adult 21, 176-182. Doi:10.1080/ 09084282.2013.782031

[57] Franks KH, Chuah MI, King AE and Vickers JC. Connectivity of Pathology: The Olfactory System as a Model for Network-Driven Mechanisms of Alzheimer's Disease Pathogenesis. Front. Aging Neurosci. 2015; 7:234. Doi: 10.3389/fnagi.2015.00234

[58] Mesholam RI, Moberg PJ, Mahr RN, & Doty RL. Olfaction in neurodegenerative disease: A meta-analysis of olfactory functioning in Alzheimer's and Parkinson's diseases. Archives of Neurology. 1998; 55, 84-90. Doi:10.1001/archneur.55.1.84

[59] Luzzi S, Snowden JS, Neary D, Coccia M, Provinciali L, Ralph MAL. Distinct patterns of olfactory impairment in Alzheimer's disease, semantic dementia, frontotemporal dementia, and corticobasal degeneration. Neuropsychologia, 2007; 45:1823-1831. Doi:10.1016/j.neuropsychologia.2006.12.008

[60] Devanand DP, Michaels-Marston KS, Liu X, et al. Olfactory deficits in patients with mild cognitive impairment predict Alzheimer's disease at follow-up. Am J Psychiatry 2000; 157:1399-405. Doi.org/10.1176/appi.ajp.157.9.1399

[61] Devanand DP, Lee S, Manly J, et al. Olfactory deficits predict cognitive decline and Alzheimer dementia in an urban community. Neurology. 2015; 84: 182-189. Doi.org/10.1212/WNL.0000000000001132

[62] McLaughlin NC, Westervelt HJ Odor identification deficits in frontotemporal dementia: a preliminary study. Arch Clin Neuropsychol. 2008; 23, 119-123. Doi:10.1016/j.acn.2007.07.008

[63] Spillantini MG and Goedert M. Tau pathology and neurodegeneration. Lancet Neurol 2013; 123, 609-622.

[64] Lafaille-Magnan ME, Poirier J, Etienne P, Tremblay-Mercier J, Frenette J, Rosa-Neto P, et al. PREVENT-AD Research Group. Odor identification as a biomarker of preclinical AD in older adults at risk. Neurology. 2017; 89:327-35. Doi 10.1212/ WNL.0000000000004159

[65] Rey NL, Wesson DW, Brundin P. The olfactory bulb as the entry site for prion-like propagation in neurodegenerative diseases. Neurobiology of Disease, 2018: 109: 226-248. Doi.org/10.1016/j.nbd.2016.12.013

[66] Fujita KA, Ostaszewski M, Matsuoka Y, et al. Integrating pathways of Parkinson's disease in a molecular interaction map. Mol Neurobiol 2014; 49:88-102. Doi 10.1007/ s12035-013-8489-4

[67] Wszolek ZK, Markopoulou K. Olfactory dysfunction in Parkinson's disease. Clin Neurosci 1998;5:94-101

[68] Doty RL, Deems DA, Stellar S. Olfactory dysfunction in Parkinsonism: a general deficit unrelated to neurologic signs, disease stage, or disease duration. Neurology. 1988; 38:1237-124.

[69] Doty RL, Stern, MB, Pfeiffer C, Gollomp, SM, Hurting HI. Bilateral olfactory dysfunction in early stage treated and untreated idiopathic Parkinson's disease. J. Neurol. Neurosurg. Psychiatry. 1992; 55, 138-142

[70] Ponsen MM, Stoffers D, Booij J, van Eck-Smit BLF, Wolters EC, Berendse HW. Idiopathic hyposmia as a preclinical sign of Parkinson's disease. Ann Neurol. 2004; 56:173-181. Doi: 10.1002/ana.20160

[71] Doty RL. Olfactory dysfunction in Parkinson disease. Nat.Rev.Neurol. 2012a; 8:329-339. Doi:10.1038/ nrneurol.2012.80

[72] Doty RL. Olfaction in Parkinson's disease and related disorders. Neurobiol. Dis. 2012b; 46, 527-552. Doi. org/10.1016/j.nbd.2011.10.026

[73] Fullard ME, Morley JF, Duda JE. Olfactory dysfunction as an early biomarker in Parkinson's disease. Neurosci Bull. 2017; 33:515-25. Doi. org/10.1007/s12264-017-0170-x

[74] Witt M, Bormann K, Gudziol V. Biopsies of olfactory epithelium in patients with Parkinson's disease. Mov Disord. 2009; 24: 906-914. Doi: 10.1002/ mds.22464

[75] Wang J, You H, Liu JF, Ni DF, Zhang ZX, Guan J. Association of olfactory bulb volume and olfactory sulcus depth with olfactory function in patients with Parkinson disease. AJNR Am J Neuroradiol. 2011; 32:677-681. Doi.org/10.3174/ajnr.A2350

[76] Luk KC, Lee VM. Modeling Lewy pathology propagation in Parkinson's disease. Parkinsonism Relat Disord. 2014; 20:S85–S87. Doi.org/10.1016/ S1353-8020(13)70022-1

[77] Del Tredici K, Rub U, De Vos RA, Bohl JR, Braak H. Where does Parkinson disease pathology begin in the brain? J Neuropathol Exp Neurol. 2002; 61: 413-426. Doi.org/10.1093/jnen/61.5.413

[78] Espay AJ, Kalia LV, Gan-Or Z, et al. Disease modification and biomarker development in Parkinson disease: Revision or reconstruction? Neurology. 2020; 94:481-494. Doi:10.1212/ WNL.0000000000009107

[79] Takeda A, Baba T, Kikuchi A., Hasegawa T, Sugeno N, Konno M., Miura E. & Mori E. Olfactory dysfunction and dementia in Parkinson's disease. J. Parkinsons Dis. 2014; 4: 181-187. Doi: 10.3233/JPD-130277

[80] Mahlknecht P, Pechlaner R, Boesveldt S, Volc D, Pinter B, Reiter E, et al. Optimizing odor identification testing as quick and accurate diagnostic tool for Parkinson's disease. Movement Disorders. 2016; 31:1408-1413. Doi: 10.1002/mds.26637

[81] Zucco, GM, Bollini F. Odour recognition memory and odour identification in patients with mild and severe major depressive disorders. Psychiatry Res. 2011; 190: 217-220. Doi:10.1016/j.psychres.2011.08.025

[82] Taalman H, Wallace C and Milev R. Olfactory Functioning and Depression: A Systematic Review. Front. Psychiatry. 2017; 8:190. Doi: 10.3389/fpsyt.2017.00190

[83] Naudin M, Atanasova B. Olfactory markers of depression and Alzheimer's disease. Neurosci. Biobehav. Rev. 2014; 45, 262-270. Doi: 10.1016/j.psychres.2014.08.050

[84] Croy I, Negoias S, Novakova L, Landis B, Hummel T. Learning about the functions of the olfactory system from people without a sense of smell. PLoS One 2012; 7, e33365.Doi: 10.1016/j.jad.2013.12.026

[85] Sivertsen H, Bjørkløf GH, Engedal K, Selbæk G, Helvik A-S. Depression and Quality of Life in Older Persons: A Review. Dement. Geriatr. Cogn. Disord. 2015; 40:311-339. Doi: 10.1159/000437299

[86] Rochet M, El-Hage W, Richa S, Kazour F, Atanasova B. Depression, olfaction, and quality of life: a mutual relationship. Brain Sci. 2018; 8: 80. Doi:10.3390/brainsci8050080

[87] Savic I, Gulyas B, Larsson M, Roland P. Olfactory functions are mediated by parallel and hierarchical processing. Neuron. 2000; 26:735-745

[88] Anderson AK, Christoff K, Stappen I, Panitz D, Ghahremani DG, Glover G, Gabrieli JDE, Sobel N. Dissociated neural representations of intensity and valence in human olfaction. Nat. Neurosci. 2003; 6:196-202. Doi.org/10.1038/nn1001

[89] Kiracanski K, Joormann J, Gotlib IH. Cognitive aspects of depression: Cognitive aspects of depression. Wiley Interdiscip. Rev. Cogn. Sci. 2012; 3:301-313. Doi: 10.1002/wcs.1177

[90] Kohli P, Soler ZM, Nguyen SA, Muus JS, Schlosser RJ. The association between olfaction and depression: a systematic review. Chem. Senses. 2016; 41: 479-86. Doi:10.1093/chemse/bjw061

[91] Negoias S, Hummel T, Symmank A, Schellong J, Joraschky P, & Croy I. Olfactory bulb volume predicts therapeutic outcome in major depression disorder. Brain imaging and behavior. 2015; Doi 10.1007/s11682-015-9400-x

[92] Wicker B, Monfardini E, & Royet J-P. Olfactory processing in adults with autism spectrum disorders. Molecular Autism. 2016; 7:1-11. Doi 10.1186/s13229-016-0070-3

[93] Geramita MA, Wen JA, Rannals, MD, Urban NN. Decreased amplitude and reliability of odor-evoked responses in two mouse models of autism Journal of Neurophysiology. 2020; 123: 1283-1294. Doi.org/10.1152/jn.00277.2019

[94] Riley JD, Delahunty, C, Alsadah A, Mazzola, S. Further evidence of GABRA4 and TOP3B as autism susceptibility genes European Journal of Medical Genetics. 2020; 63: Doi.org/10.1016/j.ejmg.2020.103876

[95] Satterstrom FK, Kosmicki JA, Wang J, Breen MS, De Rubeis S, An J-Y., Peng M, Collins, R., Grove, J., Klei L., Stevens C, Reichert J, Mulhern MS, Artomov M, Gerges S, Sheppard, B., Xu X, Bhaduri A, Norman U, Brand H, Schwartz G., Nguyen R, & Guerrero EE. Large-scale exome sequencing study implicates both developmental and functional changes in the neurobiology of autism. Cell. 2020; 180:568-584. Doi. org/10.1016/j.cell.2019.12.036

[96] Hummel T, Landis BN, Hüttenbrink KB. Smell and taste disorders. GMS Curr Top Otorhinolaryngol Head Neck Surg. 2011; 10:Doc04. Doi: 10.3205/cto000077,

[97] Cohen J, Wakefield CE, Laing DG. Smell and taste disorders resulting from cancer and chemotherapy. Curr Pharm Des 2016; 22:2253-63.

[98] Le XTPham HTN, Do PT. et al. *Bacopa monnieri* Ameliorates Memory Deficits in Olfactory Bulbectomized Mice: Possible Involvement of Glutamatergic and Cholinergic Systems. Neurochem Res. 2013; 38:2201-2215. Doi 10.1007/s11064-013-1129-6

[99] Yi LT, Li J, Li HC, Su DX, Quan, XB, He XC, Wang XH. Antidepressant like behavioral, neurochemical and neuroendocrine effects of Naringenin in the mouse repeated tail suspension test. Prog. Neuro Psychopharmacol. Biol. Psychiatry. 2012; 39:175-181. Doi. org/10.1016/j.pnpbp.2012.06.009.

[100] Bansal Y, Singh R, Saroj P, Sodhi RK, Kuhad A. Naringenin protects against oxido-inflammatory aberrations and altered tryptophan metabolism in olfactory bulbectomized-mice model of depression. Toxicol. Appl. Pharmacol. 2018; 355: 257-268. Doi.org/10.1016/j.taap.2018.07.010

[101] Leventhal AM, Gelernter J, Oslin D, Anton RF, Farrer LA, Kranzler, HR. Agitated depression in substance dependence Drug and Alcohol Dependence. 2011; 116:163-169. Doi:10.1016/j.drugalcdep.2010.12.012

[102] Saiz-Sanchez D, Ubeda-Bañon I, Flores-Cuadrado A, Gonzalez-Rodriguez M, Villar-Conde S, Astillero-LopezVandMartinez-MarcosA. Somatostatin, Olfaction, and Neurodegeneration. Front. Neurosci. 2020; 14:96. Doi: 10.3389/fnins.2020.00096

[103] Cooper KW, Brann DH, Farruggia MC, Bhutani S, Pellegrino R, Tsukahara T, Weinreb C, Joseph PV, Larson ED, Parma V, Albers MW, Barlow LA, Datta SR, and Di Pizio A. 2020 COVID-19 and the chemical senses: supporting players take center stage. Neuron, 2020; 107: 219-233 doi. org/10.1016/j.neuron.2020.06.032

[104] Parma V, Ohla K, Veldhuizen MG, Niv MY, Kelly CE, Bakke AJ, Cooper KW, Bouysset C, Pirastu N, DibattistaM,KaurR,LiuzzaMT,PepinoMY, Schopf V, Pereda-Loth V, Olsson SB, Gerkin RC, Domínguez PR, Albayay J, Farruggia MC, Bhutani S, Fjaeldstad AW, Kumar R, Menini A, Bensafi M, Sandell M, Konstantinidis I, Di Pizio A, Genovese F, Oztürk L, Thomas-Danguin T, Frasnelli J, Boesveldt S, Saatci Ö, Saraiva LR, Lin C, Golebiowski J, Hwang LD, Ozdener MH, Guàrdia MD, Laudamiel C, Ritchie M, HavlícekJ., PierronD, RouraE, NavarroM, Nolden AA, Lim J, Whitcroft KL, Colquitt LR, Ferdenzi C, Brindha EV, Altundag A, Macchi A., Nunez-Parra A, Patel ZM, Fiorucci S, Philpott CM, Smith BC, Lundström JN, Mucignat C, Parker JK, van den Brink M, Schmuker M, Fischmeister FPS, Heinbockel T, Shields VDC, Faraji F, Santamaría E, Fredborg WEA, Morini G., Olofsson JK, Jalessi M, Karni N, D'Errico A, Alizadeh R, Pellegrino R, Meyer P, Huart C, Chen B, SolerGM,AlwashahiMK,Welge-LüssenA, Freiherr J, De Groot JHB, Klein H, Okamoto M., Singh PB, Hsieh JW, GCCR

Group Author, Reed DR, Hummel T, Munger SD and Hayes JE More than smell - COVID-19 is associated with severe impairment of smell, taste, and chemesthesis. Chem Senses; 2020; bjaa041.

[105] Pellegrino R, Cooper KW, Di Pizio A, Joseph PV, Bhutani S, Parma V. Corona viruses and the chemical senses: Past, present, and future. Chem Senses. 2020. DOI: 10.1093/chemse/bjaa031

[106] Brann DH, Tsukahara T, Weinreb C, Lipovsek M, Van den Berge K, Gong B, Chance R, Macaulay IC, Chou HJ, Fletcher RB, Das D, Street K, Roux de Bezieux H, Choi YG, Risso D, Dudoit S, Purdom E, Mill J, Hachem RA, Matsunami H, Logan DW, Goldstein BJ, Grubb MS, Ngai J, Datta SR. Non-neuronal expression of SARS-CoV-2 entry genes in the olfactory system suggests mechanisms underlying COVID-19-associated anosmia. Sci. Adv; 2020; 10.1126/sciadv.abc5801

[107] Bryche B, St Albin A, Murri S, Lacôte S, Pulido, C, Ar Gouilh M, Lesellier, S, Servat A, Wasniewski, M, Picard-Meyer E. Massive transient damage of the olfactory epithelium associated with infection of sustentacular cells by SARS-CoV-2 in golden Syrian hamsters. Brain. Behav. Immun. 2020. doi.org/10.1016/j.bbi.2020.06.032

[108] Diaz D, Gomez C, Munoz-Castaneda R, et al. The olfactory system as a puzzle: playing with its pieces. Anat Rec. (Hoboken) 2013; 296: 1383-1400. Doi 10.1002/ar.22748

[109] Heinbockel T. Introductory chapter: Mechanisms and function of synaptic plasticity. In: Synaptic Plasticity. Thomas Heinbockel (ed.), Rijeka, Croatia, InTech Publisher. 2017; 3-13, Doi.org/10.5772/67891

[110] Lucassen EB, Turel A, Knehans A, Huang X, Eslinger P. Olfactory dysfunction in multiple sclerosis: a scoping review of the literature. Mult. Scler. Relat. Disord. 2016; 6:1-9. Doi.org/10.1016/j.msard.2015.12.002.

[111] Baney J. A cause of olfactory dysfunction in MS? Neurol. Rev. 2011; 19: 7.

[112] Orasji SSS, Mulder JL, de Bruijn SFTM, Wirtz PW. Olfactory dysfunction in behavioral variant frontotemporal dementia. Clin Neurol Neurosurg. 2016; 141:106-110. Doi.org/10.1016/j.clineuro.2016.01.003 0303-8467

[113] Herman AM, Critchley, H, & Duka T. Decreased olfactory discrimination is associated with impulsivity in healthy volunteers. Scientific Reports. 2018; 8. Doi: 10.1038/s41598-018-34056-9

[114] Mori I. The olfactory bulb: A link between environmental agents and narcolepsy. Medical hypotheses. 2019; 126: 66-68. doi.org/10.1016/j.mehy.2019.03.017

[115] Tan L, Li Q, Xie XS. Olfactory sensory neurons transiently express multiple olfactory receptors during development. Mol. Syst. Biol., 2015; 11:844. Doi 10.15252/msb.20156639

[116] Hanchate NK, Kondoh K, Lu Z, Kuang D, Ye X, Qiu X, Pachter L, Trapnell C, Buck LB. Single-cell transcriptomics reveals receptor transformations during olfactory neurogenesis, Science. 2015; 350:1251-1255. Doi:10.1126/science.aad2456

[117] Bashkirova E & Lomvardas S. Olfactory receptor genes make the case for inter-chromosomal interactions. Curr Opin Genet Dev. 2019; 55:106-113. Doi.org/10.1016/j.gde.2019.07.004

[118] Sedelnikova OA, Horikawa I, Zimonjic DB, Popescu NC, Bonner WM, Barrett JC. Senescing human cells and ageing mice accumulate DNA lesions with unrepairable double-strand breaks. Nat. Cell Biol. 2004; 6:168-70. Doi: 10.1038/ncb1095

[119] Petr, MA, Tulika T, Carmona-Marin LM, Scheibye-Knudsen M. Protecting the Aging Genome. Trends Cell Biol. 2020; S0962-8924. Protecting the Aging Genome. Trends Cell Biol. 2020; S0962-8924. Doi.org/10.1016/j.tcb.2019.12.001

[120] Tepe B, Hill MC, Pekarek BT, Hunt PJ, Martin TJ, Martin JF, Arenkiel BR. Single-cell RNA-Seq of mouse olfactory bulb reveals cellular heterogeneity and activity-dependent molecular census of adult-born neurons. Cell Rep. 2018; 25: 2689-2703. Doi.org/10.1016/j.celrep.2018.11.034

[121] Chou RH, Lu CY, Fan JR, Yu YL, Shyu WC. The potential therapeutic applications of olfactory ensheathing cells in regenerative medicine. Cell Transplant. 2014; 23:567-71. Doi.org/10.3727/096368914X678508

[122] Bhatia-Dey N and Heinbockel T. Endocannabinoid-Mediated Neuromodulation in the Olfactory Bulb: Functional and Therapeutic Significance. Int. J. Mol. Sci. 2020, 21: 2850. Doi:10.3390/ijms21082850

[123] Xu B, Karayiorgou M, Gogos JA. MicroRNAs in psychiatric and neurodevelopmental disorders. Brain Res. 2010; 1338:78-88. Doi.org/10.1016/j.brainres.2010.03.109

[124] Hernandez-Rapp J, Rainone S, Hébert SS. MicroRNAs underlying memory deficits in neurodegenerative disorders. Prog. Neuropsychopharmacol. Biol. Psychiatry 2017; 73:79-86. Doi.org/10.1016/j.pnpbp.2016.04.011

[125] Swarbrick S, Wragg, N, Ghosh S, and Stolzing A. Systematic review of miRNA as biomarkers in Alzheimer's disease. Mol. Neurobiol. 2019; 56: 6156-6167. Doi: 10.1007/s12035-019-1500-y

[126] Reza-Zaldivar EE, Hernández-Sápiens MA, Minjarez B, Gómez-Pinedo U, Sánchez-González VJ, Márquez-Aguirre AL and Canales-Aguirre AA. Dendritic Spine and Synaptic Plasticity in Alzheimer's disease: A Focus on MicroRNA. Front. Cell Dev. Biol. 2020; 8:255.Doi: 10.3389/fcell.2020.00255

Chapter 8

Cross-Modality Dysfunction between the Visual and Olfactory Systems in Parkinson's Disease

Motoyasu Honma

Abstract

Cross-modality in function is a fundamental ability in humans and is closely associated with the basic functions. Several studies have demonstrated that vision strongly influences other senses such as hearing, touch, taste, and smell. However, the dysfunction in this cross-modality caused by disease, is poorly understood. In addition to evidence that Parkinson's disease (PD) impairs various cognitive functions including olfaction, a recent study showed that olfactory function is unaffected by visual information in patients with PD. This finding suggests that the link between vision and olfaction is underactive in PD. This chapter reviews the cross-modal dysfunction and dwells on the possibility of a novel precursor assessment for PD.

Keywords: cross-modality, vision, olfaction, Parkinson's disease, striatum

1. Introduction

Sensory organs independently process the corresponding external stimuli such as light, sound, pressure, taste, and smell. However, one sense rarely acts alone during the perception/cognition of a given event in daily life. Our experiences are dependent on the integration of the visual, auditory, somesthetic, gustatory, and olfactory systems. For example, during the act of smelling a strawberry, the sense of smell may vary according to the color of the strawberry (whether it is bright red or green-tinged), even if the physical odorant is the same (**Figure 1**). This example demonstrates that cognition is built upon cross-modality of function. The regions associated with cross-modality are spread throughout a wide area in brain [1]. For example, the integration of vision and touch is mainly associated with the right posterior fusiform gyrus and primary somatosensory cortices [2], whereas the integration of vision and audition is mainly associated with the right frontal lobe and right superior temporal gyrus [3].

The accuracy of each of the senses is different, and vision is often prioritized over other senses during integration. Several studies have demonstrated that visual input strongly influences hearing [4] touch [5], taste [6], and smell [7, 8] (**Figure 2**); however, the reverse, in which other senses influence vision, is a rare phenomenon, excluding the auditory-vision relationships such as the McGurk effect [9] or double flash illusion [10]. For the McGurk effect, on a video of audiovisual speech, if a lip movements show a "ba-ba" sound, whereas an auditory information

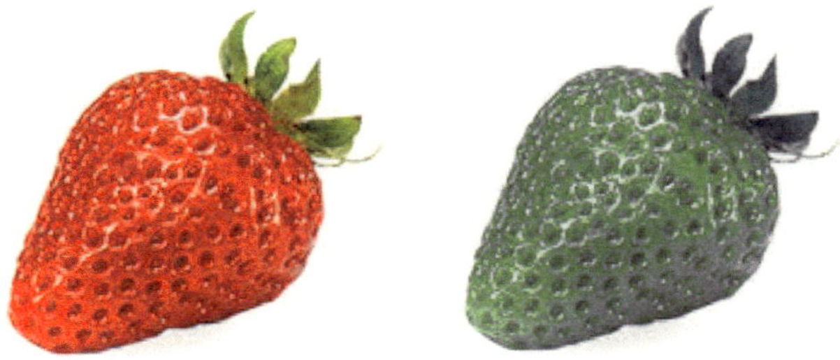

Figure 1.
An example of the effect of color effect on smell recognition. The red strawberry on the left may seem to have a more pleasant odor than the green strawberry on the right.

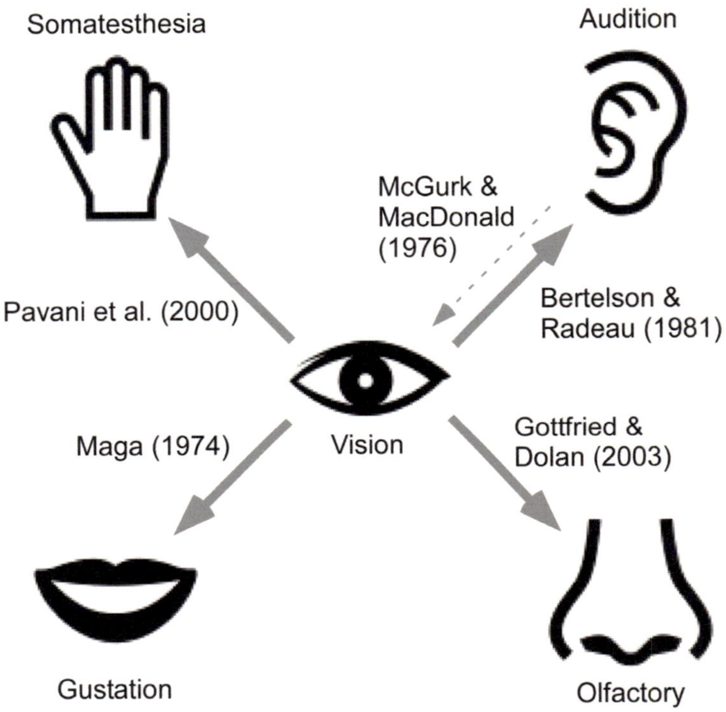

Figure 2.
Diagram representing the effective relationship among the five senses. Vision is often prioritized over the other senses during integration.

is that of "ga-ga", most people experiences an illusory sound "da-da". For the double flash illusion, if one dot flashes on the display when two beeps are sounded, most people reports experiencing two flashes. Thus, vision dominates the other senses in many cases. Although the mechanism of cross-modality has become increasingly clear in healthy persons [1–10], a function in disease states remains unclear.

2. Clinical state and cognitive dysfunction in Parkinson's disease

Parkinson's disease (PD) causes tremors of the hands, stiffness, akinesia, or inability to maintain posture. Patients with PD have decreased levels of dopamine in the striatum, which consists of the putamen and caudate nucleus, which are a part of the basal ganglia [11]. They may further develop protein-related disorders, such as the presynaptic dopamine transporter (DaT), which is responsible for the incorporation and transmission of dopamine components [12]. DaT scanning is performed with ioflupane (^{123}I-FP-CIT), a radio-iodinated cocaine analogue [13, 14]. It has a high affinity for the DaT protein located on presynaptic nerve endings in the striatum. These nerve endings are projections of dopaminergic neurons from the substantia nigra. Binding of a radiopharmaceutical agent to DaT reflects number of striatal dopaminergic neurons. The accumulation of DaT is expressed in proportion to the occipital lobe (**Figure 3**). The degree of DaT deficit is associated with the severity of the movement disorder [15].

The principal symptoms of PD are related to movement, although the non-motor symptoms are also noteworthy. For example, attention function, which demands a response speed or switching [16]; executive function, which is related to action planning or problem solving [17]; working memory function, which holds information temporarily and allocates attentional resources [18, 19]; social cognition function, which involves interpreting emotions based on others' facial expressions [20, 21]; and temporal function, which estimates duration [22, 23] were shown to be impaired in PD.

Impairment of olfaction has also been reported in patients with PD and may be a biomarker for cognitive dysfunction and early PD [24–26]. Olfactory information is projected directly to the limbic system, including the piriform (PIR), amygdala (AMG), hippocampus (HI), and entorhinal cortex (ENT). These areas determine odor detection, its emotional evaluation (pleasant or unpleasant), and memory retrieval [27]. Olfactory information finally ascends to the orbitofrontal cortex (OFC). The OFC participates in the identification or recognition of odor, filtered through emotion and memory via activation of the AMG and HI [28]. Olfactory dysfunction in PD may occur due to deficiency of dopamine and pathological changes in the ENT, AMG and HI, especially in the areas affected by early onset of PD [29].

Furthermore, the striatum is involved in various functions, which include an integration of sensory information [30–32]. Studies have demonstrated that the striatum (putamen and caudate) acts as a "hub," with specialized functional roles for different neuron types in mice [33] and humans [34, 35]. However, it was unclear whether PD affects cross-modal function.

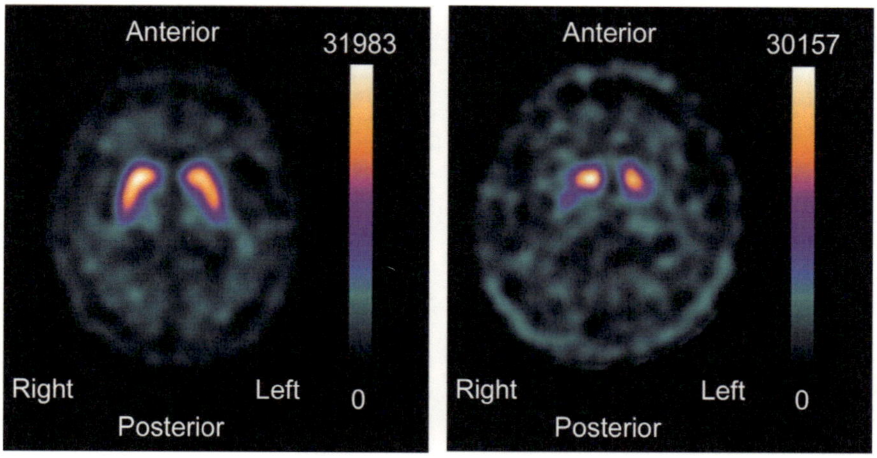

Figure 3.
Striatal DaT deficit in Parkinson's disease (coronal view). The left panel shows a binding radiopharmaceutical agent accumulation in a healthy person. The right panel shows a binding radiopharmaceutical agent accumulation in a patient with Parkinson's disease. The numbers indicate binding radiopharmaceutical agent counts on the striatum per pixel.

3. Cross-modality dysfunction in Parkinson's disease

Recently, a study showed that PD causes a decline in the cross-modal function of vision and olfaction [36]. This study conducted behavioral experiments to identify the influence of PD on cross-modal function by comparing the behavior of patients with PD with that of healthy controls. The principal aim of this study was to measure odor-strength perception and preference, while presenting smells paired with visual information, to characterize vision/olfaction integration in patients with PD.

In the experiment, odor detection thresholds in each participant were first determined using an olfactometer, which has five odorants (β-phenylethyl alcohol, methyl cyclopentenolone, isovaleric acid, γ-undecalactone, and skatole). For example, methyl cyclopentenolone smells like caramel pudding (pleasant) and skatole smells like rotten vegetables (unpleasant). The study employed detectable odorant thresholds in each of five categories and prepared five original pictures associated with the five odorants of each category. For example, the category "caramel pudding" consisted of a picture of "pudding" and the odorant "methyl cyclopentenolone," whereas "rotten vegetables" consisted of "rotten vegetables" and the odorant "skatole" (**Figure 4**). The "control" category consisted of a noise picture and an odorless liquid. Four combinations were arranged: the original picture with the original odorant (combination "A"), the control picture with the original odorant (combination "B"), and the original picture with the control odorant (combination "C"). A control combination was added: the control picture with the control odorant (combination "D") (**Figure 5**). Participants were asked take a sniff while viewing the picture, and were subsequently asked to evaluate the strength (weak – strong) and preference (pleasant – unpleasant) of each odor on a visual analog scale (VAS).

In the *caramel pudding* category, healthy controls overestimated the odor strength compared with patients with PD, when the original picture was presented (combinations A and C). Furthermore, healthy controls negatively estimated odor preference in combinations A and C in the "rotten vegetables" category (**Figure 6**). The results indicate that patients with PD accurately judged odor strength, without being distracted by visual appearance whereas odor strength/preference in healthy controls was influenced by visual appearance.

Furthermore, the study reported a possible effect of striatal DaT deficits in patients with PD on the olfaction-vision cross-modality. DaT imaging indicated that striatal DaT deficit in PD, especially that in the posterior putamen, is associated

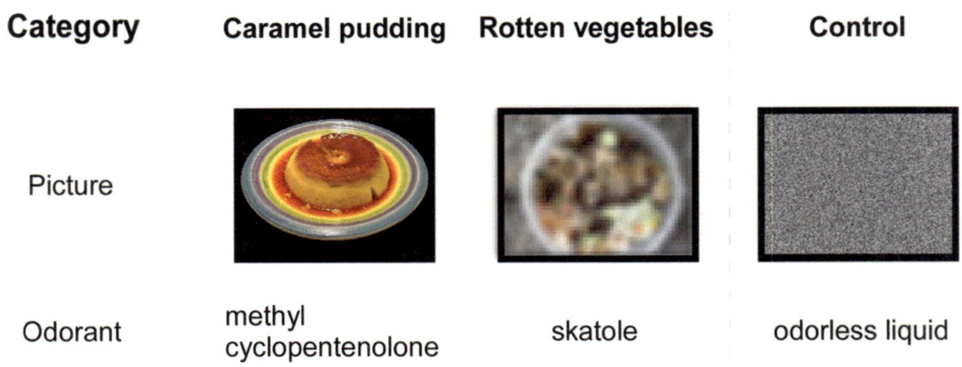

Figure 4.
Examples of the category type. Each category consists of an original odorant and an original picture corresponding to the odorant, and a control category consisting of a noise picture and an odorless liquid (this figure is cited with edit from a part of Honma et al. [36]).

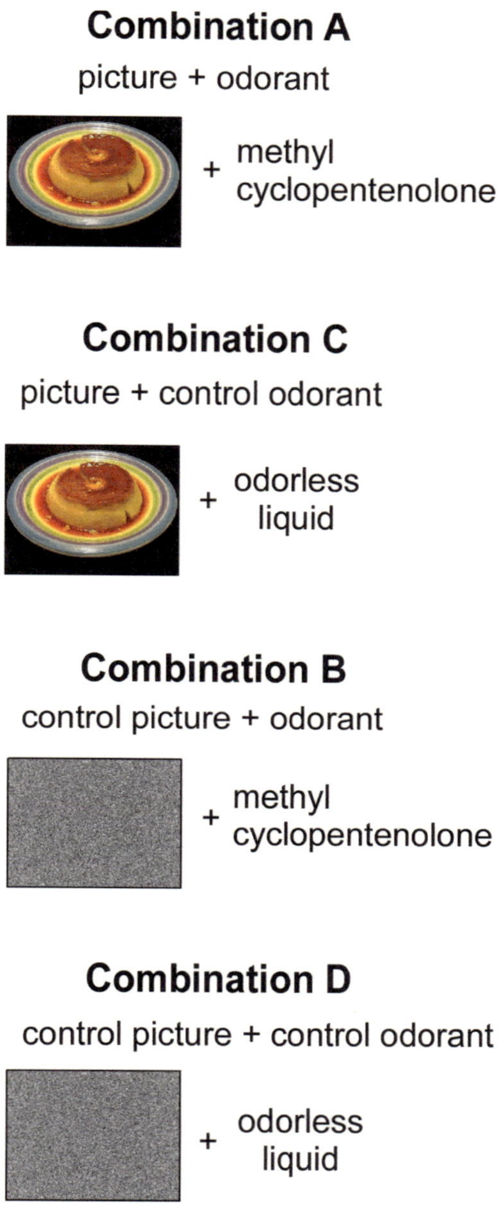

Figure 5.
Combinations of the pictures and odorants. Combination a includes the original picture and original odorant. Combination B includes the control picture and original odorant. Combination C includes the original picture and the control odorant. Combination D includes the control picture and control odorant (this figure is cited with edit from a part of Honma et al. [36]).

with the cross-modal effect of perception on odor preference, and the laterality may depend on the emotional category (pleasant or unpleasant) (**Figure** 7).

4. Possible mechanism of dysfunctional cross-modality between vision and olfaction

Honma et al. [36] showed that the olfactory function was unaffected by visual information in patients with PD, supporting the hypothesis that PD impairs cross-modality between vision and olfaction [36]. Healthy participants tend to

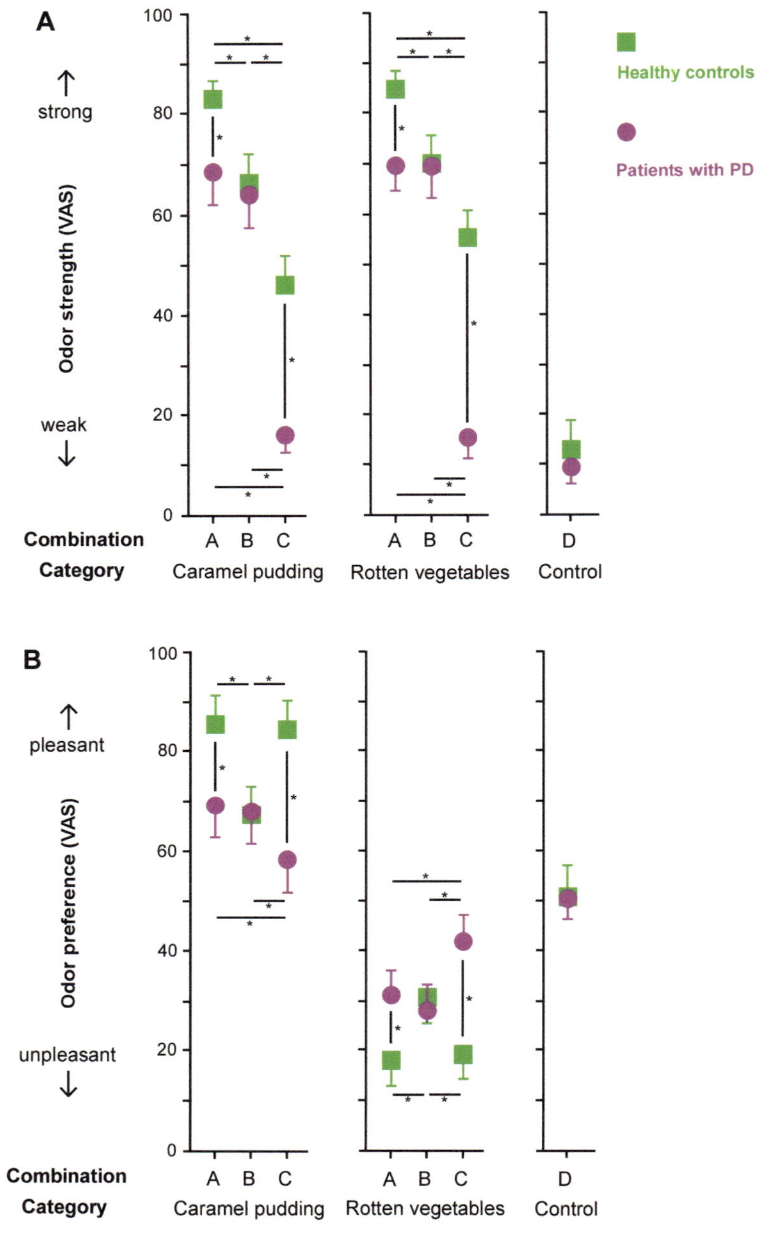

Figure 6.
(A) Strength of the odor represented on the visual analog scale. (B) Preference for odor on the visual analog scale. The visual analog scale scores of the groups (healthy controls and participants with PD) and combinations (A, B, and C) were compared for each category. The control category (combination D) was analyzed independently. Asterisks indicate significant differences. These results show that the visual input affects odor estimation in healthy controls, with little effect in PD (this figure is cited with edit from a part of Honma et al. [36]).

overestimate odor when presented with an original picture, for example, a picture of *caramel pudding* without the methyl cyclopentenolone odorant, will be perceived as pleasant. In contrast, patients with PD tend to concentrate more on smell, rather than the influence of visual stimuli. The odor estimate is independent of vision in patients with PD.

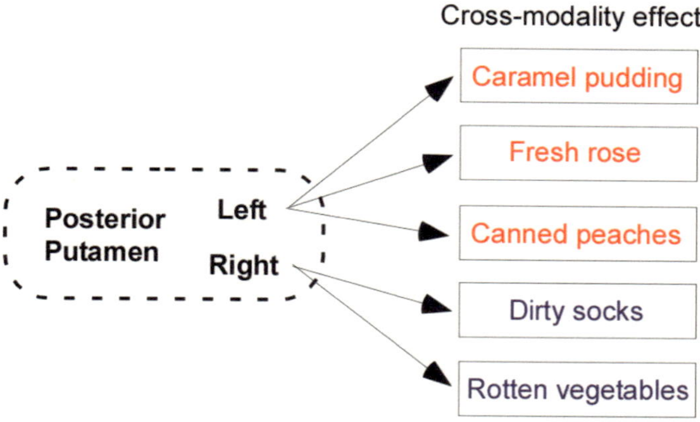

Figure 7.
Regression analysis identified the left posterior putamen as the independent variable for the cross-modal effects of pleasant categories (caramel pudding, fresh roses, and canned peaches). The right posterior putamen was identified as the independent variable for the cross-modal effects of unpleasant categories (rotten vegetables and dirty socks). The laterality in putamen may depend on emotionality.

Olfactory perception is ambiguous, and a smell may be hard to identify without verbal or visual assistance. It is true that olfaction is modulated by visual elements [7, 8]. This multimodal integration is responsible for the OFC, which receives information from visual association, and the olfactory, gustatory, somatosensory and, auditory areas [37]. Recent brain imaging studies showed that the OFC participates in vision-olfaction integration in healthy individuals [7]. Gottfried and Dolan (2003) noted higher activation of the OFC when a smell is presented with a word label [7]. Cognitive factors, such as visual stimuli modulate representations of odor at a relatively early level of cortical processing, known as the top-down cognitive influence, which directly affects emotion [38]. Healthy participants exhibited dominance of the visual sense in this study. On the other hand, patients with PD exhibited decrease dominance of visual information. They concentrated more on olfactory perception, without modulation from visual input. The OFC in patients with PD is known to be less active for all modalities during stimulation, including olfaction [39]. Decreased activation of the OFC in patients with PD may partly account for declining cross-modality. Moreover, detection and cognition levels for odor were lower than those in the controls. During olfaction, the OFC also integrates information from the AMG and HI, which play a role in emotional evaluation and memory retrieval [37]. Reduction of OFC function may lead to deficits in recognition and identification of odor. Thus, patients with PD may tend to focus more on smell detection, which may need activation of the basic primary olfactory areas, such as the ENT and PIR.

The relationship of DaT levels in PD with odor preferences demonstrated by the study is significant. However, it has been reported that administration of dopamine agonists (levodopa) does not influence the olfactory deficit. Thus, dopamine loss may not affect olfaction [40]. Here, it was not possible to establish a direct link between olfaction and dopamine levels, as measured by DaT in the putamen. However, earlier findings suggest that the putamen may play a role in sensory integration [34, 35]. Lack of dopamine linked to deficient DaT protein in the striatum leads to a decline in dopamine levels in several regions [41]. The corticostriatal loop sends signals that pass through brain regions, such as the striatum–pallidus–thalamic–cortex [42]. Dopamine regulates the prefrontal-AMG circuit, which plays an important role in emotion processing [43]. This suggests that vision-olfaction integration may be influenced by dopamine signals, via a striatum-centered network.

Dopamine deficiency in PD may affect vision-olfaction integration, including emotion and cognitive processing.

The laterality of DaT level in the putamen related to odor preference is of further interest. That is, the left is associated with pleasant smells and the right is associated with unpleasant smells. A recent study has shown that a pleasant odor is associated with bilateral or left AMG activation, and an unpleasant odor is associated with activation of the right AMG [27]. The left/right difference for smell-evoked emotion may be linked to AMG processing, because these regions are strongly connected at a fiber level [44].

5. Conclusion

It is essential to investigate the onset of cross-modality dysfunction in the future. Studies are currently focusing on early detection of PD, including signs of declining olfactory ability and rapid eye movement-related sleep disorders, as precursory biomarkers for PD [24–26, 45]. This approach may provide a new view of precursors, if the dysfunction develops before onset of movement disorders in PD (**Figure 8**). Furthermore, it is necessary to examine whether cross-modal dysfunction occurs in other diseases with striatum deficit, such as multiple system atrophy [46] and Huntington's disease [47]. Cross-modal dysfunction may also lead to diagnoses of other diseases.

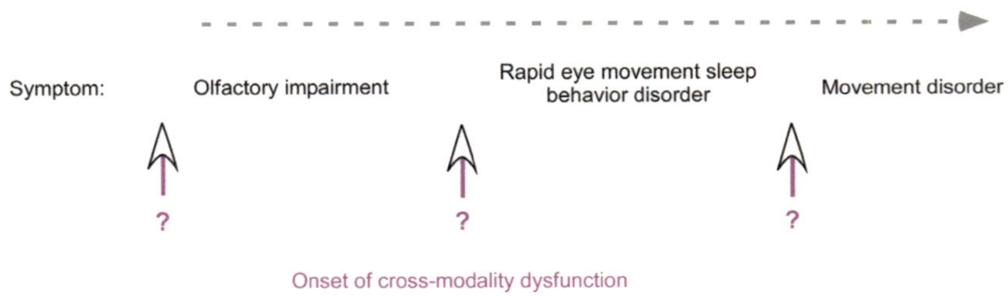

Figure 8.
Conceivable onsets of cross-modality dysfunction. Declining olfactory ability and rapid eye movement-related sleep disorder are known to be precursory biomarkers for Parkinson's disease. Cross-modality dysfunction also has the potential of becoming a novel biomarker.

Acknowledgements

The author thanks his original collaborators, Dr. Masaoka, Dr. Kuroda, Dr. Futamura, Dr. Shiromaru, Dr. Izumizaki, and Dr. Kawamura (Showa University School of Medicine). This paper was supported by Grant-in-aids for Scientific Research (C) (No. 18 K03185).

Conflict of interest

The author of this manuscript has no conflict of interest.

Author details

Motoyasu Honma
School of Medicine, Showa University, Tokyo, Japan

*Address all correspondence to: mhonma@med.showa-u.ac.jp

References

[1] Sperdin HF, Cappe C, Murray MM. The behavioral relevance of multisensory neural response interactions. Frontiers in Neuroscience. 2010;**4**:9. DOI: 10.3389/neuro.01.009.2010

[2] Helbig HB, Ernst MO, Ricciardi E, Pietrini P, Thielscher A, Mayer KM, et al. The neural mechanisms of reliability weighted integration of shape information from vision and touch. NeuroImage. 2012;**60**:1063-1072. DOI: 10.1016/j.neuroimage.2011.09.072

[3] Kawashima R, Watanabe J, Kato T, Nakamura A, Hatano K, Schormann T, et al. Direction of cross-modal information transfer affects human brain activation: A PET study. The European Journal of Neuroscience. 2002;**16**:137-144

[4] Bertelson P, Radeau M. Cross-modal bias and perceptual fusion with auditory-visual spatial discordance. Perception & Psychophysics. 1981;**29**:578-584

[5] Pavani F, Spence C, Driver J. Visual capture of touch: Out-of-the-body experiences with rubber gloves. Psychological Science. 2000;**11**:353-359

[6] Maga JA. Influence of color on taste thresholds. Chemical Senses. 1974;**1**:115-119

[7] Gottfried JA, Dolan RJ. The nose smells what the eye sees: Crossmodal visual facilitation of human olfactory perception. Neuron. 2003;**39**:375-386

[8] Luisa Demattè M, Sanabria D, Spence C. Cross-modal associations between odors and colors. Chemical Senses. 2006;**31**:531-538

[9] McGurk H, MacDonald J. Hearing lips and seeing voices. Nature. 1976;**264**:746-748

[10] Shams L, Kamitani Y, Shimojo S. Visual illusion induced by sound. Brain Research. Cognitive Brain Research. 2002;**14**:147-152

[11] Haber SN. The place of dopamine in the cortico-basal ganglia circuit. Neuroscience. 2014;**282**:248-257. DOI: 10.1016/j.neuroscience.2014.10.008

[12] Vaughan RA, Foster JD. Mechanisms of dopamine transporter regulation in normal and disease states. Trends in Pharmacological Sciences. 2013;**34**:489-496. DOI: 10.1016/j.tips.2013.07.005

[13] Kägi G, Bhatia KP, Tolosa E. The role of DAT-SPECT in movement disorders. Journal of Neurology, Neurosurgery, and Psychiatry. 2010;**81**:5-12. DOI: 10.1136/jnnp.2008.157370

[14] Tatsch K, Poepperl G. Nigrostriatal dopamine terminal imaging with dopamine transporter SPECT: An update. Journal of Nuclear Medicine. 2013;**54**:1331-1338. DOI: 10.2967/jnumed.112.105379

[15] Jaakkola E, Joutsa J, Kaasinen V. Predictors of normal and abnormal outcome in clinical brain dopamine transporter imaging. Journal of Neural Transmission. 2016;**123**:205-209. DOI: 10.1007/s00702-015-1495-0

[16] Cerasa A, Gioia MC, Salsone M, Donzuso G, Chiriaco C, Realmuto S, et al. Neurofunctional correlates of attention rehabilitation in Parkinson's disease: An explorative study. Neurological Sciences. 2014;**35**:1173-1180. DOI: 10.1007/s10072-014-1666-z

[17] Trujillo JP, Gerrits NJ, Vriend C, Berendse HW, van den Heuvel OA, van der Werf YD. Impaired planning in Parkinson's disease is reflected by reduced brain activation and connectivity. Human Brain Mapping.

2015;**36**:3703-3715. DOI: 10.1002/hbm.22873

[18] Ventre-Dominey J, Bourret S, Mollion H, Broussolle E, Dominey PF. Dissociable dorsal and ventral frontostriatal working memory circuits: Evidence from subthalamic stimulation in Parkinson's disease. Human Brain Mapping. 2014;**35**:552-566. DOI: 10.1002/hbm.22205

[19] Moustafa AA, Bell P, Eissa AM, Hewedi DH. The effects of clinical motor variables and medication dosage on working memory in Parkinson's disease. Brain and Cognition. 2013;**82**:137-145. DOI: 10.1016/j.bandc.2013.04.001

[20] Alonso-Recio L, Serrano JM, Martín P. Selective attention and facial expression recognition in patients with Parkinson's disease. Archives of Clinical Neuropsychology. 2014;**29**:374-384. DOI: 10.1093/arclin/acu018

[21] Sprengelmeyer R, Young AW, Mahn K, Schroeder U, Woitalla D, Büttner T, et al. Facial expression recognition in people with medicated and unmedicated Parkinson's disease. Neuropsychologia. 2003;**41**:1047-1057

[22] Honma M, Kuroda T, Futamura A, Shiromaru A, Kawamura M. Dysfunctional counting of mental time in Parkinson's disease. Scientific Reports. 2016;**6**:25421. DOI: 10.1038/srep25421

[23] Honma M, Murai Y, Shima S, Yotsumoto Y, Kuroda T, Futamura A, et al. Spatial distortion related to time compression during spatiotemporal production in Parkinson's disease. Neuropsychologia. 2017;**102**:61-69. DOI: 10.1016/j.neuropsychologia.2017.06.004

[24] Doty RL, Deems DA, Stellar S. Olfactory dysfunction in parkinsonism: A general deficit unrelated to neurologic signs, disease stage, or disease duration. Neurology. 1988;**38**:1237-1244

[25] Masaoka Y, Yoshimura N, Inoue M, Kawamura M, Homma I. Impairment of odor recognition in Parkinson's disease caused by weak activations of the orbitofrontal cortex. Neuroscience Letters. 2007;**412**:45-50

[26] Mahlknecht P, Pechlaner R, Boesveldt S, Volc D, Pinter B, Reiter E, et al. Optimizing odor identification testing as quick and accurate diagnostic tool for Parkinson's disease. Movement Disorders. 2016;**31**:1408-1413. DOI: 10.1002/mds.26637

[27] Patin A, Pause BM. Human amygdala activations during nasal chemoreception. Neuropsychologia. 2015;**78**:171-194. DOI: 10.1016/j.neuropsychologia.2015.10.009

[28] Rolls ET. The rules of formation of the olfactory representations found in the orbitofrontal cortex olfactory areas in primates. Chemical Senses. 2001;**26**:595-604

[29] Braak H, Del Tredici K. Neuroanatomy and pathology of sporadic Parkinson's disease. Advances in Anatomy, Embryology, and Cell Biology. 2009;**201**:1-119

[30] Chudler EH, Dong WK. The role of the basal ganglia in nociception and pain. Pain. 1995;**60**:3-38

[31] Schultz W. Reward functions of the basal ganglia. Journal of Neural Transmission. 2016;**123**:679-693. DOI: 10.1007/s00702-016-1510-0

[32] Middleton FA, Strick PL. Basal ganglia and cerebellar loops: Motor and cognitive circuits. Brain Research. Brain Research Reviews. 2000;**31**:236-250

[33] Reig R, Silberberg G. Multisensory integration in the mouse striatum.

Neuron. 2014;**83**:1200-1212. DOI: 10.1016/j.neuron.2014.07.033

[34] Gentile G, Petkova VI, Ehrsson HH. Integration of visual and tactile signals from the hand in the human brain: An FMRI study. Journal of Neurophysiology. 2011;**105**:910-922. DOI: 10.1152/jn.00840.2010

[35] von Saldern S, Noppeney U. Sensory and striatal areas integrate auditory and visual signals into behavioral benefits during motion discrimination. Journal of Neuroscience. 2013;**33**:8841-8849. DOI: 10.1523/JNEUROSCI.3020-12.2013

[36] Honma M, Masaoka Y, Kuroda T, Futamura A, Shiromaru A, Izumizaki M, et al. Impairment of cross-modality of vision and olfaction in Parkinson disease. Neurology. 2018;**90**:e977-e984. DOI: 10.1212/WNL.0000000000005110

[37] Rolls ET, Baylis LL. Gustatory, olfactory, and visual convergence within the primate orbitofrontal cortex. Journal of Neuroscience. 1994;**14**:5437-5452

[38] Rolls ET. Top-down control of visual perception: Attention in natural vision. Perception. 2008;**37**:333-354

[39] Masaoka Y, Pantelis C, Phillips A, Kawamura M, Mimura M, Minegishi G, et al. Markers of brain illness may be hidden in your olfactory ability: A Japanese perspective. Neuroscience Letters. 2013;**549**:182-185. DOI: 10.1016/j.neulet.2013.05.077

[40] Doty RL, Stern MB, Pfeiffer C, Gollomp SM, Hurtig HI. Bilateral olfactory dysfunction in early stage treated and untreated idiopathic Parkinson's disease. Journal of Neurology, Neurosurgery, and Psychiatry. 1992;**55**:138-142

[41] DeLong MR. Primate models of movement disorders of basal ganglia origin. Trends in Neurosciences. 1990;**13**:281-285

[42] Galvan A, Devergnas A, Wichmann T. Alterations in neuronal activity in basal ganglia-thalamocortical circuits in the parkinsonian state. Frontiers in Neuroanatomy. 2015;**9**:5. DOI: 10.3389/fnana.2015.00005

[43] Rey CD, Lipps J, Shansky RM. Dopamine D1 receptor activation rescues extinction impairments in low-estrogen female rats and induces cortical layer-specific activation changes in prefrontal-amygdala circuits. Neuropsychopharmacology. 2014;**39**:1282-1289. DOI: 10.1038/npp.2013.338

[44] Gattass R, Galkin TW, Desimone R, Ungerleider LG. Subcortical connections of area V4 in the macaque. The Journal of Comparative Neurology. 2014;**522**:1941-1965. DOI: 10.1002/cne.23513

[45] Chen MC, Yu H, Huang ZL, Lu J. Rapid eye movement sleep behavior disorder. Current Opinion in Neurobiology. 2013;**23**:793-798. DOI: 10.1016/j.conb.2013.02.019

[46] Cilia R, Marotta G, Benti R, Pezzoli G, Antonini A. Brain SPECT imaging in multiple system atrophy. Journal of Neural Transmission. 2005;**112**:1635-1645

[47] Rüb U, Seidel K, Heinsen H, Vonsattel JP, den Dunnen WF, Korf HW. Huntington's disease (HD): The neuropathology of a multisystem neurodegenerative disorder of the human brain. Brain Pathology. 2016;**26**:726-740. DOI: 10.1111/bpa.12426

Chapter 9

Cerebrospinal Fluid Leaks and Encephaloceles

Henry P. Barham, Harry E. Zylicz and Christian A. Hall

Abstract

Encephaloceles and cereberospinal fluid (CSF) leaks of the ventral skull base resulting from trauma (surgical and non-surgical), neoplasm, congenital, and spontaneous are a complex problem typically managed by rhinologists/skull base surgeons. Conservative management is often the first step in managing these complex problems. Endoscopic repair of CSF leaks and encephaloceles has greatly evolved with the evolution of endoscopic visualization and instrumentation. Endoscopic repairs of CSF leaks are effective and offer decreased morbidity compared to open approaches with comparative success rates. Meticulous technique is key to success in repair of skull base defects. Materials used are often less important than quality of repair.

Keywords: CSF leaks, Encephaloceles

1. Introduction

Cerebrospinal fluid (CSF) is produced by the choroid plexus in the lateral ventricles, third, and fourth ventricles at a rate of 0.35 mL/min (20 mL/hour or 350–500 mL/day) in the normal physiologic states and is reabsorbed into the dural venous sinuses through the arachnoid villi. The total volume of circulating CSF is 90–150 mL. The entire volume of CSF turns over three to five times per day. Typical intracranial pressure is 5–15 cm H2O and is considered elevated when it is greater than 15 cm H2O. The three layers of the meninges are the dura mater, arachnoid, and pia mater. The dura mater is separated into the superficial layer and the meningeal layers. Common causes of CSF leaks can be divided into trauma, both surgical and nonsurgical, neoplasm, congenital, and spontaneous [1].

An encephalocele is herniation of neural tissue through a defect in the skull base and is defined by the type of tissue that herniates through the defect. A meningocele contains herniated meninges, a meningoencephalocele contains herniated brain matter and meninges, and a meningoencephalocystocele is made up of herniated brain matter and meninges that communicate with a cerebral ventricle.

2. Etiology

2.1 Cerebrospinal fluid leak

The most common cause is nonsurgical (70–80%). 1–3% of acute head injuries result in a CSF leak. Conservative management is often the first step in managing CSF leaks resulting from acute trauma. Seventy percent of leaks close spontaneously with observation and conservative management which may include bed rest, head of bed elevation, and lumbar drainage. Overall, there is a 30–40% risk of meningitis with conservative treatment [2].

Surgical causes (planned and unplanned) make up a large portion of leaks requiring intervention. Functional endoscopic sinus surgery (FESS) carries <1% incidence of CSF leak. The most common site of skull base injury is the lateral lamella of the cribriform plate. The posterior ethmoid skull base is at greater risk when the maxillary sinus is highly pneumatized in the superior–inferior dimension, which creates a relatively decreased posterior ethmoid height. Neurologic Surgery caries an increased risk albeit typically include planned CSF leak with expected violation of the meninges. Transsphenoidal approach for sellar and suprasellar lesions carry a reported 0.5–15% incidence of CSF leak [3].

Neoplasms can result in CSF leak via direct tumor invasion and/or mass effect leading to intracranial hypertension. Congenital causes result from failure of closure of developmental spaces with resultant herniation of intracranial contents. Foramen cecum is the most common location. Spontaneous leaks are often the result of idiopathic intracranial hypertension (IIH) resulting from decreased CSF reabsorption. Patient characteristics and symptoms often include middle-age, obesity, female, pressure-type headaches, pulsatile tinnitus, and balance dysfunction.

Empty sella syndrome is a radiographic appearance of CSF-filled sella due to flattening of the pituitary gland which is an endocrine gland that resides in the sella turcica and functions to control other endocrine glands by secretion of controlling hormones. Empty sella syndrome can be seen in IIH, which typically affects obese women. Patients typically will present with headaches, pulsatile tinnitus, and diplopia. A hallmark physical exam finding is bilateral optic disc edema secondary to increased intracranial pressure (ICP). Treatment is focused on decreasing ICP with pharmacologic therapy consisting of acetazolamide and furosemide to lower ICP, and headache management, which may include amitriptyline and propranolol. In severe cases with vision problems, surgical intervention may be required, including optic nerve decompression or CSF shunting. Empty sella syndrome can be seen in conjunction with spontaneous CSF leaks.

2.2 Encephalocele

Encephaloceles can occur in both the skull and spinal column. Twenty percent occur within the cranium and 15% of these are associated with the nasal cavity. Nasal encephaloceles are divided into two types: sincipital and basal. Sincipital (anterior and superior) encephaloceles make up approximately 60% of nasal encephaloceles and typically present as a soft compressible mass over the glabella. Basal encephaloceles occur through the skull base more posteriorly and make up approximately 40% of nasal encephaloceles. They may remain hidden for many years because they are located more posteriorly than the sincipital type.

3. Clinical presentation

Clear rhinorrhea that is unilateral, watery, and salty to taste is the most common complaint in CSF leaks. It may run out of the nose in more anterior leaks, or down the back of the throat in more posterior leaks. The drainage can be exacerbated by the Dandy maneuver, which entails tilting the head forward into a chin-tuck position and straining.

Patients with an encephalocele will often present with rhinorrhea or recurrent meningitis and may have a broad nasal dorsum or hypertelorism. Encephaloceles may characteristically transilluminate, expand with the Valsalva maneuver, and demonstrate a positive Furstenberg sign (enlargement with compression of internal jugular veins). Radiologic imaging including computed tomography (CT) and magnetic resonance imaging (MRI) may be used to evaluate the size and location of encephaloceles.

4. Investigations

The most sensitive and specific test is qualitative β2-transferrin evaluation of the nasal drainage. β2-transferrin is detected in few fluids in the body including CSF, perilymph, and aqueous humor. Only 0.2 mL is needed for an adequate specimen. β2-transferrin has a sensitivity of 97% and specificity of 93%. False positive results can occur with abnormal transferrin metabolism from chronic liver disease, glycogen metabolic disease, and carcinomas; therefore, results should be verified with a negative serum β2-transferrin. β-trace protein is a newer laboratory test with higher sensitivity and specificity which offers faster results than β2-transferrin.

The radiologic evaluation of a CSF leak can be extensive and often begins with a fine cut maxillofacial CT scan to demonstrate bony abnormalities such as defects and fractures. CT is the mainstay for radiologic workup of CSF rhinorrhea with a sensitivity of 92% and a specificity of 92–96%. If the initial imaging does not show an obvious abnormality but suspicion is still high, a CT cisternogram may be useful. This study entails injection of radiopaque material through a lumbar drain into the intrathecal space to help delineate the CSF leak. Presence of contrast within the nasal space or paranasal sinuses indicates a CSF leak. CT cisternography has a sensitivity of 92% with an active leak to 40% with an intermittent leak. MRI cisternography (T2 weighted fast-spin protocol) can be helpful in cases of neoplasm, meningoencephalocele, encephalocele, and in patients with an iodine allergy.

5. Management

In patients who have a traumatic leak and normal CSF pressure, conservative treatment consists of bed rest with head of bed elevation and lumbar drainage of CSF for 5–10 days. With conservative management, there is a reported risk ranging from 7 to 30% of ascending meningitis. The incidence of spontaneous resolution with conservative management is reported to be 70%.

The general consensus among practicing otolaryngologist is that antibiotics should not be used for conservative management unless there is a very large defect with comminuted bone of the skull base as a simple CSF leak carries a 7% infection rate (meningitis, intracranial abscess, cellulitis abscess, and osteomyelitis) and prophylactic antibiotics have not been shown to decrease the risk of infection. After endoscopic repair, antibiotics are generally recommended for 24–48 hours including Cefazolin (1 gm q8), Vancomycin (1 gm q12), or Clindamycin (600 mg q8). This is done to cover possible contamination at the time of surgery in a non-sterile field with concomitant sealing of the sterile to non-sterile flushing of an active leak [4, 5].

6. Surgical Intervention

Endoscopic repair of CSF leaks is effective and offers decreased morbidity compared to open approaches. Meticulous technique is key to success in repair of skull base defects. Materials used and procedures employed are less important than the quality of the repair [6].

Advancements in the endoscopic surgical repair of CSF leaks and encephaloceles have resulted from improvements in instrumentation, visualization, access, and technique. Improved diagnostic imaging and surgical navigation have also improved management. Advancements in endoscopic reconstructive techniques of the skull base including utilization of local vascularized flaps have improved success rates with endoscopic approaches [7].

Compared to open surgery, the endoscopic approach allows for more direct visualization with less manipulation of the surrounding soft tissues. This may allow for a more precise reconstruction of the skull base due to better visualization, and minimal manipulation of nearby neurovascular structures. Compared to the traditional microscopic view, endoscopes give a dynamic operative view with the added ability to see around corners using angled endoscopes. ESBS can avoid scars, decrease hospital stays, and cause less postoperative pain [8].

Not all areas of the skull base can be visualized and safely instrumented via a transnasal endoscopic route. As a general rule, the endoscopic approach should not compromise the ability to achieve the appropriate reconstruction, and crossing major neurovascular structures is not suggested [9].

Common complications from skull base surgery include anosmia and associated taste dysfunction, epistaxis and neurologic complications such as cranial nerve injury. Major skull base surgery complications include CSF rhinorrhea, meningitis, intracranial hemorrhage, orbital complications such as diplopia or vision loss, vascular injury, stroke, and death [8–11].

Intrathecal fluorescein is often used in the surgical repair of CSF leaks. Its advantages include the ability to stain defects that may be more difficult to identify clinically, through the visible dye of CSF to a light green color. The surgeon can also use it to confirm a water-tight repair. It carries a 0% false positive rate. Its disadvantages include a moderate false negative result. It requires a lumbar puncture, and the use of fluorescein intrathecally is not FDA-approved. Rare complications including seizures (0.3%) and death have been reported; however, these have more commonly been associated with administration through a suboccipital puncture. If used to help localize a CSF leak it should be used with caution and should be dosed as 0.05–0.1 mL per 10 kg body weight up to maximum 0.1 mL 10% fluorescein. This is mixed in 10 mL of preservative-free normal saline or CSF. The surgeon should inject slowly (over 5–10 min) without paralytics in the anesthetic regimen to assess for seizure activity. Fluorescein should be avoided in patients with abnormal renal function [12].

The primary goal in endoscopic repair of CSF leaks and skull base reconstruction is to definitively identify all leaks in order to completely reconstruct all defects. After identifying the leak or leaks, the goals of reconstruction are creation of a safe barrier with separation of intracranial and sinonasal spaces and elimination of any dead space. As with any surgical intervention, meticulous surgical technique is paramount for success.

A reconstructive ladder should be used to help determine the type of repair performed. For simple, small (less than 1 cm) defects, a fat plug harvested from the earlobe or abdomen can be used to plug the defect. The next option includes a simple overlay graft harvested from the nasal floor mucosa, turbinate mucosa, or nasal septum. If a more complex, larger reconstruction is in order, a composite (underlay and overlay) graft can be used consisting of an intracranial underlay of bone or cartilage from nasal septum, auricular cartilage or turbinate bone, and an overlay graft of mucosa (free or pedicled) as above. Local pedicled flaps should include the nasoseptal flap, which is supplied by the posterior nasal septal artery, a terminal branch of the sphenopalatine artery. Additional grafts that can be useful in larger defects include temporal fascia or tensor fascia lata grafts. These grafts are often bolstered in the sinonasal cavity with abdominal fat, a nasoseptal flap or both. In complex situations of extensive defects or poor local tissue, such as in chemoradiated patients, a craniotomy with pericranial flap or free flap reconstruction of the skull base may be necessary.

Lumbar drains are often used to decrease intracranial pressure and thereby reduce the pressure applied to the skull base reconstruction; however, they may be associated with significant morbidity and potential for complications. The use of lumbar drain primarily following a repair varies from different surgeons, and should not be universally utilized in a routine fashion. When used, the duration of drainage is also up to surgeon discretion.

Most reconstructive methods appear to have similar efficacy, and therefore there is no universal "best type of reconstruction." In general, small defects (<1 cm) can be closed in a single layer, and multilayer repair is preferred for larger defects. Some surgeons prefer to use a rigid layer of bone or cartilage to reconstruct the skull base, although this is not required [13]. Vascularized mucosal tissue (e.g., nasoseptal flap) has been demonstrated to improve repair results for larger defects; however, single layer nonvascularized tissue can also be successful in this setting.

Postoperative antibiotics are an important consideration for skull base surgery because of the temporary connection between the intracranial space and external world. Rates of postoperative wound infection following ESBS are approximately 2%, and appear to be higher in open skull base surgery. Broad coverage with IV cephalosporins with or without vancomycin (or oral amoxicillin/clavulanate) is most often recommended. Studies are lacking to support the use of prolonged postoperative antibiotics, although most surgeons prefer to use systemic or topical antibiotics in some form after surgery.

7. Conclusion

A multitude of studies over the past 25 years have shown high success rates of primary repair around 90%, and secondary repair around 97%. These success rates compare favorably to traditional craniotomy approaches with reported success rates between 70 and 80% that carry a higher morbidity profile. Symptoms of failure in reconstruction include clear rhinorrhea and constant postnasal drip. Other signs may include meningitis, severe headaches, seizures, and worsening pneumocephalus.

Author details

Henry P. Barham[1,2]*, Harry E. Zylicz[1,2] and Christian A. Hall[1,2]

1 Sinus and Nasal Specialists of Louisiana, Baton Rouge, Louisiana, United States of America

2 Rhinology and Skull Base Research Group, Baton Rouge General Medical Center, Baton Rouge, Louisiana, United States of America

*Address all correspondence to: hbarham@sinusandnasalspecialists.com

References

[1] Kennedy DW, Hwang PH. Rhinology: Disease of the Nose, Sinuses and Skull Base. New York: Thieme; 2012

[2] Lund VJ, Stammberger H, Nicolai P, et al. European position paper on endoscopic management of tumours of the nose, paranasal sinuses and skull base. Rhinology Supplement. 2010;**1**(22):1-143

[3] Bleier BS. Comprehensive techniques in CSF leak repair and skull base reconstruction. Advances in Oto-Rhino-Laryngology. 2013;**74**:1-11

[4] Bernal-Sprekelsen M, Alobid I, Mullol J, et al. Closure of cerebrospinal fluid leaks prevents ascending bacterial meningitis. Rhinology. 2005;**43**(4):277-281

[5] Brown SM, Anand VK, Tabaee A, et al. Role of perioperative antibiotics in endoscopic skull base surgery. Laryngoscope. 2007;**117**(9):1528-1532

[6] Hegazy HM et al. Transnasal endoscopic repair of cerebrospinal fluid rhinorrhea: A meta-analysis. Laryngoscope. 2000;**110**(7):1166-1172

[7] Lanza DC, O'Brien DA, Kennedy DW. Endoscopic repair of cerebrospinal fistulae and encephaloceles. Laryngoscope. 1996;**106**(9 Pt 1):1119-1125

[8] May M, Levine HL, Mester SJ, et al. Complications of ESS: Analysis of 2,018 patients. Laryngoscope. 1994;**104**:1080-1083

[9] Suh JD, Ramakrishnan VR, Chi JJ, et al. Outcomes and complications of endoscopic approaches for malignancies of the paranasal sinuses and anterior skull base. The Annals of Otology, Rhinology, and Laryngology. 2013;**122**(1):54-59

[10] Schlosser RJ, Bolger WE. Nasal cerebrospinal fluid leaks. The Journal of Otolaryngology. Supplement. 2002;**1**:S28-S37

[11] Suwanwela C, Suwanwela N. A morphological classification of sincipital encephalomeningoceles. Journal of Neurosurgery. 1972;**36**:201-211

[12] Wolf G et al. Endoscopic detection of cerebral spinal fistulas with a fluorescence technique. Report of experiences with over 925 cases. Laryngorhinootogie. 1997;**76**(10):588-594

[13] Zweig JL et al. Endoscopic repair of cerebrospinal fluid leaks to the sinonasal tract: Predictors of success. Otolaryngology and Head and Neck Surgery. 2000;**123**(3):195-201

Chapter 10

Optical Fiber-Based Sleep Apnea Syndrome Sensor

Seiko Mitachi, Ken Satoh, Kumiko Shimoyama, Makoto Satoh and Takeshi Sugiyama

Abstract

A noninvasive sleep apnea syndrome (SAS) sensor using optical fibers, the "F-SAS sensor," has been evaluated in a clinical application ranging in age from 13 to 78 years and with BMIs of 19.2–39.3. The respiratory disturbance index (RDI) from the F-SAS sensor corresponded well with the apnea hypopnea index (AHI) from polysomnography (PSG). Concurrent measurement of the RDI and the AHI had a correlation coefficient of 0.71. This means that the F-SAS is well-suited for preliminary SAS screening. They would also be useful for screening potential SAS sufferers during normal sleep at home. Then, we have succeeded in downsizing F-SAS sensor and have recognized that it is highly correlated with PSG and pulse oximetry. Next, we applied the compact F-SAS sensor to examining SAS diagnosis in a child patient (2–12 years) and report on improved pediatric analysis. The analysis results revealed the correlation value to be R = 0.87 was a significant improvement over the correlation value of R = 0.697 between the AHI obtained by a sleep apnea syndrome examination apparatus (SAS 2100) and RDI obtained by the conventional F-SAS sensor.

Keywords: optical fiber sensors, sleep apnea syndrome, SAS, F-SAS sensor, noninvasive, plastic optical fiber

1. Ordinal size of F-SAS sensors and application to adults

1.1 Introduction

Sleep apnea syndrome (SAS) has been identified as a risk factor for traffic accidents because it can cause excessive daytime sleepiness. As shown in **Figure 1**, the probability of a traffic accident for ordinary people is about 5% while that for SAS sufferers range from about 7–25% depending on the level of the apnea–hypopnea index (AHI), which indicates the severity of sleep apnea. Given this finding, the Japanese government requires train drivers and airplane pilots to get periodic SAS check-ups.

The prevalence of SAS sufferers in Japan is estimated to be 4%: 2.0 million and 2.8 million yet to be identified. The polysomnography (PSG) test commonly used for diagnosing SAS is a bothersome and uncomfortable examination as shown in **Figure 2**.

In contrast, a previously developed sleep apnea syndrome (SAS) sensor using optical fibers, the "F-SAS sensor," is non-invasive and non-restrictive [1–4].

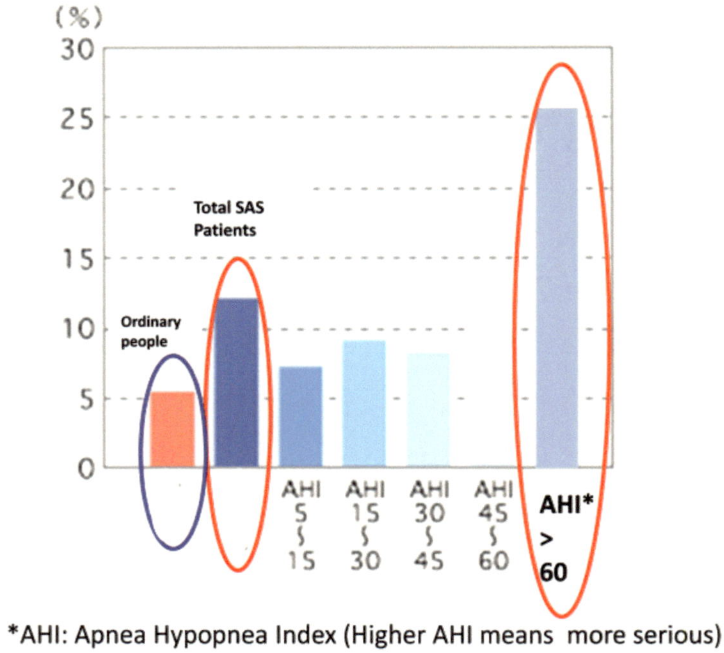

Figure 1.
Probability of traffic accident for various AHI levels of Japanese adults.

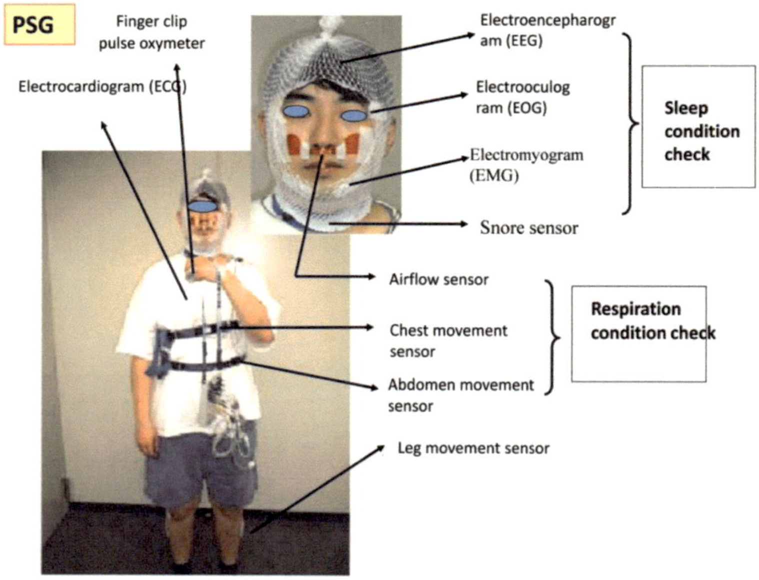

Figure 2.
Subjects ready for PSG test.

It is both quiet and compact and thus potentially useful for screening potential SAS sufferers during normal sleep at home.

This paper describes the F-SAS sensor and the measurement principle. It then describes its application in a hospital setting and in hotels [5, 6]. Under the assistance of the "Beautiful Fukushima Next-Generation Medical Industry Agglomeration Project," in Japan, we have succeeded in downsizing the F-SAS sensor and have recognized that it highly correlates with polysomnography (PSG) and pulse oximetry (PLSX). The F-SAS sensor is promising for screening latent SAS patients (Sleep Apnea Syndrome patients) during usual sleep.

On the other hands, obstructive sleep apnea syndrome (OSAS) in children is a disease in which respiratory arrest during sleep is frequently observed due to narrowing of the upper airways, such as due to tonsil hypertrophy, growth disorders, and a lowered quality of life (QOL) such as from having a decreased ability to learn. We reviewed the improvement made to pediatric analysis software by using the F-SAS sensor and report it [7–11]. Further, we report on a comparison of sleep events with the conventional F-SAS sensor and polysomnography (PSG) in children [9].

1.2 F-SAS sensor system

Figure 3 shows plastic optical fiber sheets and physics of measurement. Fibers interspaces are narrower one and wider one within several centimeters. Commercially available SI plastic optical fibers (CK10) were used. Physical principle is to measure the deviation of output optical power from fiber sheet by micro-bending loss and/or bending loss. **Figure 4** is the experimental response for intentional apnea. One pulse wave form means one breath in and out. Flat parts indicate the apnea after breath in or out. Narrower fiber interspaces POF sheet is more sensitive than the wider one. As shown in **Figure 5**, a plastic optical fiber (POF) sensor sheet is simply placed under the bottom bed sheet. There is no need for the subject to wear any special clothing or devices. The measurement data is transmitted to a remote location for analysis and diagnosis. The measurement principle is illustrated in **Figure 3**. The deviation in the output optical power from the POF sheet due to micro-bending loss and/or bending loss caused by the lateral pressure change created by the motion of the person's chest during respiration is measured.

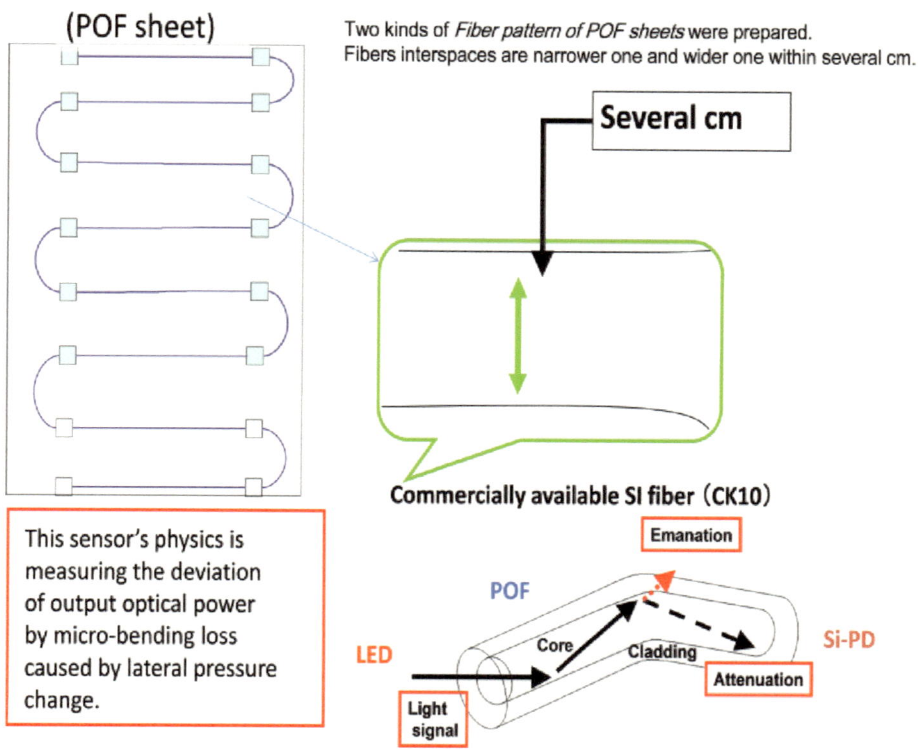

Figure 3.
Measurement principle.

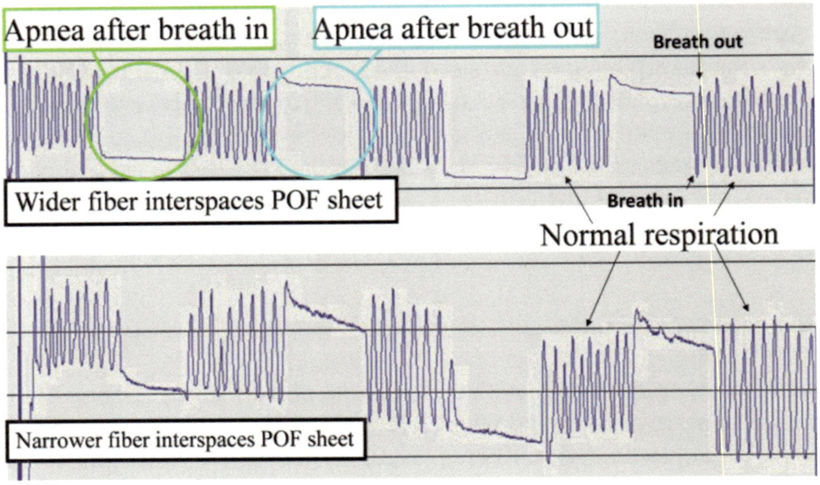

Figure 4.
Example measurement results for intentional apnea.

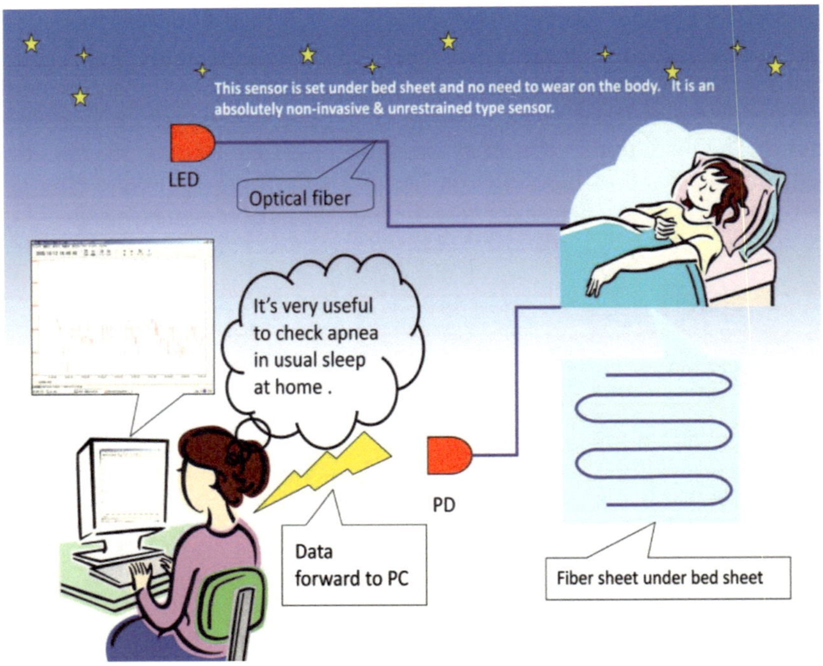
This sensor is set under bed sheet and no need to wear on the body. It is an absolutely non-invasive & unrestrained type sensor.
LED
Optical fiber
It's very useful to check apnea in usual sleep at home .
PD
Data forward to PC
Fiber sheet under bed sheet

Figure 5.
Overview of F-SAS sensor system.

The theoretical formula for irregular bending loss of multimode optical fibers was given by Furuya and Suematsu [12]. As shown by Eq. (1), R_1 decreases/increases depending on the stress increase/decrease with expansion/contraction of the chest by respiration. Therefore, the stress increases/decreases, and transmission loss L_m increases/decreases.

$$L_m = 2500\, N\overline{(1/R_1)^2 W^2}\,\frac{1}{\Delta}\exp\left[-\left(\frac{\overline{W}}{d}\right)^2\Delta\right](dB/km) \qquad (1)$$

N: Average number of bends par meter, $\overline{(1/R_1)^2}$: Mean square of fiber curvature, $\overline{W}$: Correlation length, d: core diameter, Δ: Relative refractive index difference.

Example measurement results for intentional apnea are shown in **Figure 4**. One pulse wave-form corresponds to one breath in and out. The flat parts indicate apnea after breathing in or out. Results are shown for a POF sheet with narrow fiber spacing and for one with wider spacing. The one with narrower spacing was more sensitive. As shown in **Figure 6**, the sensor system comprises a SI-POF (240/250 micron, NA = 0.5) sheet, an optical power meter (9 V DC) with a Si photodiode, an LED (650 nm) built-in controller, a microcomputer (5 V DC), a memory card, and a small liquid crystal display panel. Input power is 12 V DC from AC commercial power.

Commercially available Si plastic fibers (ESCA CK10, Mitsubishi Rayon Co., Ltd.) are used. The sheet is packed between the bottom sheet and the bed. The user initiates operation by simply pushing the SW button and then sleeps on the bed as usual without wearing any electrodes. While sleeping, the user can freely roll over, change body position, and go to the toilet. The user ends operation upon awaking by again pushing the SW button. The measurement data are automatically stored on the memory card (SD card), which is attached to the side of the controller. The data for more than 200 nights can be stored; the data for each night is stored in a separate file with an automatically generated sequential file name. As necessary, the data can be analyzed at remote site or on site by inserting the SD card into a PC running a specially developed data analysis program. For one night's data file, it takes about 1 second to plot the signals for normal respiration, apnea, hypopnea, body motion, rolling over, and sleeping body position, and to generate the respiratory disturbance index (RDI).

A clinical application of this F-SAS sensor system was conducted at JR Sendai Hospital and in Tsukuba University Hospital in Japan using 20 subjects with ages from 13 to 78 and with BMIs of from 19.2 to 39.3. The POF sheet and PSG were used concurrently. The F-SAS sensor data were automatically analyzed by using the specially developed data analysis program to plot the signals for normal respiration,

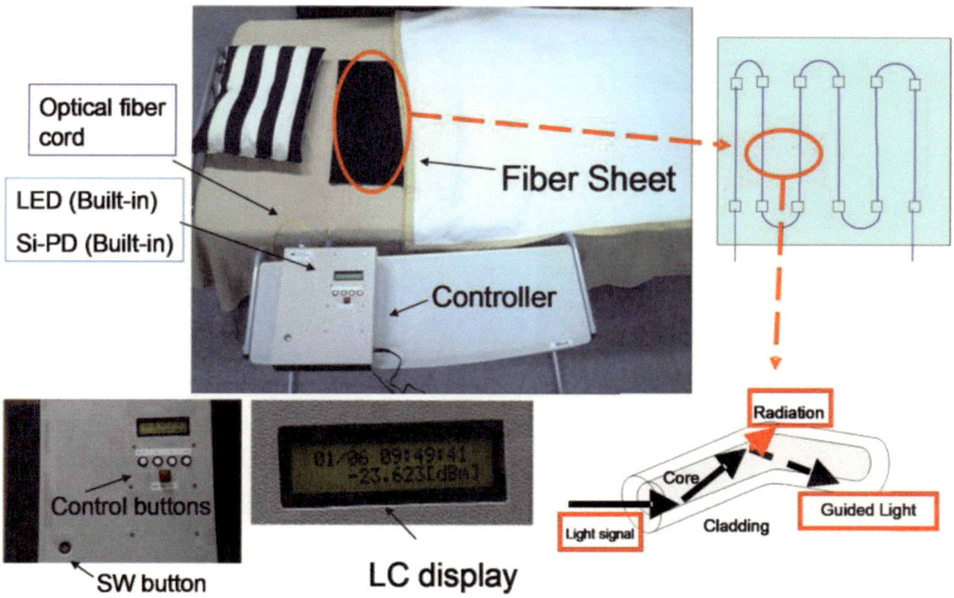

Figure 6.
Sensor system components and configuration.

apnea, hypopnea, body motion and rolling over independently from the PSG analysis. The example respiration waveforms for the F-SAS sensor and PSG are shown in **Figure 7** exhibits good consistency. The correlation coefficient between the AHI from the PSG and the RDI from the F-SAS was 0.71 in the region of AHI from 0 to 85.9 as shown in **Figure 8**. For AHI values from 0 to 20, the correlation coefficient was much better 0.89. In contrast, it was 0.57 for AHI values from 20 to 85.9. This means that the F-SAS sensor is more accurate and sensitive for milder degrees of SAS. The RDI from the F-SAS sensor was smaller than the AHI from the PSG for moderate and severe degrees of SAS because of the bigger difference between the sleeping time and the time in bed. This means that the F-SAS sensor is better suited for screening than for diagnosis. In fact, in a separate study of at-home use, potential SAS sufferers from among 19 ordinary people were identified by using this

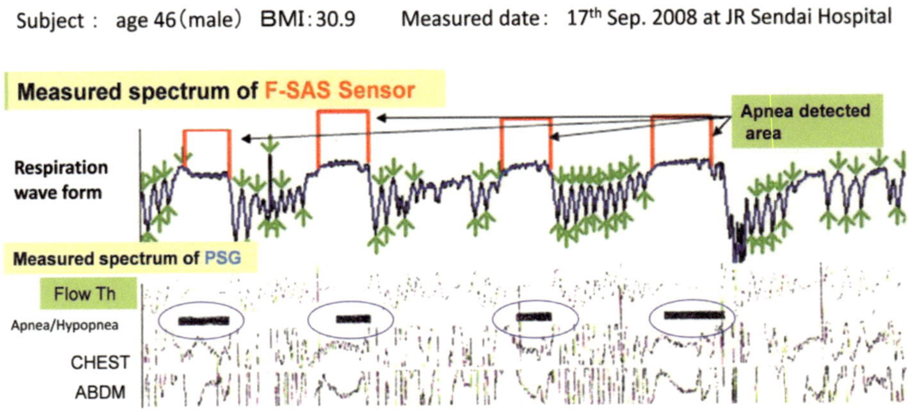

Figure 7.
Example respiration waveforms for F-SAS sensor and PSG [3] from 0 to 85.9 (R = 0.71).

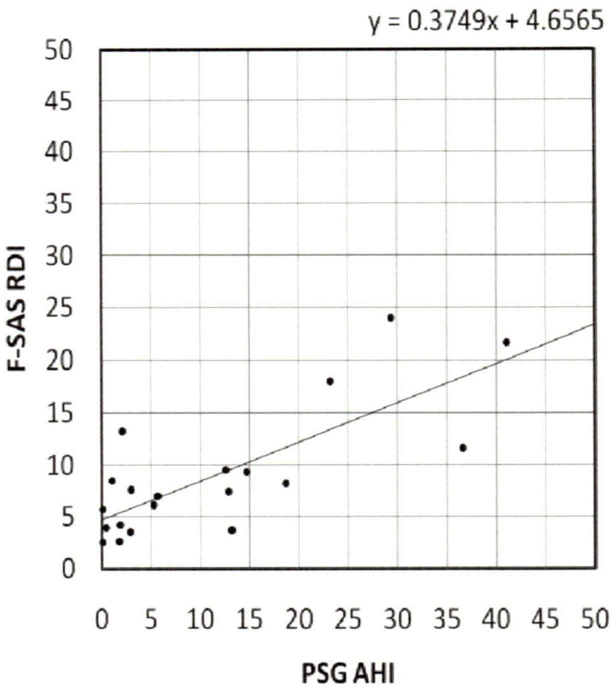

Figure 8.
Correlation between AHI by PSG and RDI from F-SAS for AHI values.

F-SAS sensor system. Definitive diagnoses made in the JR Sendai Hospital for the four potential sufferers were that three had mild cases and one had a moderate case.

The apnea and hypopnea distributions from the PSG and the F-SAS sensor for one night for a severe SAS sufferer (**Figure 9**) show good accordance. **Table 1** shows the reliability of the F-SAS sensor in comparison with PSG under the American Academy of Sleep Medicine (AASM) criteria published in 2001 [13]. It had good sensitivity of 0.909.

1.3 Application to other areas

A multi-channel F-SAS sensor system has been developed and done field test in a hotel, full medical check-up and clinical test in pediatrics. **Figure 10** shows the

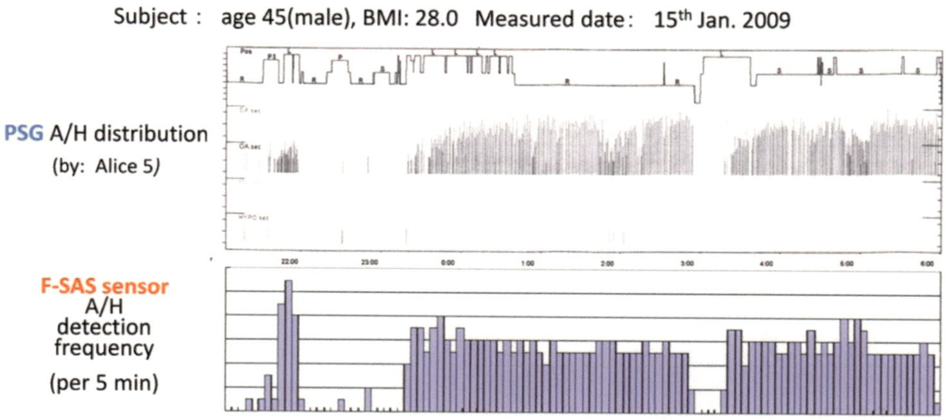

Figure 9.
Apnea and hypopnea distributions from PSG and F-SAS sensor for one night for severe SAS sufferer.

	PSG(AD)	PSG(NAD)	Total
F-SAS (AD)	10	4	14
F-SAS (NAD)	1	5	6
Total	11	9	20

POF sheet (400x900mm: 20 Subjects)

Sensitivity	0.909
Specifity	0.111
False negative rate	0.091
False positive rate	0.444
Positive predictive value	0.714
Negative predictive value	0.833
Likelihood ratio for a negative finding	1.023

PSG(AD): AHI≧5
F-SAS (AD): RDI≧5
AD: Appreciable Disease
NAD: No Appreciable Disease

Table 1.
Reliability of F-SAS sensor in comparison with PSG under AASM criteria published in 2001 [13].

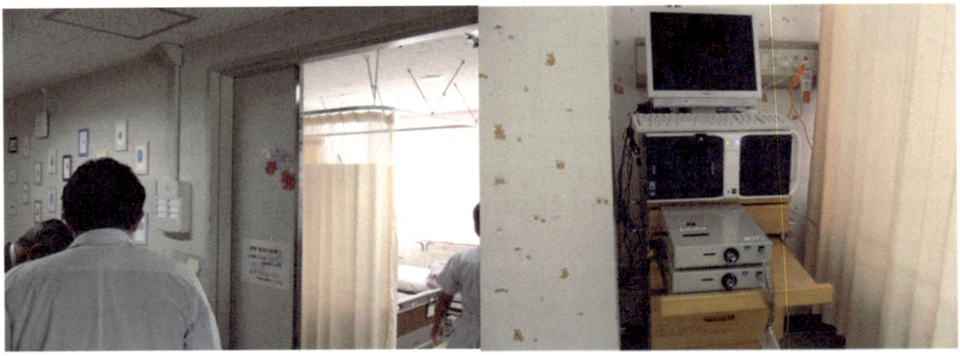

Figure 10.
Clinical test of multichannel system of F-SAS sensor in pediatrics.

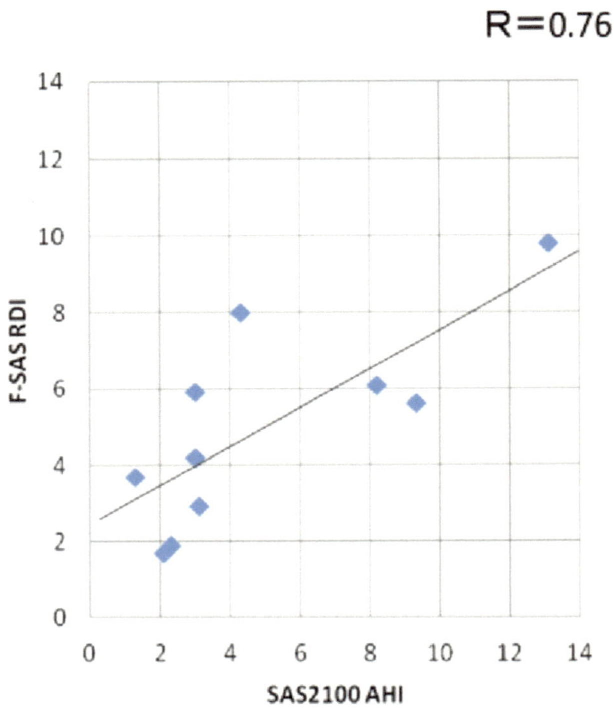

Figure 11.
Correlation between AHI of SAS2100 of the Yamanashi University Hospital (subjects: 11 children of age 2~10 y) as a reference and RDI of F-SAS sensor [11].

installation of the system in the pediatric ward. A correlation coefficient of 0.76 was obtained for 11 infantile subjects (**Figure 11**).

2. Downsizing the F-SAS sensor

Under the assistance of the "Beautiful Fukushima Next-Generation Medical Industry Agglomeration Project," in Japan, we have succeeded in downsizing the F-SAS sensor as shown in **Figure 12** and have recognized that it highly correlates with polysomnography (PSG) and pulse oximetry (PLSX). The F-SAS sensor is promising for screening latent SAS patients (Sleep Apnea Syndrome patients) during usual sleep.

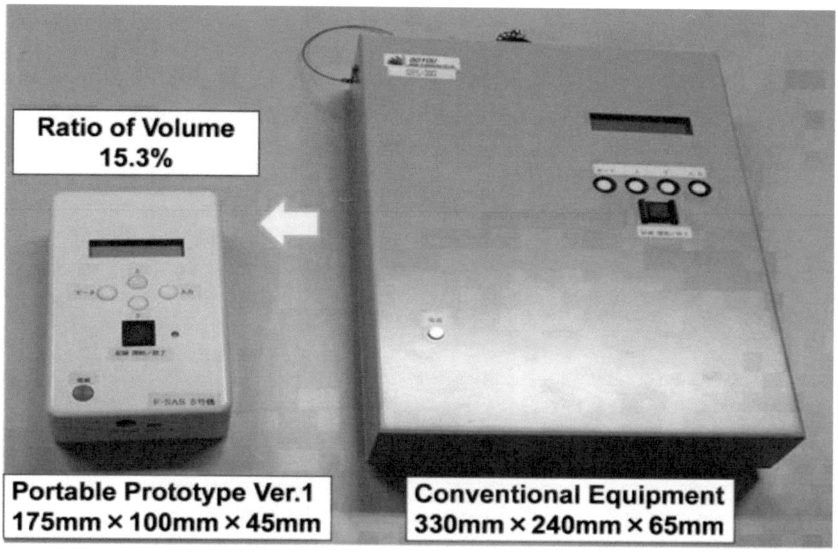

Figure 12.
Portable prototype and original F-SAS sensor.

2.1 Measuring procedure

Under the agreement of the ethical committee of Tohoku Rosai Hospital in Japan and the following two conditions, coincident measurements of PLSX and F-SAS sensors were taken for an overnight medical checkup screening.

1. Subjects were 33 men and 8 women (age: 55.7 ± 7.49, BMI: 25.6 ± 4.2, ESS: 6.9 ± 3.5), and as shown in **Figures 6** and **13–16**, an optical fiber sheet was set under the bed pad, respiratory motion of the chest was measured, and arterial blood oxygen saturation was measured by PLSX from February 16, 2012 to September 7, 2016 in Tohoku Rosai Hospital, Sendai in Japan.

2. Next, conditions for 68 men and 8 women (age: 52.5 ± 20.5, BMI: 24.8 ± 6.8, ESS: 6 ± 6) were measured by using the downsized F-SAS sensor (controller is 16.8% and weight is 19% less than before) with a conventional PLSX from March 12, 2013 to Januray 11, 2016, in Tohoku Rosai Hospital, Sendai in Japan.

3. Finally, the clinical examination was carried out in the Department of Sleep Medicine, University of Tsukuba in Japan. Candidates were chosen from both healthy subjects and those suspected to be severe SAS patients who were definitive diagnosed by PSG and complied with F-SAS sensor clinical tests. Clinical test periods were from September 25, 2013 to February 12, 2014, and measurements were taken for 35 SAS patients including healthy subjects. Simultaneously parallel used measurements were taken with a PSG system, Alice 5, and a compact F-SAS sensor system-Ver. 1 and 2, as shown in **Figures 15** and **16**.

2.2 Results and discussion

The analytical results of RDI (Respiratory disturbance index, Pro-AHI; Provisional Apnea Hypopnea Index) by the conventional F-SAS sensor and ODI3% (oxygen desaturation index: 3%) of PLSX [5] are shown in **Figure 17**.

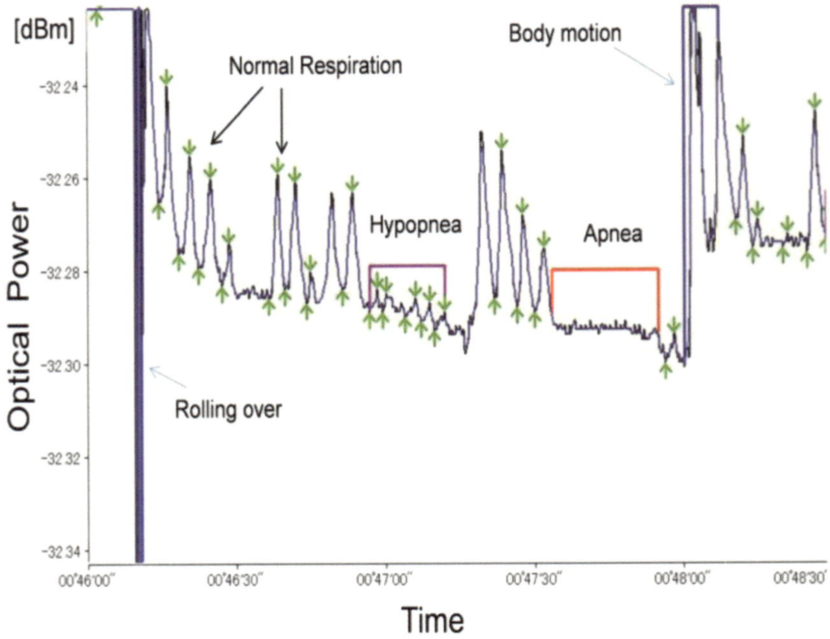

Figure 13.
A measured example by conventional F-SAS sensor.

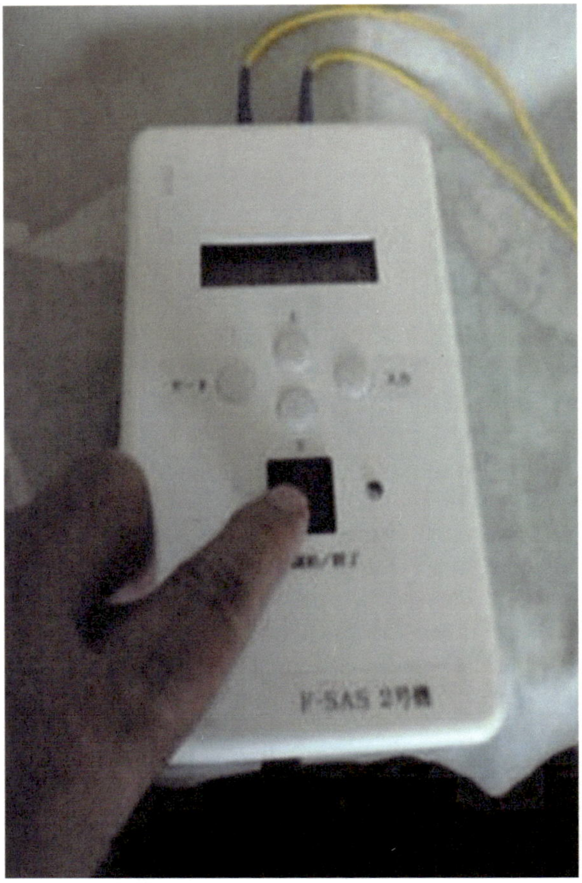

Figure 14.
F-SAS sensor for used.

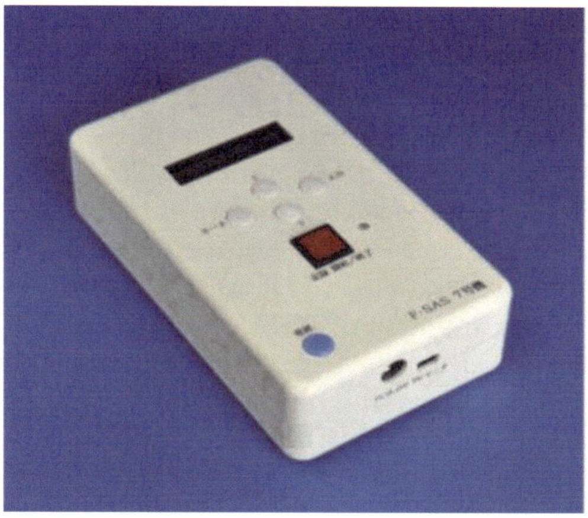

Figure 15.
Compact F-SAS sensor system (175 × 100 × 45 mm, 390 g, voltaic drive during electric outage) (before improvement).

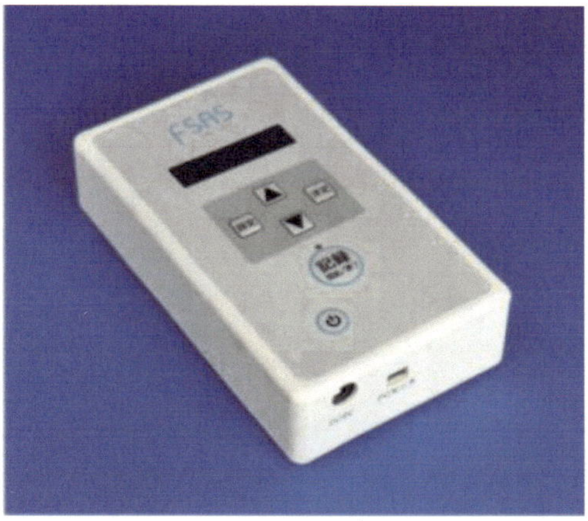

Figure 16.
Compact F-SAS sensor system (175 × 100 × 45 mm, 390 g, voltaic drive during electric outage) (after improvement).

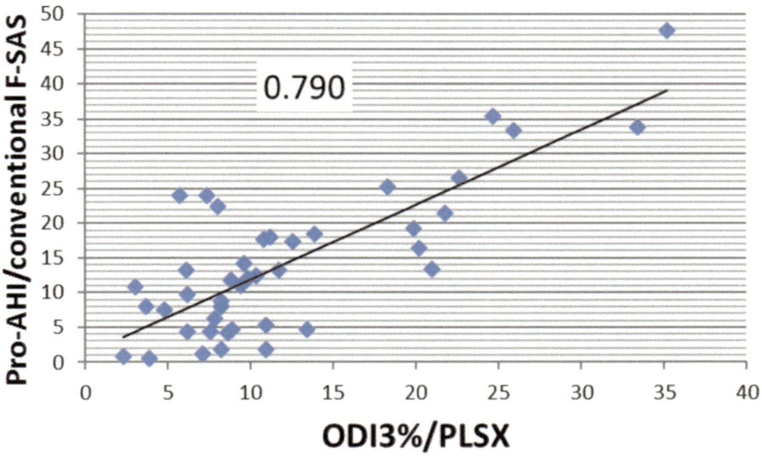

Figure 17.
Correlation between conventional F-SAS sensor's pro-AHI and ODI3% of PLSX.

Thirty-eight of the 42 examinees show Pro-AHI > 5 and were suspected of SAS. The coincident measurement of ODI3% and Pro-AHI shows significant correlation (r = 0.79, p < 0.01). Seventeen examinees with Pro-AHI were over 10 and were eventually given SAS outpatient consultation. Four of them received a complete checkup by PSG and were given CPAP (Continuous Positive Airway Pressure) therapy. Next, a comparison of the analytical data of RDI (Pro-AHI) by the compact F-SAS sensor system and the coincident measurement of ODI3% by PULSOX are shown in **Figure 18**. Out of 76 examinees, 56 were Pro-AHI > 5 and were suspected of SAS. The coincident measurement of PULSOX, Pro-AHI, and ODI3% shows good correlation (r = 0.796, p < 0.01). The 32 examinees were consulted during SAS outpatient screening. In this manner, both the conventional type and the compact

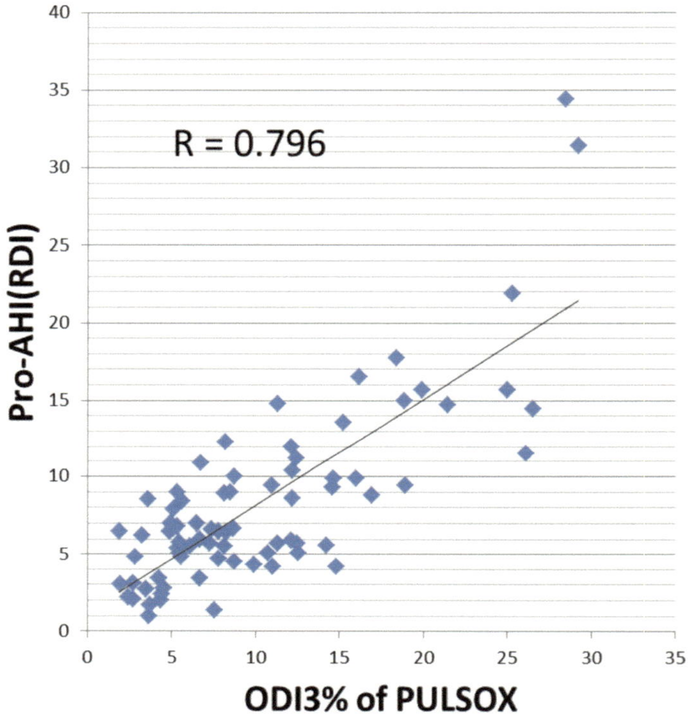

Figure 18.
Correlation between the portable F-SAS sensor's pro-AHI and ODI3% of PULSOX.

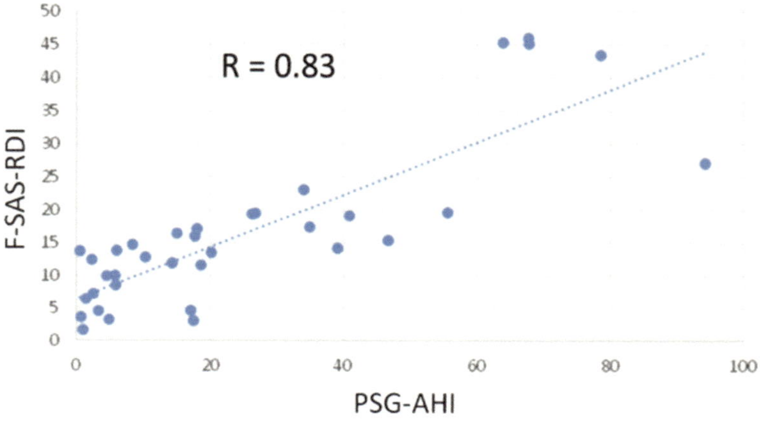

Figure 19.
Correlation between the portable F-SAS sensor's pro-AHI and AHI of PSG.

type F-SAS sensors are very useful for SAS screening during a complete medical checkup.

Finally, we demonstrate the results of simultaneous measurement with the portable F-SAS sensor and PSG (Alice5). Healthy subjects and SAS patients diagnosed by full PSG were included as examinees. There is a significant correlation between AHI by PSG, the gold standard for diagnosis of SAS, and Pro-AHI by the compact F-SAS sensor, as shown in **Figure 19** (r = 0.83).

3. Application to children

The compact F-SAS sensor is made portable by it having only 15.3% of the volume of a conventional F-SAS sensor, as is shown in **Figure 20**. Under the approval of the Ethics Committee at the Dept. of Pediatrics at the University of Yamanashi, the subject wore a portable sleep apnea syndrome examination apparatus (SAS 2100) while a plastic optical fiber sheet was placed under the subject's bed. The subject's apnea/hypopnea index (AHI) was measured by the SAS 2100 and the respiratory disturbance index (RDI) was measured with new analysis software developed for the compact F-SAS sensor.

Further, this type of F-SAS sensor and Alice PDX of Philips-Respironics GK, a PSG device used to inspect sleep for OSAS diagnosis, were used for measurement. **Figure 21** below shows a diagram of the F-SAS sensor and PSG (Alice PDX).

3.1 Results

Their correlation value was then obtained. The new analysis software was made up of a new algorithm that is difficult to use when the number of body movements per hour exceeds a certain number, and it analyzes the RDI by checking both the gasping judgment and weakness judgment against the data from a seriously ill patient. In this study, we improved the algorithm for severe markers in children (2–12 years old) and aimed to expand the application area to the compact F-SAS sensor. We compared severe markers obtained with the compact F-SAS sensor and existing simple polysomnography (PSG) (SAS 2100 manufactured by Nihon Kohden).

In this study, 27 data collected by the compact F-SAS sensor were analyzed by using the new analysis software, which were a severe marker caused by RDI, severe markers with periodic distribution, severe markers due to gasping respiratory

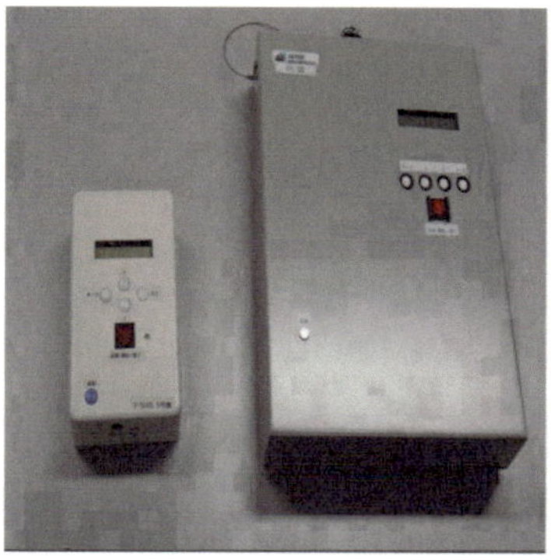

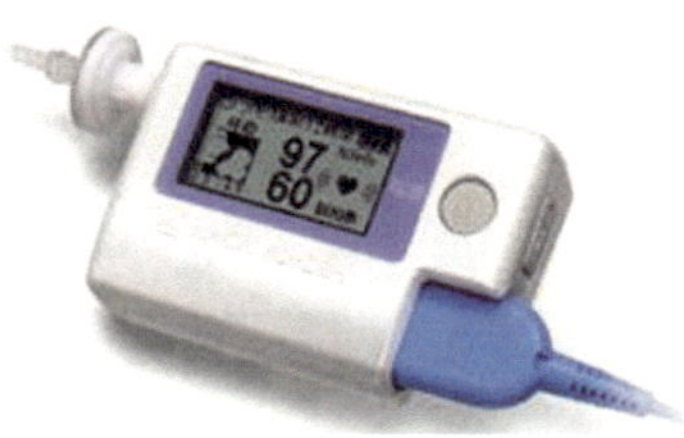

Compact type 175×100×45mm — Conventional type 330×240×65 mm — SAS 2100

Figure 20.
Comparison of compact F-SAS sensor and conventional one (left) and SAS 2100 (right).

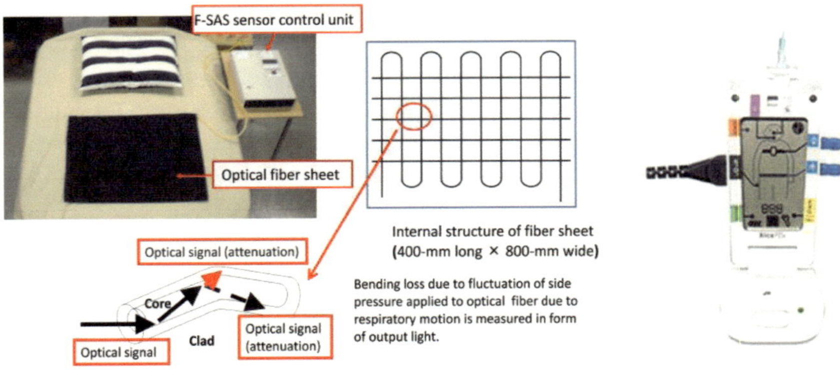

Figure 21.
F-SAS sensor (left) and PSG (right).

frequency, severe markers due to hypopnea, and severe marker due to body movement frequency. The results are shown below. Before introducing the markers, the correlation value of R was 0.697 as shown in **Figure 22**.

After introducing the severe markers obtained by RDI, R = 0.58 as shown in **Figure 23**. RDI 10 or more was considered as a serious patient and examined.

After introducing the severe markers due to gasping respiratory frequency, R = 0.76 as shown in **Figure 24**. We divided the total number of detected low respiration times by total landing time, and assumed that one with a high number of low respirations per hour is a serious one.

After introducing the severe markers due to hypopnea, and R = 0.87 after introducing the severe markers due to body movement frequency, as shown in **Figure 25**.

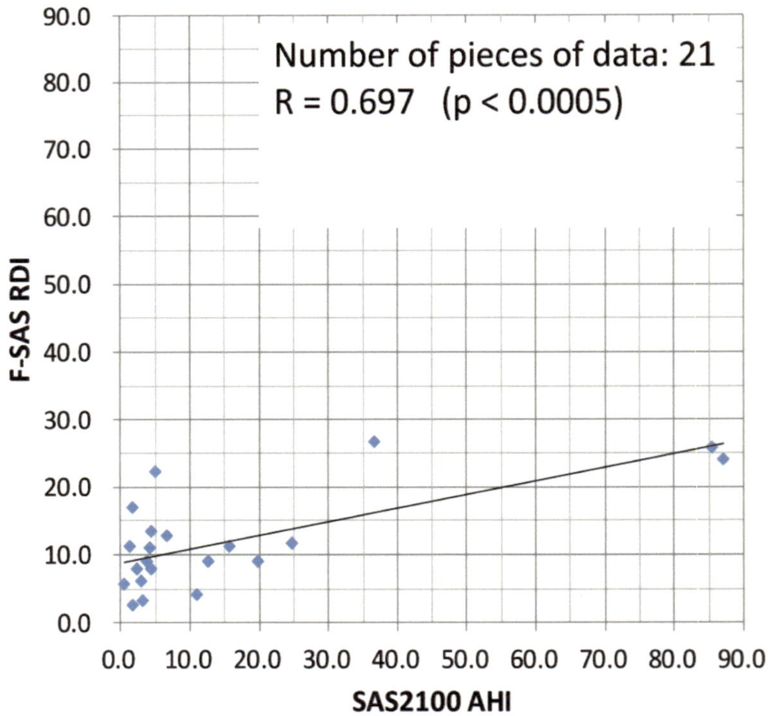

Figure 22.
Scatter diagram of F-SAS RDI and SAS 2100 AHI of severe marker algorithm by RDI before introduction of severe marker.

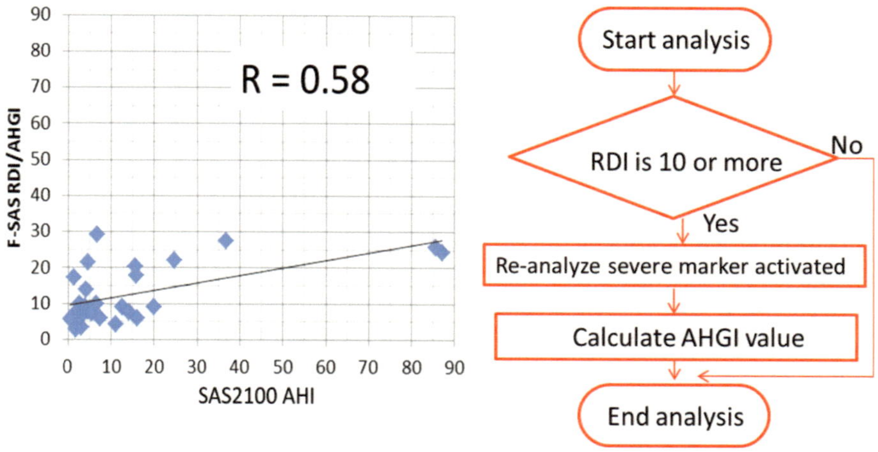

Figure 23.
Scatter diagram of F-SAS RDI/AHGI and SAS 2100 AHI after introduction of severe marker that is RDI 10 or more was considered as a serious patient and examined.

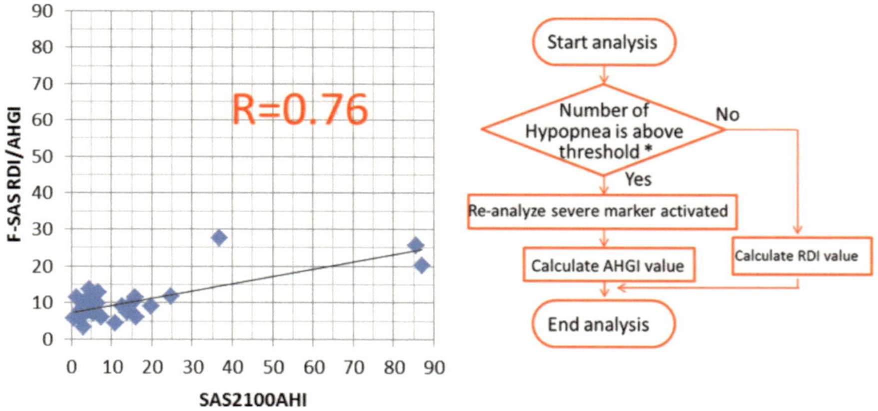

Figure 24.
Scatter diagram of F-SAS RDI/AHGI and SAS 2100 AHI of severe marker algorithm with the number of hypopnea.

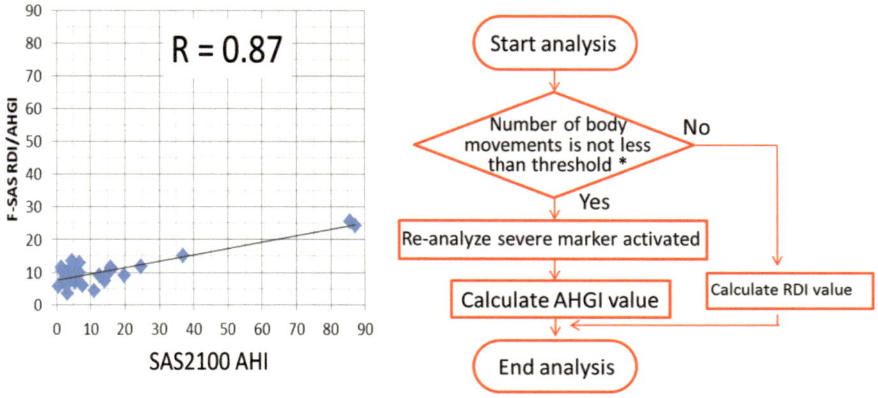

Figure 25.
Scatter diagram of F-SAS RDI/AHGI and SAS 2100 AHI of severe marker algorithm based on body movement frequency.

We divided the total number of detected body movements by total bedtime, and assumed that one with more body movements per hour is a serious one.

Finally, we summarized as shown in **Table 2**. Sever markers were as *RDI*, *Periodic distribution*, *Candle breathing frequency*, *Low breathing frequency* and *Number of body movements*. As a result, *Number of body movements* showed best data of correlation value is 0.87.

The analysis results revealed the correlation value to be R = 0.87, which is a significant improvement over the correlation value of R = 0.697 between AHI obtained by SAS 2100 and RDI obtained by the conventional F-SAS sensor. From this, the software using the new algorithm effectively analyzes the RDI. In the future, to further improve the sensitivity of the compact F-SAS sensor, the remaining gap between the AHI and RDI in seriously ill patients must be bridged. To do this, algorithms will need to be developed that allow the analysis software of F-SAS sensors to capture highly disturbed respiration in seriously ill patients.

We improve the accuracy of the software used for analysis with the F-SAS sensor for child development. This was done for the development of PSG equipment of Philips Respironics GK used in a pediatric clinical trial at Yamanashi University School of Medicine for the purpose of comparing apneic events between the pediatric F-SAS sensor and PSG. That is, the respiratory events were judged and compared from the waveform data at bedtime, which is the analysis result of the F-SAS sensor and PSG. On the basis of the definition of the scoring rule of children for sleeping respiratory events, proposed by the American Academy of Sleep

Severe marker	Correlation value
RDI	0.58
Periodic distribution	0.67
Candle breathing frequency	0.52
Low breathing frequency	0.76
Number of body movements	0.87

Table 2.
Correlation value in each severe marker.

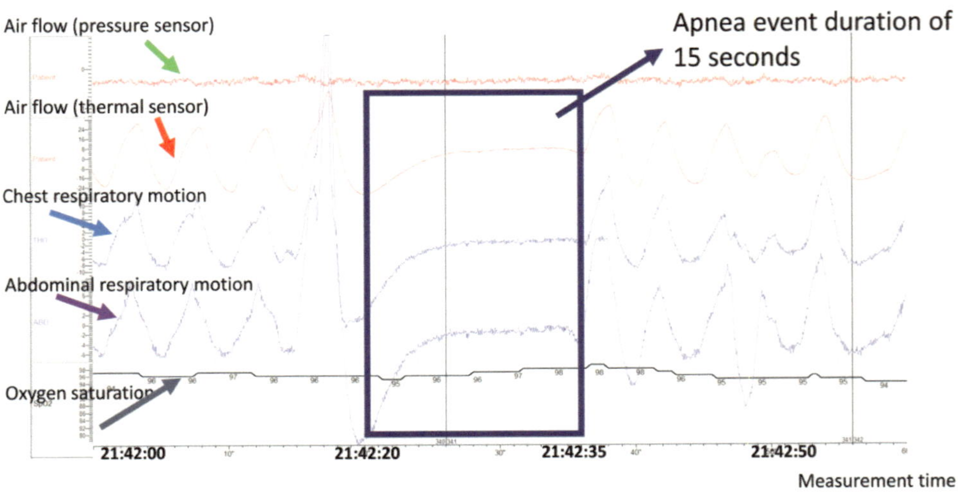

Figure 26.
Measurement analysis result of PSG (apnea waveform).

Apnea event start time (F-SAS)	Apnea event duration (F-SAS) [sec]	Apnea event start time (PSG)	Apnea event duration (PSG) [sec]
21:30:12	18	21:23:20	18
21:49:12	15	21:42:20	15
22:02:12	13	21:55:20	13
22:52:50	12	22:45:58	12
22:56:54	12	22:50:02	12

Table 3.
Results of apnea events comparison between F-SAS sensor and PSG.

Medicine (AASM) in 2007, apnea events were judged from the waveforms of PSG. The analysis results are as shown in **Figure 26**.

The subject was a boy, aged 4 years and 0 months. The measurement comparison time was 21:18:39 to 23:36:24. His height was 99.1 cm, and his weight was 16.6 kg. The respiration cycle was 6 seconds/turn. Concerning the maximum amplitude of the thermal sensor, which was 24 (unit unknown), a drop of 90% or more can be seen for 15 seconds. **Table 3** shows that all five apnea event durations of F-SAS and PSG were consistent. As a result of comparing apneic events between F-SAS sensor and PSG, five apneic events in five out of five matched. In this subject, all apnea events could be detected by the F-SAS sensor.

4. Conclusions

Clinical application of the F-SAS sensor showed that the respiratory disturbance index (RDI) from the F-SAS sensor corresponded well with the apnea-hypopnea index (AHI) from polysomnography under the AASM criteria published in 2001. The concurrently measured RDI and AHI had a correlation coefficient of 0.71. This means that the F-SAS sensor is well suited for preliminary SAS screening. The sensor would also be useful for screening potential SAS sufferers during normal sleep at home and for SAS screening of and monitoring of the respiration and heartbeat of neonates. Also we demonstrated through a detailed examination by PLSX and PSG (Alice5) that PLSX data and PSG (Alice5) data are well correlated with those of the F-SAS sensor. The F-SAS sensor is effective for SAS screening during a full overnight medical check-up.

Further, a good correlation value of 0.87 was obtained between the RDI calculated by a new compact F-SAS sensor analysis system using an algorithm for severely ill children and AHI calculated by using the SAS 2100. Also, by comparing the sleep-event results of the F-SAS sensor with those of the PSG, it was observed that apnea sleep events matched. This suggests that it might be valid applied to diagnosing sleep apnea with the pediatric F-SAS sensor. We further analyze the subject data for further improvement.

Acknowledgements

This research was supported by the Japanese Ministry of Education, Science, Sports and Culture, Grant-in-Aid for Scientific Research, 19,656,101, in fiscal year 2007–2008 and partially supported by the Japan Science and Technology Agency, Grant-in-Aid for A-STEP High-risk Challenge, JST (A-STEP, #AS2114072A), in fiscal year 2009–2011. For the portable prototype manufacturing, I am grateful for the Fukushima Grants of the Next-Generation Medical Industry Agglomeration Project, in fiscal year 2012–2014, Arena Co. Ltd., Honda Tsushin Kogyo Co., Ltd., and GOYO Design & Engineering Co., Ltd. for fabricating the compact F-SAS sensor systems.

Author details

Seiko Mitachi[1]*, Ken Satoh[2], Kumiko Shimoyama[3], Makoto Satoh[4] and Takeshi Sugiyama[5]

1 Graduate School of Bionics, Computer and Media Sciences of Tokyo University of Technology, Tokyo, Japan

2 Ohu University, Koriyama, Japan

3 University of Tsukuba Hospital, Tsukuba, Japan

4 Sleep Center of University of Tsukuba, Tsukuba, Japan

5 Ichinomiyanishi Hospital, Japan

*Address all correspondence to: mitachi@stf.teu.ac.jp

References

[1] Mitachi S, Shiroishi D, Nakagawa M, Satoh K. Development of a sleep apnea syndrome sensor using optical fibers. In: IEEE LEOS 2007, TuQ1; October, 21–25, 2007; Lake Buena Vista, Florida. pp. 294-295

[2] Mitachi S, Shiroishi D. Development of portable sleep apnea syndrome sensor using POF and measurement results in sleeping. In: 2006 Electronics Society Conference of IEICE, C-3-65; September, 2006; Kanazawa, Japan

[3] Mitachi S, Kamo T, Kagami N, Sato K. Development of a simple operational SAS sensor using optical fibers and comparison with PSG. In: 9th World Cong Sleep Apnea, Paper No.114; March, 2009; Seoul

[4] Mitachi S, Ikarashi H, Kikuchi N, Satoh M, Yanagihara M, Shimiyama K et al. Comparison between optical fiber type SAS sensor and PSG by combined measurement. In: Sleep 2010 (24th Annual Meeting of the Associated Professional Sleep Societies), Vol. 33 (No.0403); June 7, 2010; San Antonio Texas. p. A139

[5] Mitachi S, Ikarashi H, Amano J, Imamura Y. Field test results of 4ch optical fiber type sleeping apnea sensor system in hotel. 2012 IECE, C-3-63; March 20, 2012; Okayama. p. 212

[6] Satoh K, Mitachi S. Screening of sleep apnea syndrome during full medical check-up. In: 5th WASM, at Valencia, Tuesday-S-Board #190, Valencia; September 28 to October 2, 2013

[7] Hayashi M, Mitachi S, Sugiyama T. The software improvement of pediatric analysis for portable F-SAS sensor. In: The Institute of Electronics, Information and Communication Engineers, C-3-13, Electronics Presentation paper I; Kusatu; March 10–13, 2015. p. 137

[8] Hasegawa N, Mitachi S, Sugiyama T. Application of a portable F-SAS sensor system to pediatric sleep apnea syndrome. C-3-6, Electronics Presentation Paper I; Niigata; March 18–21, 2014. p.161

[9] Saito R, Mitachi S, Sugiyama T. Comparison of apnea event by pediatric F-SAS sensor and polysomnography. In: The Institute of Electronics, Information and Communication Engineers, C-3-26, Electronics Presentation Paper I; Fukuoka; March 15–18, 2016. p. 164

[10] Mitachi S, Kameyama T, Kamiyama Y, Shimoyama K, Satoh M. Comparison between automated analysis by F-SAS sensor system and diagnosis by polysomnography. In: The Institute of Electronics, Information and Communication Engineers, C-3-70, Electronics Presentation Paper I; March 19–22, 2013; Gifu. p. 230

[11] Mitach S, Ikarashi H, Sugiyama T. Application of diagnosis with pediatric sleep apnea syndrome of F-SAS sensor. In: Proceedings of the 58th JASAP Spring Meeting, 2011, pp. 05-156, 25a-KB-11; 2011

[12] Furuya K, Suematsu Y. Random-bend loss in single-mode and parabolic-index multi-mode optical Fiber cables. Applied Optics. 1980;**19**(9):1493-1500

[13] American Academy of Sleep Medicine Taskforce. Sleep-related breathing disorders in adults: Recommendations for syndrome definition and measurement techniques in clinical research. Sleep. 1999;**22**:667-689

Chapter 11

2D- and 3D-QSRR Studies of Linear Retention Indices for Volatile Alkylated Phenols

Assia Belhassan, Samir Chtita, Tahar Lakhlifi and Mohammed Bouachrine

Abstract

In this study, 29 volatile alkylated phenols were subjected to a quantitative structure retention relationships (QSRR) studies; we have developed two- and three-dimensional quantitative structure retention relationships (2D- and 3D-QSRR) for this series; and these molecules were subjected to a 2D-QSRR analysis for their retention property using stepwise multiple linear regression (MLR) and 3D-QSRR analysis using partial least squares (PLS). The 28 descriptors are calculated for the 29 molecules using the ChemOffice and ChemSketch software to construct 2D-QSRR model. The 3D-QSRR models were constructed using comparative molecular field analysis (CoMFA) method. The models were used to predict the linear retention indices of the test set compounds, and agreement between the experimental and predicted values was verified. The statistical results indicate that the predicted values are in good agreement with the experimental results (r^2 = 0.980; r^2_{CV} = 0.977 and r^2 = 0.998; r^2_{CV} = 0.959 for MLR and CoMFA methods, respectively). To validate the predictive power of the resulting models, external validation multiple correlation coefficient was calculated; in addition to a performance prediction power, this coefficient has a favorable estimation of stability for the two methods (r_{test} = 0.938 and r_{test} = 0.955 for MLR and CoMFA methods, respectively).

Keywords: quantitative structure retention relationship, linear retention indices, multiple linear regression, molecular field analysis, external validation, alkylated phenols

1. Introduction

Phenols are widely present in the environment as building blocks for plants [1]. They are formed naturally from decomposition of leaves and wood as well as through human activity like water purification processes [2]. Alkylphenols are a family of organic compounds obtained by the alkylation of phenols. The term is usually reserved for major industrial compounds such as propylphenol, amylphenol, heptylphenol, octylphenol, nonylphenol, dodecylphenol, and other long-chain carbon compounds. Methylphenols and ethylpenols are also alkylphenols, but are more often referred to by their specific names, cresols and xylenols, respectively. The alkylated phenols have a good ability to be adsorbed on solid materials and some are toxic to fish and other forms of aquatic environment. Very low concentrations of these molecules have unfavorable effects on the taste and odor of water and fish [3].

All phenolic compounds can be considered as important parameters of the organoleptic (color, flavor, and aroma) and nutritional qualities of food products. The phenolic compounds which participate in the vegetable aroma are relatively simple volatile compounds whose odors can be pleasant or unpleasant. Vanilla, for example, is the most popular aroma in the world, and its production is estimated at 1500 tons per year [4]. Approximately 250 compounds are responsible for vanilla aroma and among these are about 20 phenolic compounds, the most abundant of which are vanillin, p-hydroxybenzaldehyde, and vanillic acid [5]. The spices we use to enhance taste and flavor of food contain volatile compounds characterized by the presence of a methoxyl group. 4-vinyl guaiacol is responsible for the pleasant odors that occur during the manufacture and storage of citrus juices (orange and grapefruit in particular). This compound is formed from the degradation of ferulic acid, and the quality of the orange juice aroma is directly related to changes in free ferulic acid and 4-vinyl guaiacol contents [6]. These two compounds are also produced during the thermal degradation of lignin. With their derivatives (4-methyl guaiacol, 4-ethyl guaiacol, vanillin, vanillic acid, etc.), they are at the origin of the aroma developed by the smoking techniques used in meat and fish conservation [7].

Some alkylated phenols represent another group of compounds with a constantly weak odor. In addition, some individual odorants in this group have been described in several studies as having various sensory properties. Because of their obviously high odor potency, the odor thresholds of the alkylated phenols have been extensively evaluated.

The multidimensional quantitative structure-activity/property relationship (multidimensional-QSAR/QSPR) analysis is a computational method used to predict biological activities or chemical properties of existing or supposed chemical compounds. With incessant development, the multidimensional-QSAR/QSPR analyses have made notable achievement in diverse fields, such as toxicology and medicinal chemistry [8, 9]. Through the fast progress of computer science and theoretical study, it can quickly and accurately find molecular information (chemical descriptors) of compounds by computation. These chemical descriptors used in the construction of the QSAR/QSPR models can increase the interpretability and can predict the activity/property of new molecules [10].

The release of odorant molecules from a solid or liquid medium and their passage in the vapor phase is the first step before a possible perception due to the activation of the olfactory receptors present in the nasal cavity followed by a series of complex neurophysiological reactions, in order to code a particular smell, that's why in this study, a series of 29 volatile alkylated phenols, including monoalkylated phenols and di- and trimethylphenols, were subjected to a quantitative structure retention relationships (QSRR) studies, we have developed two- and three-dimensional quantitative structure retention relationships (2D- and 3D-QSRR) for a series of 29 molecules odorants based on phenol. We construct 2D-QSRR model using 28 descriptors. The 3D-QSAR/QSPR models were constructed using the comparative molecular field analysis (CoMFA) [11] tools that collect and interpret complex data from series of bioactive molecules to construct computational models that correlate chemical properties with biological activity/propriety [12]. Through this approach, molecular features responsible for the retention property of the investigated compounds (alkylated phenols) were identified using the CoMFA contour plots. Furthermore, the statistical consistency of the developed models was evaluated on the basis of their correlation ability for the training set, as well as their predictive power for an external test set. We accordingly propose quantitative models, using stepwise multiple linear regression (MLR) for 2D-QSRR analysis and the partial least squares (PLS) for 3D-QSRR model, and we try to interpret the retention property of the compounds relying on the multidimensional-QSRR analyses [13].

2. Material and methods

2.1 2D-QSRR study

2.1.1 Data set

The reliability of the 2D-QSRR analysis is depending on the available data set, and the method of analysis and the validations. In the present analysis, a series of 29 selected alkylated phenols that have been evaluated for their linear retention indices was taken from literature, and as reported in the literature [14], high-resolution GC/O (HRGC/O) analyses were performed with a type 5160 gas chromatograph (Carlo Erba), and the analyses were accomplished using DB-1701, as demonstrated by Czerny et al. [14]. We considered to carry out the 2D-QSRR analysis: 24 molecules are selected to propose the quantitative model (training set) and 5 compounds that have been selected randomly and were not used in training set have served to test the performance of the proposed model (test set). **Table 1** shows the studied compounds and the experimental linear retention indices values (LRI).

No.	Compound	LRI	Log(LRI)	No.	Compound	LRI	Log(LRI)
1[a]	Phenol	1167	3.067	16	4-n-hexylphenol	1784	3.251
Monoalkylated phenols				17	4-n-heptylphenol	1886	3.276
2	2-Methylphenol	1244	3.095	18	4-n-octylphenol	1994	3.300
3	3-Methylphenol	1270	3.104	**Dimethylated phenols**			
4	4-Methylphenol	1269	3.103	19	2,3-Dimethylphenol	1387	3.142
5	2-Ethylphenol	1330	3.124	20	2,4-Dimethylphenol	1344	3.128
6	3-Ethylphenol	1371	3.137	21	2,5-Dimethylphenol	1342	3.128
7	4-Ethylphenol	1369	3.136	22	2,6-Dimethylphenol	1300	3.114
8	2-n-propylphenol	1415	3.151	23	3,4-Dimethylphenol	1406	3.148
9[a]	3-n-propylphenol	1463	3.165	24	3,5-Dimethylphenol	1369	3.136
10	4-n-propylphenol	1463	3.165	**Trimethylated phenols**			
11[a]	2-Isopropylphenol	1414	3.150	25	2,3,5-Trimethylphenol	1483	3.171
12	3-Isopropylphenol	1418	3.152	26	2,3,6-Trimethylphenol	1440	3.158
13	4-Isopropylphenol	1419	3.152	27	2,4,5-Trimethylphenol	1472	3.168
14	4-n-Butylphenol	1571	3.196	28[a]	2,4,6-Trimethylphenol	1400	3.146
15	4-n-Pentylphenol	1678	3.225	29[a]	3,4,5-Trimethylphenol	1551	3.191

LRI: linear retention indices.
[a]*Test set.*

Table 1.
Alkylated phenols used in this study and their experimental linear retention indices.

2.1.2 Molecular descriptors generation

Twenty-eight molecular descriptors were calculated using ACD/ChemSketch and ChemOffice programs [15, 16] to predict the correlation between these descriptors and the retention property of studied compounds and to develop a linear model [17]. The descriptors used in this study are displayed in **Table 2**.

2.1.3 Statistical analysis

To explain the structure-property relationship, 28 descriptors are calculated for the 29 molecules using the ChemOffice and ChemSketch software, and they were subjected to a stepwise multiple linear regression (MLR) available in the SPSS software [18]. The stepwise MLR was generated to predict retention property values Log(LRI). Equation was justified by the correlation coefficient (r), the root mean square of the errors (RMSE), the Fishers F-statistic (F), and the significance level (*P*-value) [19].

The final stage of this 2D-QSRR analysis consists of statistical validation in order to assess the significance of the model and hence its ability to predict property of other compounds. In this chapter, the model was validated internally by the cross-validation test. The cross validations are statistical techniques in which different proportions of chemicals are iteratively held out from the training set used for model development. In this chapter, the leave-one-out procedure is used; this process sequentially removes one compound from the training set containing 24 compounds. A 2D-QSRR model is created on a "23" set of molecules, and the molecule removed is predicted by the constructed model. This process is repeated "24" times in order to predict the retention property of all compounds [20].

2.2 3D-QSRR study

2.2.1 Minimization and alignment

Chemical structures of studied compounds were sketched with sketch module in SYBYL [21] and minimized using Tripos force field [22] with the Gasteiger-Hückel charges [23] and conjugated gradient method, and gradient convergence criteria of 0.01 kcal/mol. Simulated annealing on the energy minimized structures was performed with 20 cycles.

Molecular alignment is one of the most sensitive parameters in 3D-QSRR methods. In this work, all studied compounds were aligned on the common core (compound no. 1), using the simple alignment method in Sybyl [24]. Compound

Software	Descriptors
ChemOffice	Melting point T (Kelvin); molecular weight MW (g/mol); critical temperature CT (Kelvin); heat of formation H° (kJ mol^{-1}); boiling point TB (Kelvin); Gibbs free energy G (kJ mol^{-1}); critical pressure CP (Bar); Connolly solvent-excluded volume V $(A°)^3$; shape coefficient I; total connectivity TC; Log P; number of rotatable bonds NRB; winner index (W); number of H-bond acceptors (NHA); molecular topological index MTI; number of H-bond donors (NHD); partition coefficient PC; Balaban index (J); Henry's law constant KH; polar surface area PSA $(A°)^2$; total valence connectivity TVC; sum of valence degrees SVD
ChemSketch	Percent ratios of nitrogen, hydrogen, oxygen, and carbon atoms ($H_{\%}$; $O_{\%}$; $C_{\%}$); surface tension γ (dyne/cm); index of refraction (n); density (d)

Table 2.
Descriptors selected and software packages used in the calculation of descriptors.

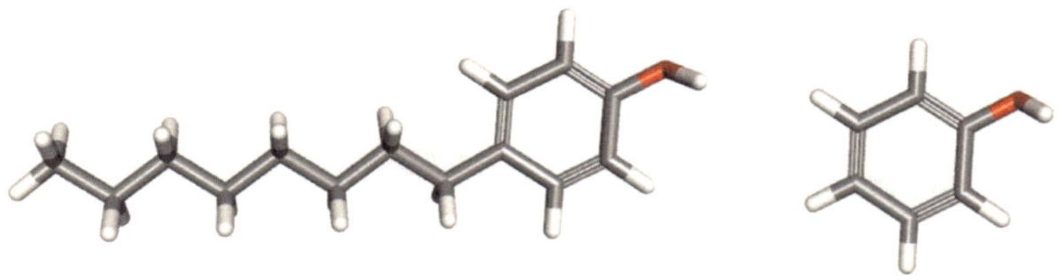

Figure 1.
3D structure of the core (molecule no. 1) and the template (molecule no. 18).

no. 18, which was the most active compound (with highest Log(LRI)), was used as template (**Figure 1**).

2.2.2 CoMFA studies

Based on the molecular alignment, CoMFA studies were performed to analyze the specific contributions of steric and electrostatic effects. These interactions were calculated using the Tripos force field with a distance-dependent dielectric constant at all interactions in a regularly spaced (2 Å) grid taking a sp^3 carbon atom as steric probe and a +1 charge as electrostatic probe. The cutoff was set to 30 kcal/mol [25]. With standard options for scaling of variables, the regression analysis was carried out using the fully cross-validated partial least squares (PLS) method (leave one out) [26]. The final model that is non–cross-validated conventional analysis was developed with the optimum number of components to yield a non–cross-validated r^2 value.

2.2.3 Partial least squares analysis (PLS) and validation

The 3D-QSRR models were generated using a training set of 24 molecules. Predictive power of the resulting models was evaluated using a test set of five molecules (**Table 1**). The test compounds have been selected randomly. PLS analysis used to construct the 3D-QSRR models is an extension of multiple regression analysis in which the initial variables are replaced by optimum number of components of their linear combinations. PLS statistical method with leave-one-out (LOO) cross-validation procedure was used in this work to determine the optimal numbers of components considering cross-validated coefficient r_{CV} for the training set of 24 molecules. The external validation of created models was determined using five compounds (test set). The final analysis (non-cross-validated analysis) was carried out using the optimum number of components obtained from the cross-validation analysis to get correlation coefficient r^2 [27, 28].

3. Results and discussions

3.1 2D-QSRR study

3.1.1 Data set for analysis

A 2D-QSRR study was carried out for a series of 29 alkylated phenols, as indicated above, to determine a quantitative relationship between the structure and the retention property. The values of the 28 descriptors are shown in Table S1 (in Supplementary Material).

3.1.2 Stepwise multiple linear regression MLR

The stepwise multiple linear regression (MLR) procedure based on the forward selection and backward elimination method (including the critical probability: *P*-value <0.05 for all descriptors and for the model complete) was employed to determine the best regression model.

The 2D-QSRR model built using stepwise MLR is represented by the following equation:

$$Log(LRI) = 2.935 + 1.682 \times 10^{-3} \times V \quad (1)$$

N = 24; r = 0.990; r^2 = 0.980; RMSE = 0.008; F = 1085.981; $P < 0.0001$.

In this equation, V is the Connolly solvent-excluded volume, N is the number of compounds, r is the correlation coefficient, r^2 is the coefficient of determination, RMSE is the root mean square of the errors, F is the Fisher's criterion, and *P* is the significance level.

It is observed that the coefficient of correlation r is high, and RMSE is low, which makes it possible to indicate that the model is reliable. A *P* value much smaller than 0.05 indicates that the regression equation is statistically significant; thus, we can conclude, with confidence, that the model provides a significant amount of information [29, 30].

The predicted Log(LRI) values calculated from equation are given in **Table 4** in comparison to the observed values. The correlation between the predicted and observed Log(LRI) is shown in **Figure 2**.

3.1.3 Internal validation (cross-validation)

The 2D-QSRR model expressed by the equation of stepwise MLR method is validated by its appreciable value of r^2_{CV} obtained using the leave-one-out (LOO) procedure. The value of r^2_{CV} greater than 0.5 is the basic condition for qualifying a

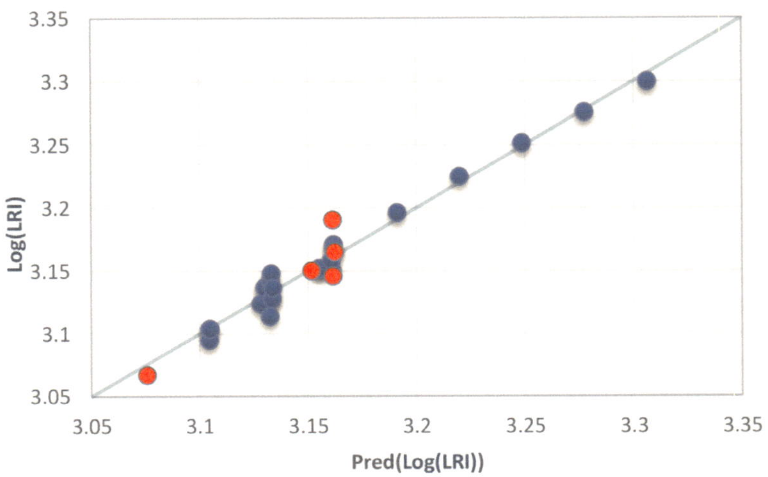

Figure 2.
Correlations of observed and predicted Log(LRI) with MLR stepwise (training set in blue; test set in red).

2D-QSRR model as valid. The model's performance was good and was characterized by r^2_{CV} value of 0.977 with the descriptor (V) proposed by the stepwise MLR.

3.1.4 External validation

The model created in the calculation process using the alkylated phenols is used to predict the retention property values (Log(LRI)) of the remaining (five molecules). The results obtained by stepwise MLR model are very sufficient to conclude the performance of models; it is confirmed by the test done with the five compounds (r_{test} = 0.938; r^2_{test} = 0.880).

3.1.5 Domain of applicability

Evaluation of the applicability domain of the 2D-QSRR model is considered as an important step to establish that the model is reliable to make predictions within the chemical space for which it was developed [31]. In this chapter, we used leverage approach [20]. Leverage of a given chemical compound h_i is defined as follows:

$$h_i = x_i^T (X^T X)^{-1} x_i (i = 1 \ldots n) \quad (2)$$

where x_i is the descriptor row of the query compound and X is the descriptor matrix of the training set compounds used to develop the model. As a prediction tool, the warning leverage h* is defined as follows:

$$h^* = 3(P + 1)/n \quad (3)$$

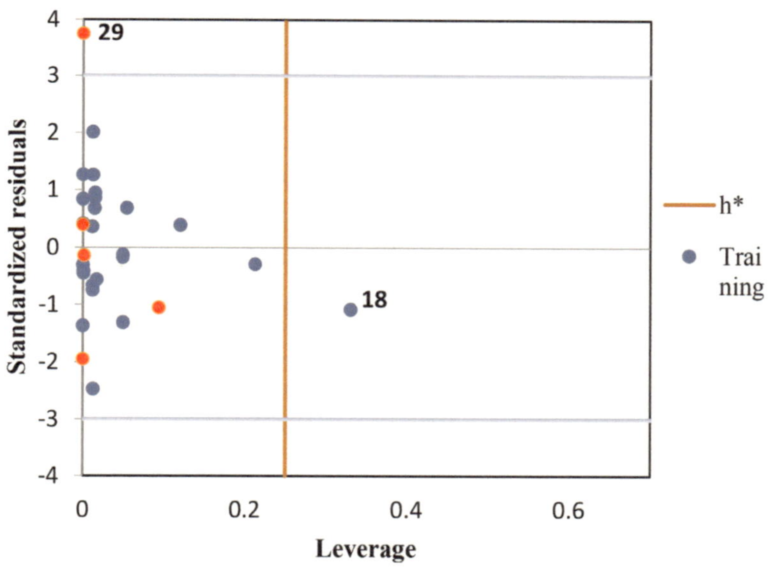

Figure 3.
Williams plot to evaluate the applicability domain of stepwise MLR model.

	r^2_{CV}	r^2	SE	F-t	N	r^2_{test}
CoMFA	0.959	0.998	0.003	2937.327	7	0.913

Table 3.
Statistical parameters of CoMFA model.

where n is the number of training compounds and *P* is the number of descriptors in the model.

From the Williams plot (**Figure 3**), it is obvious that all the compounds in the data set are within the applicability domain of the model (the warning leverage limit is 0.250) except one training compound (no. 18); these compounds have their

No	Log(LRI) (obs.)	Log(LRI) (calc.)			
		2D-QSRR		3D-QSRR	
		MLR	Residual	CoMFA	Residual
1[a]	3.067	3.076	−0.009	3.062	0.005
2	3.095	3.104	−0.010	3.094	0.001
3	3.104	3.105	−0.001	3.103	0.001
4	3.103	3.105	−0.001	3.100	0.003
5	3.124	3.128	−0.004	3.124	0.000
6	3.137	3.130	0.007	3.141	−0.004
7	3.136	3.130	0.006	3.137	−0.001
8	3.151	3.161	−0.010	3.149	0.002
9[a]	3.165	3.162	0.003	3.150	0.015
10	3.165	3.162	0.003	3.163	0.002
11[a]	3.150	3.152	−0.001	3.150	0.000
12	3.152	3.155	−0.003	3.147	0.005
13	3.152	3.155	−0.003	3.150	0.002
14	3.196	3.191	0.005	3.196	0.000
15	3.225	3.220	0.005	3.226	−0.001
16	3.251	3.249	0.003	3.250	0.001
17	3.276	3.277	−0.002	3.280	−0.004
18	3.300	3.306	−0.007	3.298	0.002
19	3.142	3.133	0.009	3.137	0.005
20	3.128	3.133	−0.005	3.132	−0.004
21	3.128	3.133	−0.006	3.127	0.001
22	3.114	3.132	−0.018	3.128	−0.014
23	3.148	3.133	0.015	3.144	0.004
24	3.136	3.134	0.003	3.136	0.000
25	3.171	3.162	0.010	3.168	0.003
26	3.158	3.161	−0.002	3.170	−0.012
27	3.168	3.162	0.006	3.167	0.001
28[a]	3.146	3.161	−0.015	3.164	−0.018
29[a]	3.191	3.161	0.029	3.175	0.016

LRI: linear retention indices.
[a]*Test set.*

Table 4.
Actual and predicted Log(LRI) along with residual of training and test sets using stepwise MLR and CoMFA models.

leverage values greater than the warning h^* value and could be high leverage compound influencing the performance of the model. However, their standard residual values are very low and within the established limit [32]. As a result, this compound could be considered as influential in fitting the model performance but not necessarily outliers to be deleted from the training dataset, and thus, the model can be applied with confidence within the defined applicability domain.

For all the compounds in the training and test sets, their standardized residuals are smaller than three standard deviation units ($3 \pm \delta$) except one test compound (No 29). Thus, compound no. 29 can be as outlier. Because this compound is one of the test set compounds, there is no need to remove this compound from the data set.

Therefore, the predicted of linear retention indices values (Log(LRI)) by the developed stepwise MLR model is reliable.

3.2 3D-QSRR study

3.2.1 Molecular alignment

All other compounds were aligned on the basis of the common structure (compound no. 1). Alignment of training and test set compounds using distill module is shown in **Figure 4**.

3.2.2 CoMFA result

The 3D-QSRR models were obtained from the CoMFA analysis, and its statistical parameters are listed in **Table 3**. The values of predicted Log(LRI) are calculated by CoMFA model, and the observed values are given in **Table 4**. The correlations of predicted and observed Log(LRI) values are illustrated in **Figure 5**.

We use cross-validation as an internal test of the quality of the PLS models. And to evaluate the predictive power of a QSRR model (external test), the Log(LRI) of the remained set of five molecules (test set) are deduced from the constructed model with the 24 compounds (training set) by CoMFA model (**Table 3**).

where r^2_{CV} is the square of the LOO cross-validation (CV) coefficient; r^2 is the square of the non-CV coefficient; SE is the standard error of prediction; F is the F-test value; N is the optimum number of components; and r^2_{test} is the external validation correlation coefficient for test set compounds.

The 3D-QSRR models gave good statistical results in terms of r^2 value ($r^2 = 0.998$) for the CoMFA model. This approach has good predictive capability

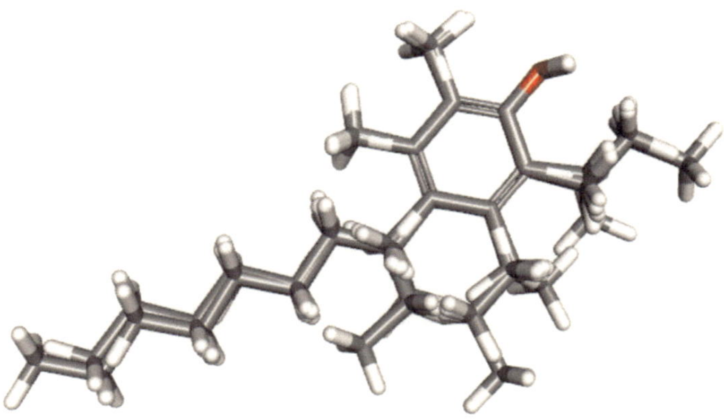

Figure 4.
3D-QSRR structure superposition and alignment of training set using molecule no. 18 as a template.

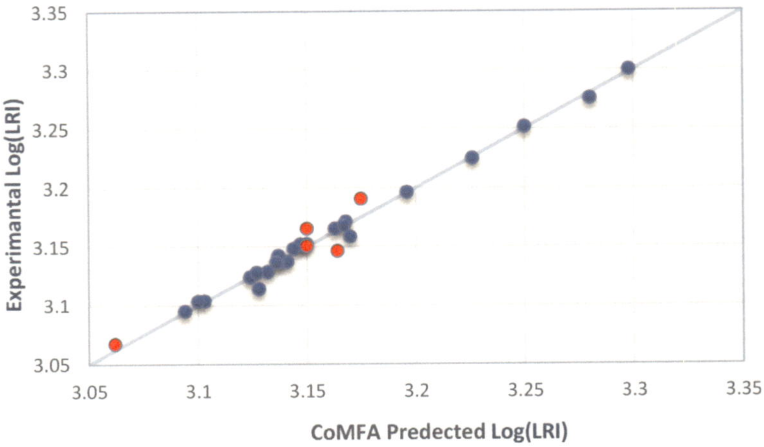

Figure 5.
Correlations of observed and predicted Log(LRI) derived from CoMFA model (training set in blue; test set in red).

2D-QSRR	3D-QSRR
MLR Stepwise	PLS CoMFA
$r = 0.990$; $r^2 = 0.980$ $r_{CV} = 0.988$; $r^2_{CV} = 0.977$ $r_{test} = 0.938$; $r^2_{test} = 0.880$	$r = 0.999$; $r^2 = 0.998$ $r_{CV} = 0.979$; $r^2_{CV} = 0.959$ $r_{test} = 0.955$; $r^2_{test} = 0.913$

Table 5.
Statistical parameters for the stepwise MLR and PLS models using multidimensional-QSRR analyses.

gives good results ($r^2_{CV} = 0.956$). The model was able to establish a satisfactory relationship between the molecular descriptors and the linear retention indices of the studied compounds. The results obtained by CoMFA analysis are sufficient to conclude the performance of the model; it is confirmed by the test done with the five compounds (**Table 3**).

3.3 Comparison between 2D- and 3D-QSRR results and design of novel alkylated phenols

Aiming to provide a comparison among the stepwise MLR and CoMFA models, **Table 5** lists the main statistical indicators for 2D- and 3D-QSRR models.

A comparison of the quality of stepwise MLR and CoMFA model (**Table 5**) shows that the two approaches stepwise MLR and CoMFA have better predictive capability gives better results. Stepwise MLR and CoMFA models were able to found a suitable relationship between the chemical descriptors and the linear retention indices of the studied molecules.

Multidimensional-QSRR correlates retention property with the physicochemical and structural descriptors of a series of molecules. It has been habitually used to predict retention of new molecules and to propose molecules with preferred properties. The constructed models can be used for the designing of new alkylated phenols with higher or lower property values (Log(LRI)).

In this way, we can design new compounds by adding suitable substituents and calculate their property using stepwise MLR equation. The stepwise MLR equation indicated the positive correlation of the Connolly solvent-excluded volume (V).

The obtained results show that, to increase propriety of alkylated phenols, we will increase Connolly solvent-excluded volume (V) value of these molecules. Moreover, to decrease property, we will decrease the descriptor (V) value, by adding suitable substituents, and calculate their property using the regression equation. This study consists of the first step explored to code a particular odor of this group of molecules, followed by docking molecular study that allows understand the mechanism of activation of olfactory receptor present in the nasal cavity by this type of molecules.

We can also use the results of 3D-QSRR to design new alkylated phenols with higher or lower retention property values (Log(LRI)). The CoMFA contour plots were able to identify that molecular fragments, functional groups, and physicochemical properties strongly correlated with the linear retention indices of this series. CoMFA steric and electrostatic contours are shown in **Figure 6**.

The steric interaction is represented by green and yellow contours, while electrostatic interaction is denoted by red and blue contours. The green region around the 2, 3, 4, 5, and 6 positions (the carbon to which the initial —OH is bonded is counted as the first position) (**Figure 6a**) indicates that bulky groups are favored and they might increase the property. That can explain very well why the property of the alkylated phenols with a group bigger than Et group (case of compounds 8, 9, 10, 11, 12, 13, 14, 15, 16, 17, and 18) is higher than those of other compounds. We can also explain, that for the alkylated phenols with a group smaller than Pr group, on the one hand, the property of dimethylated phenols is higher than those of monoalkylated phenols and, on the other hand, the property of the trimethylated phenols is higher than those of dimethylated phenols and monoalkylated phenols. The bigger green region is observed around the four positions in comparison with the other positions, suggesting that groups with steric tolerance are required at this position to reach the green area, which means to increase the property, this fact can

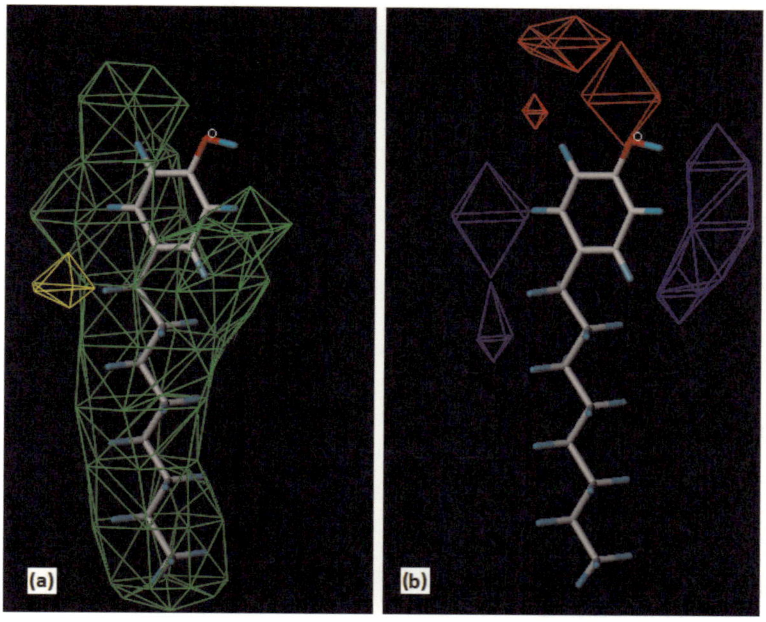

Figure 6.
(a) Std coeff. contour maps of CoMFA analysis with 2 Å grid spacing in combination with compound 18. Steric fields: green contours (80% contribution) indicate regions where bulky groups increase property, while yellow contours (20% contribution) indicate regions where bulky groups decrease property. (b) Std* coeff. contour maps of CoMFA analysis with 2 Å grid spacing in combination with compound 18. Electrostatic fields: blue contours (80% contribution) indicate regions where groups with positive charges increase property, while red contours (20% contribution) indicate regions where groups with negative charges increase property.*

be used to further explain why compounds 14, 15, 16, 17, and 18 have highest property than those of all other compounds.

The CoMFA electrostatic contour plot is displayed in **Figure 6b**. A blue contour indicates that substituents should be electron deficient, and red color indicates that substituents should be electron rich. The blue contour near the 2, 3, 4, and 5 positions (**Figure 6b**) indicates that electron-donating substituents (such Alkyl group) are beneficial for propriety in this area. The electrostatic contour map displays a region of red contours neighbor to the 1 and 6 positions indicating that groups with negative charges may increase the property.

All these findings may be used to design improved compounds with higher or lower retention property, as observed in the CoMFA maps, by adding suitable substituents.

4. Conclusion

In this study, 2D- and 3D-QSRR analyses were used to predict the linear retention indices of a set of alkylated phenols. The multidimensional-QSRR models gave good statistical results in terms of r_{CV} and r values. The stepwise MLR and CoMFA models showed high internal and external consistency; this is verified using different validation methods to evaluate their statistical quality. External validation using a test series verified the capacity of these models to estimate with appropriate precision the linear retention indices of alkylated phenols. In addition, the stepwise MLR equation and CoMFA contour plots can identify that physicochemical properties, organic functional groups, and chemical molecular fragments strongly correlated with the linear retention indices of this studied compounds. The highlighted features are important information for delineating the chemical space, which can be used to design new volatile alkylated phenols. This study consists of the first step explored to code a particular odor of this group of molecules, followed by docking molecular study that allows understand the mechanism of activation of olfactory receptor present in the nasal cavity by this kind of chemical compounds.

Acknowledgements

We are grateful to the "Association Marocaine des Chimistes Théoriciens" (AMCT) for its pertinent help concerning the programs.

Conflict of interest

"The authors declare that they have no competing interests."

Supplementary material

Table S1. Molecular descriptors computed by ChemOffice and ChemSketch software.

No	MW	H^o	G	V	T	CT	TB	CP	KH	TVC	PC	MTI	NRB	I	SVD	TC	H%	O%	C%	n	γ	D	log P	W	NHA	NHD	J	PSA
1[a]	94,113	−96.48	−23.94	83.387	282.50	677.45	439.20	59.26	4.64	0.014	1.475	360	0	0	24	0.102	0.064	0.170	0.766	1.553	40.9	1.071	1.64	42	1	1	2050	20.23
2	108,140	−128.59	−34.15	100.414	306.29	692.39	467.06	50.30	4.60	0.012	1.924	506	0	0	26	0.083	0.075	0.148	0.777	1.545	38.8	1.038	2.13	60	1	1	3818	20.23
3	108,140	−128.59	−34.15	100.612	306.29	692.39	467.06	50.30	4.60	0.012	1.974	512	0	0	26	0.083	0.075	0.148	0.777	1.545	38.8	1.038	2.13	61	1	1	3882	20.23
4	108,140	−128.59	−34.15	100.611	306.29	692.39	467.06	50.30	4.60	0.012	1.974	518	0	0	26	0.083	0.075	0.148	0.777	1.545	38.8	1.038	2.13	62	1	1	3942	20.23
5	122,167	−149.23	−25.73	114.476	317.56	707.14	489.94	44.09	4.47	0.009	2.453	714	1	0	28	0.059	0.083	0.131	0.787	1.536	37.6	1.012	2.55	86	1	1	6909	20.23
6	122,167	−149.23	−25.73	115.630	317.56	707.14	489.94	44.09	4.47	0.009	2.503	726	1	0	28	0.059	0.083	0.131	0.787	1.536	37.6	1.012	2.55	88	1	1	7069	20.23
7	122,167	−149.23	−25.73	115.634	317.56	707.14	489.94	44.09	4.47	0.009	2.503	738	1	1	28	0.059	0.083	0.131	0.787	1.536	37.6	1.012	2.55	90	1	1	7222	20.23
8	136,194	−169.87	−17.31	134.066	328.83	720.74	512.82	38.97	4.35	0.006	2.982	992	2	1	30	0.042	0.089	0.117	0.794	1.529	37.1	0.992	2.97	121	1	1	11,979	20.23
9[a]	136,194	−169.87	−17.31	134.747	328.83	720.74	512.82	38.97	4.35	0.006	3.032	1010	2	1	30	0.042	0.089	0.117	0.794	1.529	37.1	0.992	2.97	124	1	1	12,277	20.23
10	136,194	−169.87	−17.31	134.751	328.83	720.74	512.82	38.97	4.35	0.006	3.032	1028	2	0	30	0.042	0.089	0.117	0.794	1.529	37.1	0.992	2.97	127	1	1	12,562	20.23
11[a]	136,194	−175.15	−19.75	128.458	313.83	709.69	512.38	39.36	4.35	0.007	2.702	938	1	0	30	0.048	0.089	0.117	0.794	1.525	35.7	0.987	2.88	114	1	1	11,308	20.23
12	136,194	−175.15	−19.75	130.527	313.83	709.69	512.38	39.36	4.35	0.007	2.902	956	1	0	30	0.048	0.089	0.117	0.794	1.525	35.7	0.987	2.88	117	1	1	11,607	20.23
13	136,194	−175.15	−19.75	130.529	313.83	709.69	512.38	39.36	4.35	0.007	2.902	974	1	1	30	0.048	0.089	0.117	0.794	1.525	35.7	0.987	2.88	120	1	1	11,891	20.23
14	150,221	−190.51	−8.89	151.962	340.10	733.30	535.70	34.68	4.23	0.004	3.561	1396	3	1	32	0.029	0.094	0.107	0.800	1.522	36.7	0.977	3.38	174	1	1	20,809	20.23
15	164,248	−211.15	−0.47	169.037	351.37	744.89	558.58	31.07	4.10	0.003	4.090	1850	4	0	34	0.021	0.098	0.097	0.804	1.518	36.4	0.965	3.8	232	1	1	33,013	20.23
16	178,275	−231.79	7.95	186.175	362.64	755.62	581.46	27.99	3.98	0.002	4.619	2398	5	1	36	0.015	0.102	0.090	0.808	1.514	36.2	0.954	4.22	302	1	1	50,439	20.23
17	192,302	−252.43	16.37	203.315	373.91	765.54	604.34	25.35	3.86	0.002	5.148	3048	6	0	38	0.010	0.105	0.083	0.812	1.510	36.0	0.946	4.64	385	1	1	74,587	20.23
18	206,329	−273.07	24.79	220.457	385.18	774.71	627.22	23.07	3.74	0.001	5.677	3808	7	1	40	0.007	0.107	0.078	0.815	1.507	35.8	0.939	5.05	482	1	1	107,219	20.23
19	122,167	−160.70	−35.36	117.217	330.08	706.16	494.92	43.23	4.55	0.011	2.373	682	0	0	28	0.068	0.083	0.131	0.787	1.540	37.2	1.014	2.62	82	1	1	6599	20.23
20	122,167	−160.70	−35.36	117.634	330.08	706.16	494.92	43.23	4.55	0.011	2.423	696	0	0	28	0.068	0.083	0.131	0.787	1.540	37.2	1.014	2.62	84	1	1	6756	20.23
21	122,167	−160.70	−35.36	117.636	330.08	706.16	494.92	43.23	4.55	0.011	2.423	698	0	0	28	0.068	0.083	0.131	0.787	1.540	37.2	1.014	2.62	84	1	1	6756	20.23
22	122,167	−160.70	−35.36	117.077	330.08	706.16	494.92	43.23	4.55	0.011	2.373	684	0	0	28	0.068	0.083	0.131	0.787	1.540	37.2	1.014	2.62	82	1	1	6599	20.23
23	122,167	−160.70	−35.36	117.406	330.08	706.16	494.92	43.23	4.55	0.011	2.423	694	0	0	28	0.068	0.083	0.131	0.787	1.540	37.2	1.014	2.62	84	1	1	6756	20.23
24	122,167	−160.70	−35.36	117.845	330.08	706.16	494.92	43.23	4.55	0.011	2.473	696	0	0	28	0.068	0.083	0.131	0.787	1.540	37.2	1.014	2.62	84	1	1	6759	20.23
25	136,194	−192.81	−36.57	134.437	353.87	718.88	522.78	37.55	4.51	0.009	2.872	906	0	0	30	0.056	0.089	0.117	0.794	1.535	36.1	0.996	3.11	110	1	1	10,919	20.23

No	MW	$H°$	G	V	T	CT	TB	CP	KH	TVC	PC	MTI	NRB	I	SVD	TC	H%	O%	C%	n	γ	D	log P	W	NHA	NHD	J	PSA
26	136,194	−192.81	−36.57	133.873	353.87	718.88	522.78	37.55	4.51	0.009	2.822	900	0	0	30	0.056	0.089	0.117	0.794	1.535	36.1	0.996	3.11	109	1	1	10,821	20.23
27	136,194	−192.81	−36.57	134.435	353.87	718.88	522.78	37.55	4.51	0.009	2.872	912	0	0	30	0.056	0.089	0.117	0.794	1.535	36.1	0.996	3.11	111	1	1	11,015	20.23
28[a]	136,194	−192.81	−36.57	134.301	353.87	718.88	522.78	37.55	4.51	0.009	2.872	906	0	0	30	0.056	0.089	0.117	0.794	1.535	36.1	0.996	3.11	110	1	1	10,919	20.23
29[a]	136,194	−192.81	−36.57	134.214	353.87	718.88	522.78	37.55	4.51	0.009	2.872	902	0	0	30	0.056	0.089	0.117	0.794	1.535	36.1	0.996	3.11	110	1	1	10,919	20.23

[a] *Test set.*

Author details

Assia Belhassan[1,2], Samir Chtita[3], Tahar Lakhlifi[1] and Mohammed Bouachrine[1,2]*

1 MCNS Laboratory, Faculty of Science, Moulay Ismail University, Meknes, Morocco

2 Materials, Environment and Modeling Laboratory, ESTM, Moulay Ismail University, Meknes, Morocco

3 Laboratory Physical Chemistry of Materials, Faculty of sciences Ben M'Sik, Hassan II University of Casablanca, Casablanca, Morocco

*Address all correspondence to: m.bouachrine@est-umi.ac.ma

References

[1] Baltussen E, David F, Sandra P, Janssen H, Cramers C. Automated sorptive extraction-thermal desorption-gas chromatography-mass spectrometry analysis: Determination of phenols in water samples. Journal of Microcolumn Separations. 1999;**11**:471-474. DOI: 10.1002/(SICI)1520-667X(1999)11:6<471::AID-MCS9>3.0.CO;2-9

[2] Mahugo Santana C, Sosa Ferrera Z, Esther Torres Padrón M, Juan Santana Rodríguez J. Methodologies for the extraction of phenolic compounds from environmental samples: New approaches. Molecules. 2009;**14**:298-320. DOI: 10.3390/molecules14010298

[3] Czaplicka M. Determination of phenols and chlorophenols in bottom sediments. Chromatographia. 2001;**53**:S470-S473. DOI: 10.1007/BF02490380

[4] Fleuriet A, Uhel C, Dédaldéchamp F. Les composés phénoliques et la qualité des produits d'origine végétale consommés par l'homme. Acta Botanica Gallica. 1996;**143**:493-500. DOI: 10.1080/12538078.1996.10515346

[5] Hartman TG, Karmas K, Chen J, Shevade A, Deagro M, Hwang H-I. Determination of vanillin, other phenolic compounds, and flavors in vanilla beans: Direct thermal desorption—gas chromatography and—gas chromatography—mass spectrometry analysis. ACS Publications. 1992;**506**:60-76. DOI: 10.1021/bk-1992-0506.ch004

[6] Naim M, Zehavi U, Nagy S, Rouseff RL. Hydroxycinnamic acids as off-flavor precursors in citrus fruits and their products. ACS Publications. 1992;**506**:180-191. DOI: 10.1021/bk-1992-0506.ch014

[7] Maga JA. Contribution of phenolic compounds to smoke flavor. ACS Publications. 1992;**506**:170-179. DOI: 10.1021/bk-1992-0506.ch013

[8] Wang T, Yuan X, Wu M-B, Lin J-P, Yang L-R. The advancement of multidimensional QSAR for novel drug discovery-where are we headed? Expert Opinion on Drug Discovery. 2017;**12**:769-784. DOI: 10.1080/17460441.2017. doi: 10.1080/17460441.2017.1336157

[9] De Souza AS, Ferreira LG, Andricopulo AD. 2D and 3D QSAR studies on a series of antichagasic fenarimol derivatives. International Journal of Quantitative Structure-Property Relationships. 2017;**2**:44-63. DOI: 10.4018/IJQSPR.2017010104

[10] Belhassan A, Chtita S, Lakhlifi T, Bouachrine M. QSRR study of linear retention indices for volatile compounds using statistical methods. Chemical Science Transactions. 2018;7:558-575. DOI: 10.7598/cst2018.1501

[11] Cramer RD, Patterson DE, Bunce JD. Comparative molecular field analysis (CoMFA). 1. Effect of shape on binding of steroids to carrier proteins. Journal of the American Chemical Society. 1988;**110**:5959-5967. DOI: 10.1021/ja00226a005

[12] Klebe G, Abraham U, Mietzner T. Molecular similarity indices in a comparative analysis (CoMSIA) of drug molecules to correlate and predict their biological activity. Journal of Medicinal Chemistry. 1994;**37**:4130-4146. DOI: 10.1021/jm00050a010

[13] Vaidya A, Jain S, Jain S, Jain AK, Agrawal RK. Quantitative structure-activity relationships: A novel approach of drug design and discovery. Journal of Pharmaceutical Sciences and Pharmacology. 2014;**1**:219-232. DOI: 10.1166/jpsp.2014.1024

[14] Czerny M, Brueckner R, Kirchhoff E, Schmitt R, Buettner A. The influence of molecular structure on odor qualities and odor detection thresholds

of volatile alkylated phenols. Chemical Senses. 2011;**36**:539-553. DOI: 10.1093/chemse/bjr009

[15] ACD/LABS. 10 Advanced Chemistry Development, Inc. Toronto, ON, Canada; 2015. Available from: www.acdlabs.com

[16] ChemBioOffice. PerkinElmer Informatics. 2010. Available from: http://www.cambridgesoft.com

[17] Belhassan A, Chtita S, Lakhlifi T, Bouachrine M. QSPR study of the retention/release property of odorant molecules in water, dairy and pectin gels. Materials Today: Proceedings. 2019;**13**:621-629. DOI: 10.1016/j.matpr.2019.04.021

[18] SPSS 19.0. Available from: http://www.ibm.com/analytics/fr/fr/technology/spss/

[19] Chtita S, Ghamali M, Ousaa A, Aouidate A, Belhassan A, Taourati AI, et al. QSAR study of anti-human African trypanosomiasis activity for 2-phenylimidazopyridines derivatives using DFT and Lipinski's descriptors. Heliyon. 2019;**5**:e01304. DOI: 10.1016/j.heliyon.2019.e01304

[20] Gramatica P. Principles of QSAR models validation: Internal and external. QSAR and Combinatorial Science. 2007;**26**:694-701. DOI: 10.1002/QSPR.200610151

[21] Zaki H, Belhassan A, Aouidate A, Lakhlifi T, Benlyas M, Bouachrine M. Antibacterial study of 3-(2-amino-6-phenylpyrimidin-4-yl)-N-cyclopropyl-1-methyl-1H-indole-2-carboxamide derivatives: CoMFA, CoMSIA analyses, molecular docking and ADMET properties prediction. Journal of Molecular Structure. 2019;**1177**:275-285. DOI: 10.1016/j.molstruc.2018.09.073

[22] Clark M, Cramer IIIRD, Van Opdenbosch N. Validation of the general purpose tripos 5.2 force field. Journal of Computational Chemistry. 1989;**10**:982-1012

[23] Purcell WP, Singer JA. A brief review and table of semiempirical parameters used in the Hueckel molecular orbital method. Journal of Chemical & Engineering Data. 1967;**12**:235-246

[24] AbdulHameed MDM, Hamza A, Liu J, Zhan C-G. Combined 3D-QSAR modeling and molecular docking study on indolinone derivatives as inhibitors of 3-phosphoinositide-dependent protein kinase-1. Journal of Chemical Information and Modeling. 2008;**48**:1760-1772. DOI: 10.1021/ci800147v

[25] Ståhle L, Wold S. 6 multivariate data analysis and experimental design in biomedical research. Progress in Medicinal Chemistry. 1988;**25**:291-338

[26] Bush BL, Nachbar RB. Sample-distance partial least squares: PLS optimized for many variables, with application to CoMFA. Journal of Computer-Aided Molecular Design. 1993;**7**:587-619

[27] Belhassan A. 3D-QSAR study of biodegradability in water for aromatic compounds. RHAZES: Green and Applied Chemistry. 2018;**1**:21-30

[28] Srivastava V, Kumar A, Mishra BN, Siddiqi MI. CoMFA and CoMSIA 3D-QSAR analysis of DMDP derivatives as anti-cancer agents. Bioinformation. 2008;**2**:384

[29] Belhassan A, Chtita S, Lakhlifi T, Bouachrine M. QSPR study of the retention/release property of odorant molecules in water using statistical methods. Orbital: The Electronic Journal of Chemistry. 2017;**9**:234-247. DOI: 10.17807/orbital.v9i4.978

[30] Chtita S, Ghamali M, Hmamouchi R, Elidrissi B, Bourass M,

Larif M, et al. Investigation of antileishmanial activities of acridines derivatives against promastigotes and amastigotes form of parasites using quantitative structure activity relationship analysis. Advances in Physical Chemistry. 2016;**2016**:16. DOI: 10.1155/2016/5137289

[31] Eriksson L, Jaworska J, Worth AP, Cronin MT, McDowell RM, Gramatica P. Methods for reliability and uncertainty assessment and for applicability evaluations of classification-and regression-based QSARs. Environmental Health Perspectives. 2003;**111**:1361-1375

[32] Garg R, Smith CJ. Predicting the bioconcentration factor of highly hydrophobic organic chemicals. Food and Chemical Toxicology. 2014;**69**: 252-259. DOI: 10.1016/j.fct.2014.03.035

Chapter 12

Smelling "Zuko": Incense Rubbing into the Hands and Smelling the Hands Activates Specific Brain Regions

Mitsuo Tonoike

Abstract

The purpose of this study is to clarify the effects of the smelling "Zuko", incense rubbing into hands and putting the hands for the human brain. From our previous studies on the smelling an incense odor with putting the hands together, the activities of "Zuko" incense are also considered to be promoted as the imitation of habitual behaviors by mirror neurons and the default mode network in our brain. In this experiment, the brain activation was measured in 10 healthy adult volunteers who did or did not have a habit of putting their hands together and magnetoencephalography (MEG) data were recorded while the participants smelled "Zuko" incense and putting their hands together. The peak response of MEG P300m for the "auditory odd-ball paradigm" was also measured for a rare auditory pulse stimulation and was more enforced by the smelling "Zuko" incense. We used alpha-amylase value as an index of the stress state measured in the state before and after smelling "Zuko" and MEG experiments. From these results it can be considered that smelling "Zuko" promote the excitation of the higher activities to human brain and make changing the specific brain areas such as OFC, F5 and V1.

Keywords: "Zuko" rubbing into the hands, OFC, P300m, alpha-amylase, MEG, spatiotemporal dipole fit, time-varying analysis

1. Introduction

In general, incense can be classified mainly into two groups, one of which is a kind of smelling the odor of stick by burning it and another is smelling the odor of "Zuko" rubbing into the hands. There are two major types of incense in Japan, one of which is direct burning incense of sticks and another is not burning and called "Zuko," smelling incense rubbed into the hands by using small pieces of powders [1, 2].

In Japanese smelling "Zuko" rubbed into the hands has been recently often applied to the usage as a kind of smelling incense in daily life. The special meaning of "Zuko" is known as directly smelling the hands with rubbed incense and cleaning the self by the hands with cleaning his/her emotion at the same time.

In these experiments, we are trying to study how "Zuko" has the effects to the human brain.

It is known that olfactory neuronal processing was found in the orbitofrontal cortex (OFC) in the human brain from the previous studies [3–5]. In the recent researches, sniffing and smelling were important function of the "active olfaction" [6, 7]. On the other hand, imitation of smelling hands and the behavior of putting the hands together were investigated as an activation of mirror neurons and an operation of the default-mode network [8–12].

In the analysis of brain activity, fMRI, PET, EEG, and MEG are usually applied. In general fMRI and PET are suitable to measure the metabolism of physiological activities but not suitable to measure the real-time changes of neuronal activities. On the other hand, it is known that the advantage of MEG is suitable to obtain the real-time changes of the presiding neural activities in the brain by millisecond time resolution [13, 14]. MEG method is more excellent than EEG method because no distortion of an electro-resistance in the brain was found. So, we applied MEG experiments to this study for the estimation of signal source in the brain.

In our MEG experiments, we used to trace the cortical current by the first-order differential planar type of DC-SQUID sensors. This MEG sensor system has the greatest advantage of using the differential planar type of device.

The determination of a current source is very precise and useful because the current source exists in the maximum of absolute magnetic field values [15]. This estimated main current source was the largest dipole, and the second and the third current dipoles were smaller and weaker than the first main dipole.

To improve up fittingness of the estimation, we applied "spatiotemporal dipole fit theory" introduced by Scherag et al. [16] in which the time-varying amplitude of each dipole was applied at every 50 ms intervals. For the estimation of the signal source, we applied time-varying analysis method to obtain the most suitable MEG dipole which is called equivalent current dipole. From this time-varying analysis, we obtained the most suitable single dipole at every 50 ms in real-time analysis continuously.

The event-related responses (ERPs) in the human brain were studied as an inner mental state or the various psychological factors having an inner origin in the brain, for example, using measuring brain waves and so on. A P300 response peak in brain waves was researched as a response of "cognitive function" by using "oddball paradigm" experiment [17–19]. This P300m response (the magnetic P300 response peak is called as P300m in the MEG experiment) was investigated for the olfactory cognitive function, too. From these reasons, we can study P300m response to test the cognitive ability of olfaction [20].

The alpha-amylase value in the saliva is known as a kind of marker and an index of stress states in human [21, 22]. So we can have alpha-amylase in the saliva to test the stress state for the response of olfactory function in human before or after smelling "Zuko" incense.

The purpose of this study is to clarify that smelling "Zuko" incense rubbing into the hands and putting the hands together more activate the human brain than smelling incense odors using sticks burned such as the responses obtained from our previous study and to show how specific areas in the brain are activated.

2. Materials and methods

2.1 Materials

In this MEG experiment, "Zuko" incense rubbing the powder into the hands is used.

These materials were produced especially by Nippon Kodo Co. Ltd. in Japan as follows. This new material is called as a code name "Nou-Katsu-Gassho-Ko" (in Japanese) including the following three basic materials:

1. Agarwood (*Aquilaria agallocha*, *Aquilaria agallocha* Roxburgh)

2. Sandalwood (*Santalum album*, *Santalum album* L)

3. Benzoin (*Styrax tonkinensis*, *Styrax tonkinensis* Craib et Hortwick)

2.2 Subjects

From the previous 11 Japanese volunteer subjects, in this analysis 10 subjects (5 males, 5 females) between the ages of 22 and 58 years (mean age 41 ± 11 years) were chosen. These subjects were tested by using the previous two types of incense sticks for the effects of the simultaneous smelling incense odor and putting the hands together. However, for only one subject N1 in the previous 11 subjects, it was tested how his brain showed the response to smelling a "Zuko" incense into the hands and putting the hands together by using the analyses of MEG and MRI experiment [23].

On the other hand, in this experiment new other 10 subjects (5 males, 5 females) between the ages of 31 and 73 years (mean age 54.1 ± 7.8 years) who were selected with higher ages than the above subjects participated. They were tested by using "Zuko," an incense which were rubbed into their hands for the effects of simultaneous smelling."

All subjects had no significant smell loss, and they were given the informed consent perfectly by the ethical committee on human studies under Helsinki treaty in both AIST and Aino University in Japan.

2.3 Methods of MEG experiments and algorithms of source estimation

2.3.1 Signal source estimation using the theory of "spatiotemporal dipole fit"

In this study, we applied to the signal source an estimation by using "spatiotemporal dipole fit" theory [16]. We obtained the value of an estimated current dipole continuously using a unit time step by step at every 50 ms, in turn. From these time-varying analyses, the most suitable dipole was obtained at the most reliable time for MEG data in the experiment. This "time-varying analysis" is the method using time-varying covariate (also called time-dependent covariate) in statistics, particularly in survival analyses. It reflects the phenomenon that a covariate is not necessarily constant through the whole study to get the suitable higher goodness of fit (GOF) for the estimation [24].

In this study, we were selecting the most suitable dipole from these dipoles estimated in time varying at every 50 ms. In these single dipoles for this time-varying estimation method, the most reliable ECD was of course obtained as a very higher goodness of fit (GOF) more than 80% by using the above time-varying analysis. These ECDs were fitted using iterative algorithms which estimated the source parameters in order to explain the MEG data as accurate as possible [25, 26]. A smoothing spline is also used to propose a novel model for the time-varying quantile of the univariate time series using a state-space approach. A correlation is further incorporated between the dependent variable and its one-step-ahead quantile. Using a Bayesian approach, an efficient Markov chain Monte Carlo algorithm is described where we use the multi-move sampler, which generates simultaneously latent time-varying quantiles [27].

In our source reconstruction analysis, three main components were characterized. The first was related to the definition of the solution space, and the second was reconstructed by the information of the physical and geometrical characteristics of the head. The third was treated by modeling the propagation of the source electromagnetic fields through various tissues in the brain [28, 29]. In these inverse operations, a forward model was used according to some criterion, a unique source distribution to get the unique inverse solution.

2.3.2 Data acquisition

Our planar type DC-SQUD system is useful for the determination of the current dipole of brain activity source where it exists at the maximum of absolute magnetic field value. Data acquisition was applied after starting the signal during the time of 500 ms by using MATLAB software. In our MEG experiment, the subjects sniff an incense odor by using his own nose, and when he starts to sniff, he pushed the optical sensor button as a trigger. To record time-varying MEG amplitude value, we used a sampling interval every 50 ms.

2.3.3 ICA algorithms

This independent component analysis (ICA) program [30] was applied to our input data of MEG experiments. ICA is one method of blind source separation and a computational method for separating a multivariate signal into additive subcomponents. In ICA algorithms, if the subcomponents are non-Gaussian signals, they are statistically independent from each other. The number of components was five for the estimation. The criteria of ICA estimation on the total five components for selecting are determined to 85% (independent rate) to all other components (non-Gaussian components) of data.

As a general definition of ICA algorithms, the MEG data are represented by the observed random vector: x = $(x_1,...,x_m)T$ and the hidden components as the random vector s = $(s_1,...,s_n)^T$. The task is to transform the observed data x, using a linear static transformation W as $s = Wx$ into an observable vector of maximally independent components s measured by some function $F(S_1,...S_n)$ of independence.

2.3.4 MRI system

This MRI system is a 0.4 T Hitachi open type MRI system (AIRIS-Light MRI system, permanent magnetic type, made in Hitachi Co. Ltd. in Japan). These experiments were performed in the Kansai center in Ikeda city, National Institute of Advanced Industrial Science and Technology (AIST) in Japan.

2.3.5 Measurements of the stress state using alpha-amylase activity by sipping the subject's saliva

In general, the stress state in human is evaluated using salivary alpha-amylase activity (sAA) to evaluate the change of the autonomic nervous function by sipping the subject's saliva [31–33]. We used a sheet of polyethylene terephthalate as a chip to collect the subject's saliva by putting it under the subject's tongue during about 30 s. After the collection of the subject's saliva, this chip was soon inserted in an enzyme analyzer (NIPRO Co. Ltd.: type T-110-N in Japan) to detect salivary alpha-amylase activity (sAA) during about 60 s.

In these experiments, magnetoencephalography (MEG) was performed, and for the experiments of the stress state using the alpha-amylase activity by sipping, the subject's saliva was measured at the second times (the first measure, before experiments of MEG, and the second measure, after smelling "Zuko" incense rubbing into the hands and measuring the response of the brain using MEG experiments).

2.4 An MEG experiment for the previous smelling "Zuko" incense and putting the hands together for one subject in the previous 11 subjects

For only one subject N1 in the previous 11 subjects, it was tested how his brain showed the response to smelling "Zuko" incense into the hands and putting the hands together by using the analyses of MEG and MRI experiment [23].

2.5 MEG experiments for five mode states

MEG response data were measured at the following five mode states, (1) control state, (2) cognitive testing mode using "auditory oddball paradigm" without smelling "Zuko" incense rubbing into the hands, (3) smelling "Zuko" incense into the hands mode without putting the hands together, (4) the mode of smelling "Zuko" incense rubbing into the hands and putting the hands together, and (5) cognitive testing mode using "auditory oddball paradigm" with smelling "Zuko" incense into the hands.

1. MEG experiments for control state

Control state was measured under no smelling "Zuko" and no putting the hand together.

2. For the next mode, cognitive testing mode using "auditory oddball paradigm" without smelling "Zuko" incense rubbing into the hands, regardless of whether the subject did or did not have the habit of putting his or her hands together or praying in daily life.

During this cognitive testing mode using "auditory oddball paradigm" without smelling "Zuko" incense rubbing into the hands, the subject held the optical sensor by a hand and pushed the button with the right thumb quickly when he/she caught a rare tone. The averaged MEG response was measured by adding the raw MEG data collected about 100 times by pushing the optical sensor button. By using the above mode, we tried to measure the subject's cognitive ability on the peak of the so-called P300m of cognitive MEG response and own singular characteristic active area for cognition, and we have examined to compare how the brain activity is different for the habit and no habit behavior of putting the hand together in daily life.

3. Next, in the mode of smelling "Zuko" incense into the hands without putting the hands together, the subject rubbed "Zuko" incense into his/her both hands in advance at the preparation room. In this MEG experiment, he/she smelled "Zuko" incense of his/her one hand and at random time pushed the optical sensor button with his/her thumb by another hand. We measured the MEG response of "Zuko" incense into the hand and obtained the active brain area and have examined to compare how the brain activity is different for the habit and no habit behavior of putting the hand together in daily life. The averaged MEG response was measured by adding the raw MEG data collected about 100 times by pushing the optical sensor button.

4. In the next mode that included smelling "Zuko" incense into the hands and putting the hands together, we measured the MEG response and active brain area of both brain activities: smelling "Zuko" incense into the hands in synchronization with active inspiration (i.e., sniffing and smelling "Zuko" incense odor) and the behavior of putting the hands together [30]. In this

MEG experiment, when the subject smelled "Zuko" incense with putting both hands, he/she pushed the optical sensor button by his/her thumb with holding the optical fiber among both hands, and also we have examined to compare how the brain activity is different for the habit and no habit behavior of putting the hand together in daily life.

5. This cognitive testing mode is "auditory oddball paradigm" with smelling "Zuko" incense rubbing into the hands.

During this cognitive testing mode using "auditory oddball paradigm" with smelling.

"Zuko" incense rubbing into the hands, the subject smelled "Zuko" incense into one hand and held the optical sensor by another hand and pushed the button with the right thumb quickly when he/she caught a rare tone. The averaged MEG response was measured by adding the raw MEG data collected about 100 times by pushing the optical sensor button. By using the above mode, we tried to measure the subject's cognitive ability on the peak of the so-called P300m of cognitive MEG response at the state of smelling "Zuko" incense into the hand and own singular characteristic active area for the cognition with smelling "Zuko" incense, and we have examined to compare how the brain activity is different for the habit and no habit behavior of putting the hand together in daily life.

3. Results

3.1 Result of signal source estimation of control state mode with no smelling and no putting the hands in the MEG experiments

Figure 1 shows the result of real-time MEG wave forms in the brain measured at a control state.

Figure 1a shows MEG response waves of all 122ch in the whole head regions with no smelling and no putting the hands together. The figure shows all MEG

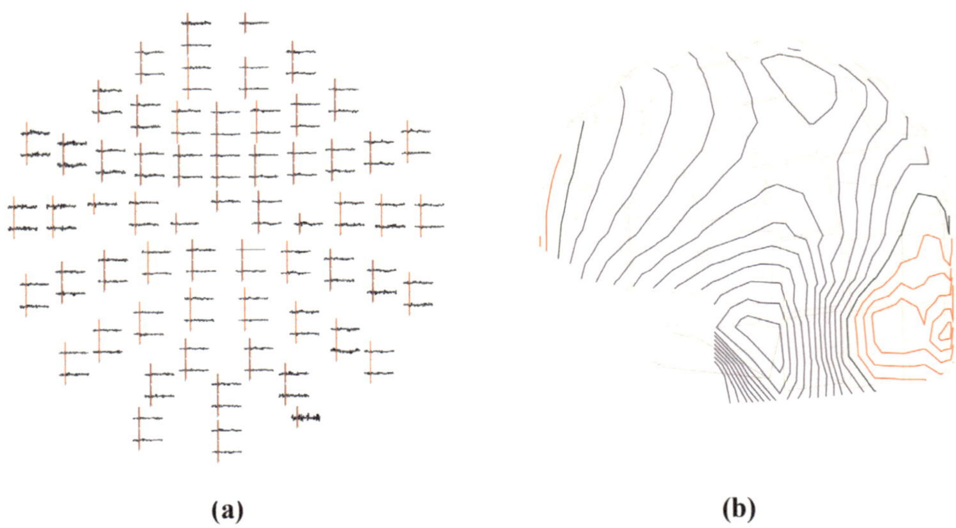

Figure 1.
An example of real-time active state at a control in our brain. (a) Over view of 122ch MEG wave forms on the whole head at a control state. (b) Contour map of equivalent magnetic fields on the head at a control state.

waves from overview. The red vertical line shows the starting time. We can find no remarkable wave peaks in over all around the brain regions.

Figure 1b shows the contour mapping of real-time MEG response at a control state. We could not almost obtain a constricted dipole completely, and then we could not find out the active brain area generally in this control state.

From this result of a control state with no smelling and no putting hands together, we can find no remarkable wave peaks in all around brain regions and no active brain areas in this control state.

3.1.1 The result of the previous MEG and MRI experiment for one subject N1 to smelling "Zuko" incense into the hand and putting the hands together

Only one in the previous 11 subjects was classified in neither the A- nor B-group, and this only one subject (N1) was used by "Zuko" incense into the hand-coating smell method [23]. He had the left priority brain type. His estimated current dipole in his brain was drawn in MRI map coordinates. The X-axis is the horizontal line of the right to left ear, the Y-axis is the line from nasion to inion, and the Z-axis is the upper to lower line of the vertical line of the brain. In this case, we found a vector at the right OFC in the brain.

In our system, MEG data were superimposed to the MRI system on the head data which was obtained from the same subject, and the estimated source was drawn into the brain of MRI imaging as a vector (showed as green vector in MRI **Figure 2b**) of the estimated current dipole(ECD) [34, 35].

Figure 2a shows a vector of single current dipole estimated in the brain using a 3-D model.

Figure 2b shows MRI images and an estimated dipole (red line) in the brain mapping,

In four panels in **Figure 2b**, the upper left panel shows the plane imaging in the coronal plane section, the upper right panel shows the plane imaging in the sagittal plane section, the left lower panel shows the plane imaging in the horizontal plane section, and the right lower panel shows the mapping method by 3-D axis in the brain in the MRI imaging system.

The red line shows a vector of single current dipole estimated in the brain by MRI imaging.

3.1.1.1 P300m mode of MEG response for an "auditory oddball paradigm"

P300m MEG peak of the cognitive response for a rare auditory stimulation without smelling. In this experimental task on an "auditory oddball paradigm," a subject concentrates his attention to the rare auditory pulse stimulation which was given without smelling. The subject must push he optic fiber button quickly when he caught the rare auditory tone. In this "auditory oddball paradigm," two kinds of auditory pulse stimuli were used (1ch, rare stimulation, 1 kHz tone burst, 2ch, frequent stimulation, 2 kHz tone burst). Two auditory pulse stimuli were given to the subject in the duration of 300 millisecond pulse tone burst at random intervals which were controlled at the rates of 1:3 for rare stimuli (1 kHz tone): frequent stimuli (2 kHz tone). We obtained P300 peak response of the subject's type as an individual variation for the priority of brain laterality regarding for "auditory odd-ball paradigm" without smelling.

Figure 3 shows an example of P300m MEG response to an "auditory oddball paradigm" for subject B2 without smelling "Zuko" incense into the hands. The active area in the brain was obtained with the single current dipole tracing method for this MEG experimental condition. We analyzed the estimated active areas

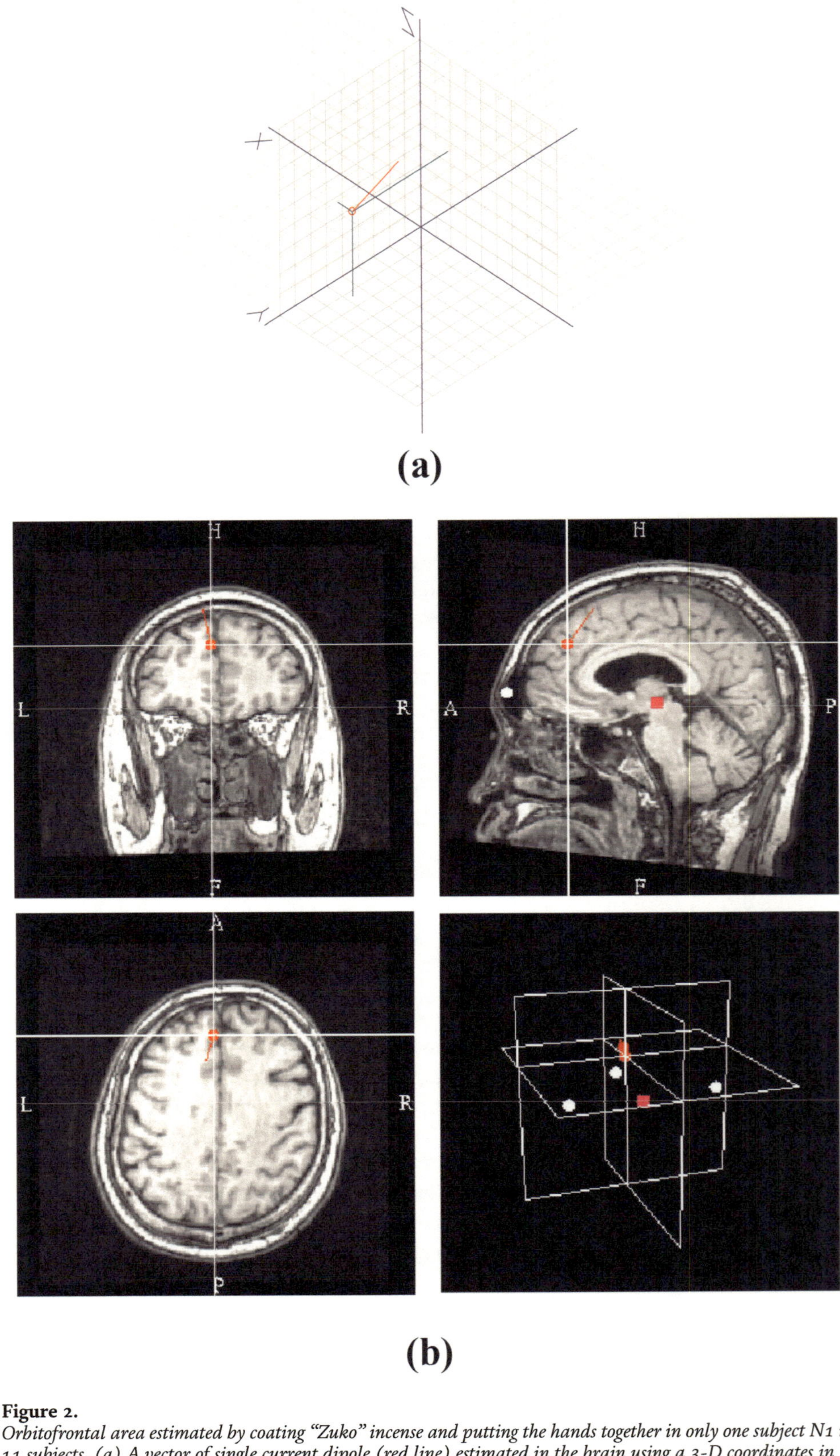

Figure 2.
Orbitofrontal area estimated by coating "Zuko" incense and putting the hands together in only one subject N1 in 11 subjects. (a) A vector of single current dipole (red line) estimated in the brain using a 3-D coordinates in subject N1. (b) MRI imagings and an estimated dipole (red line) in each fault brain images.

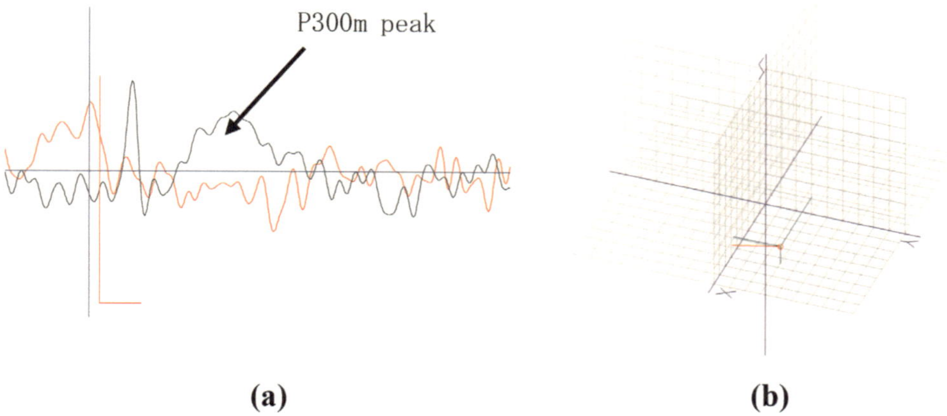

Figure 3.
An example of P300m MEG response for an "auditory oddball paradigm" in subject B2. (a) An example of P300m MEG wave (black wave line) in subject B2. (b) A vector of single current dipole (red line) estimated in the brain using a 3-D coordinates.

continuously using a real-time estimation method. **Figure 3a** shows an example of P300m of MEG wave (black wave line) response to "auditory oddball paradigm" for subject B2 without smelling "Zuko" incense into the hands. **Figure 3b** shows a vector of single current dipole estimated in the brain using 3-D coordinates. In this case, we obtained that active area was at the right anterior temporal area in the brain when he recognized a rare tone at the "auditory oddball paradigm" without smelling "Zuko" incense into the hands.

Figure 3a shows that the value of the maximum peak height of P300m was 26.4 fT/cm and the size of the peak area was S = 14.3 $(fT/cm)^2$ as the latency time of P300m at T = 344.2 ms.

Figure 4 shows another male example of P300m MEG response to an "auditory oddball paradigm" for subject B1 without smelling "Zuko" incense into the hands.

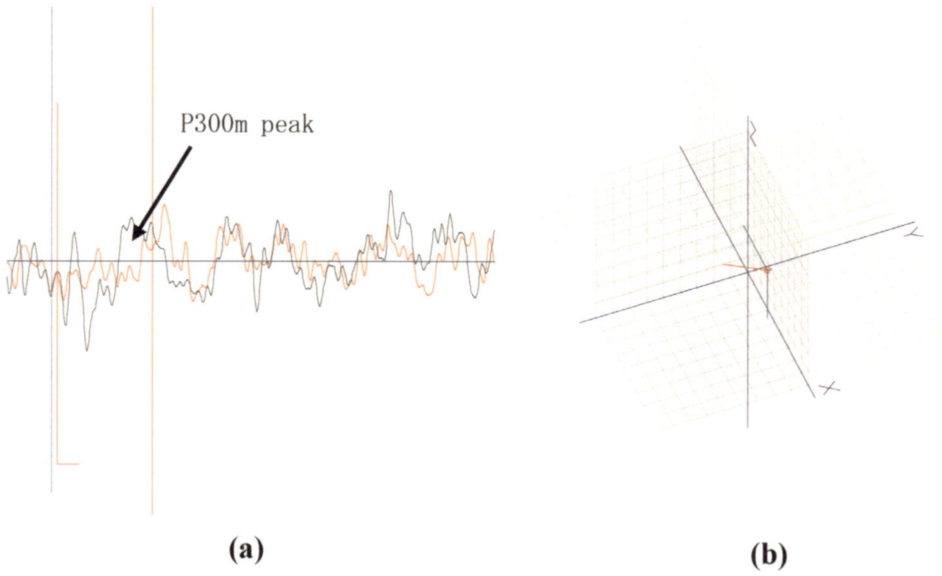

Figure 4.
An example of P300m MEG response for an "auditory oddball paradigm" in subject B1. (a) An example of P300m MEG wave (black wave line) in subject B1. (b) A vector of single current dipole (red line) estimated in the brain using a 3-D coordinates.

In this case, this male subject B1 had the characteristic no habit of putting the hands in daily life. **Figure 4a** shows an example of P300m of MEG wave (black wave line) response to "auditory oddball paradigm" for subject B1 without smelling "Zuko" incense into the hands. **Figure 4b** a vector of single current dipole estimated in the brain using 3-D coordinates. In this case, we obtained that active area was right anterior temporal area in the brain when he recognized a rare tone at the "auditory oddball paradigm" without smelling "Zuko" incense into the hands.

Figure 4a shows that a value of the maximum cognitive peak height of P300m was 11.8 fT/cm and a size of the peak area was S = 7.5 $(fT/cm)^2$ as the latency time of P300m at T = 364.2 ms. **Figure 4b** shows that a vector of single current dipole was estimated in the right superior temporal cortex of brain.

3.1.1.2 The mode of smelling "Zuko" incense rubbing into the hands without putting the hands

Figure 5 shows an example result of MEG response for the mode of smelling "Zuko" incense rubbing into the hands without putting the hands together. In this case, this male subject A5 had the characteristic habit of putting the hands in daily life. **Figure 5a** shows the result of response of a vector by single current dipole estimation method for smelling "Zuko" incense. **Figure 5b** shows also a vector of single current dipole estimated in the brain using 3-D coordinates. From these estimations we obtained the result of which a right inner frontal gyrus was activated by smelling "Zuko" incense without putting the hands together.

Figure 5a shows the contour mapping of real-time MEG responses in the state of smelling "Zuko" incense rubbing into the hands without putting the hands together. The red curves show equivalent positive magnetic fields, and the blue curves show equivalent negative magnetic fields on the subject's head surface. A green arrow shows an estimated single current dipole obtained from these contour mapping by the computer.

Figure 6 shows another example of MEG response or the mode of smelling "Zuko" incense rubbing into the hands without putting the hands together. In this case, a female subject B5 had the characteristic of no habit of putting the hands in daily life. **Figure 6a** shows the result of the response of a vector by single current dipole estimation method for smelling "Zuko" incense. **Figure 6b** shows also a

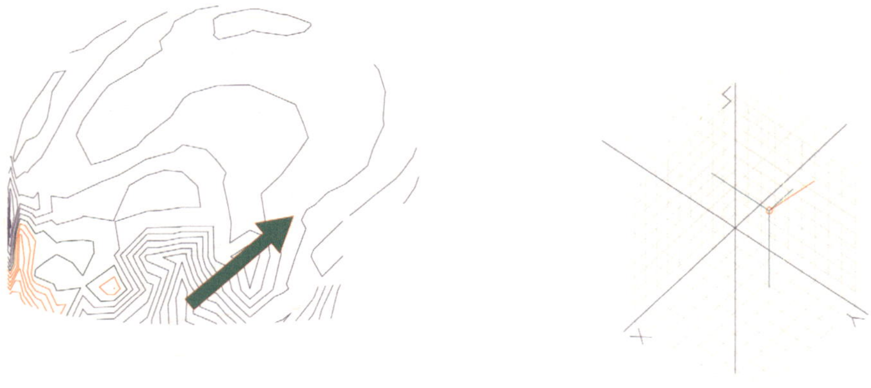

(a) **(b)**

Figure 5.
An example of MEG responses to smelling "Zuko" incense rubbing into the hands without putting the hands together in subject A5. (a) Contour map of equivalent magnetic fields and an estimated current dipole (green arrow) on the head for the smelling "Zuko" incense without putting the hand in subject A5. (b) A vector of single current dipole (red line) estimated in the brain using a 3-D coordinates.

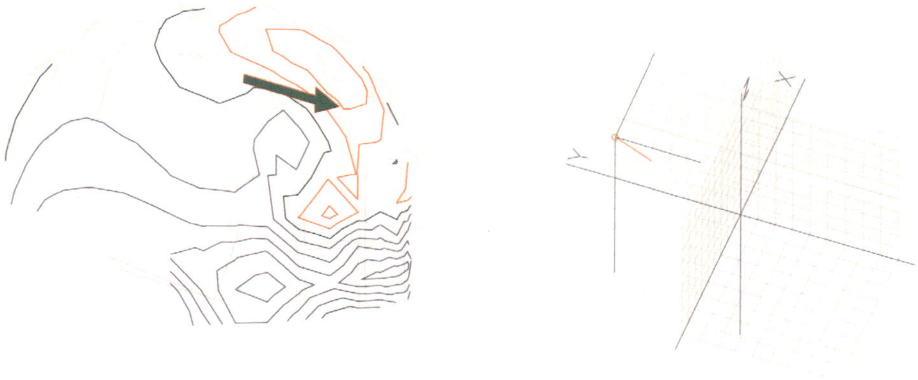

(a) **(b)**

Figure 6.
An example of MEG responses to smelling "Zuko" incense rubbing into the hands without putting the hands together in subject B5. (a) Contour map of equivalent magnetic fields and an estimated current dipole (green arrow) on the head for the smelling "Zuko" incense without putting the hand in subject B5. (b) A vector of single current dipole (red line) estimated in the brain using a 3-D coordinates.

vector of single current dipole estimated in the brain using 3-D coordinates. From these estimations we obtained the result of which a left inner frontal gyrus (F5 language area) was activated by smelling "Zuko" incense without putting the hands together.

Figure 6a shows the contour mapping of real-time MEG responses in the state of smelling "Zuko" incense rubbing into the hands without putting the hands together. The red curves show equivalent positive magnetic fields, and the blue curves show equivalent negative magnetic fields on the subject's head surface. A green arrow shows an estimated single current dipole obtained from these contour mapping by the computer.

Figure 7 shows another example of MEG response for the mode of smelling "Zuko" incense rubbing into the hands without putting the hands together. In this

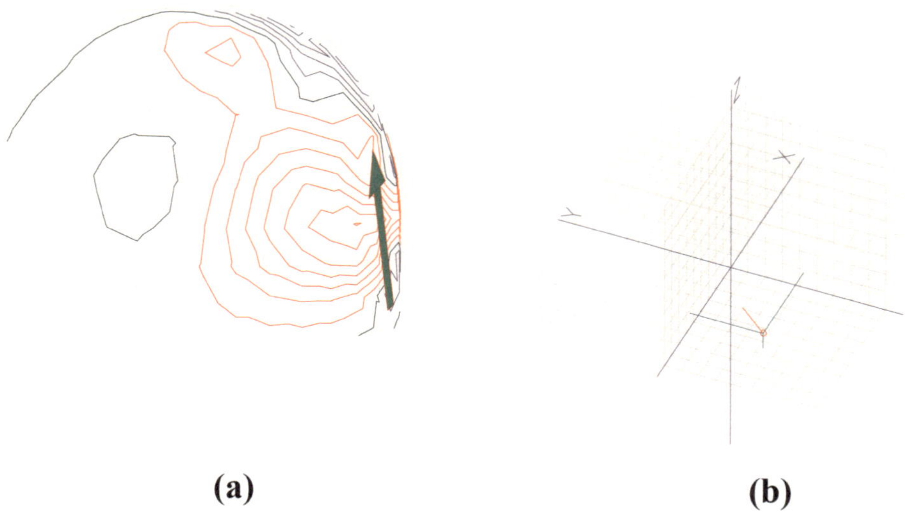

(a) **(b)**

Figure 7.
An example of MEG responses to smelling "Zuko" incense rubbing into the hands without putting the hands together in subject A3. (a) Contour map of equivalent magnetic fields and an estimated current dipole (green arrow) on the head for the smelling "Zuko" incense without putting the hand in subject A3. (b) A vector of single current dipole (red line) estimated in the brain using a 3-D coordinates.

case, another female subject A3 had the characteristic habit of putting the hands in daily life. **Figure 7a** shows also the result of response of a vector by single current dipole estimation method for smelling "Zuko" incense. **Figure 7b** shows also a vector of single current dipole estimated in the brain using 3-D coordinates. From these estimations we obtained the result of which a left occipital gyrus (V1 visual region) was especially activated by smelling "Zuko" incense without putting the hands together. This subject A3 had especial remember impressions of visual image for this "Zuko" incense because of her smelling "Zuko" incense with putting the hands in usual daily life.

Figure 7a shows the contour mapping of real-time MEG responses in the state of smelling "Zuko" incense rubbing into the hands without putting the hands together. The red curves show equivalent positive magnetic fields, and the blue curves show equivalent negative magnetic fields on the subject's head surface. The green arrow shows an estimated single current dipole obtained from these contour mapping by the computer.

3.1.1.3 The mode of smelling "Zuko" incense rubbing into the hands and putting the hands together

Figure 8 shows an example of MEG response for the mode of smelling "Zuko" incense rubbing into the hands with putting the hands together. In this case, a female subject A3 had the characteristic habit of putting the hands in daily life. **Figure 8a** shows also the result of response of a vector by single current dipole estimation method for smelling "Zuko" incense. **Figure 8b** shows also a vector of single current dipole estimated in the brain using 3-D coordinates.

Figure 8a shows the contour mapping of real-time MEG responses in the state of smelling "Zuko" incense rubbing into the hands with putting the hands together. The red curves show equivalent positive magnetic fields, and the blue curves show equivalent negative magnetic fields on the subject's head surface. A green arrow shows an estimated single current dipole obtained from these contour mappings by the computer.

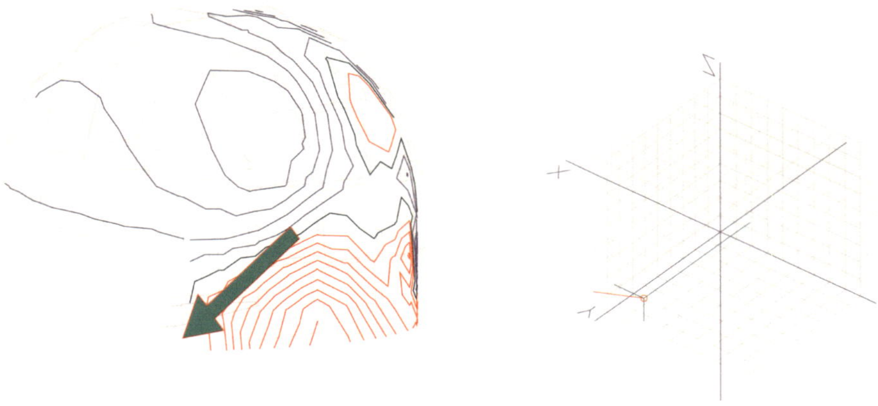

(a) (b)

Figure 8.
An example of MEG responses to smelling "Zuko" incense rubbing into the hands and putting the hands together in subject A3. (a) Contour map of equivalent magnetic fields and an estimated current dipole (green arrow) on the head for the smelling "Zuko" incense with putting the hand in subject A3. (b) A vector of single current dipole (red line) estimated in the brain using a 3-D coordinates.

From these estimations of **Figure 8**, we obtained the result of which a left orbitofrontal cortex (OFC) was activated by smelling "Zuko" incense with putting the hands together.

Next, **Figure 9** shows also another example of a different female subject B5 who had no habit with putting the hands in daily life. **Figure 9a** shows the result of response of a vector by single current dipole estimation method for smelling "Zuko" incense with putting the hands together. **Figure 9b** shows also a vector of single current dipole estimated in the brain using 3-D coordinates.

In this case, a left inner frontal area (F5 language region) was activated. She told that she had the especial impressions for the recall of a few words of the language on the praying when she smelled "Zuko" incense with putting the hands during this MEG experiment.

Figure 9a shows the contour mapping of real-time MEG responses in the state of smelling "Zuko" incense rubbing into the hands with putting the hands together. The red curves show equivalent positive magnetic fields, and the blue curves show equivalent negative magnetic fields on the subject's head surface. A green arrow shows an estimated single current dipole obtained from these contour mapping by the computer.

Figure 10 shows the result of another example of MEG response for the mode of smelling "Zuko" incense rubbing into the hands with putting the hands together. In this case, a female subject A4 who had the habit of putting the hands in daily life hold the especial strong impressions of visual image of praying when she smelled "Zuko" incense with putting the hands during the MEG experiments.

Figure 10a shows the result of response of a vector by single current dipole estimation method for smelling "Zuko" incense with putting the hands together. **Figure 10b** shows also a vector of single current dipole estimated in the brain using 3-D coordinates. From these above estimations, a left occipital area (V1 visual region) in the brain was activated.

Figure 10a shows the contour mapping of real-time MEG responses in the state of smelling "Zuko" incense rubbing into the hands with putting the hands together. The red curves show equivalent positive magnetic fields, and the blue curves show

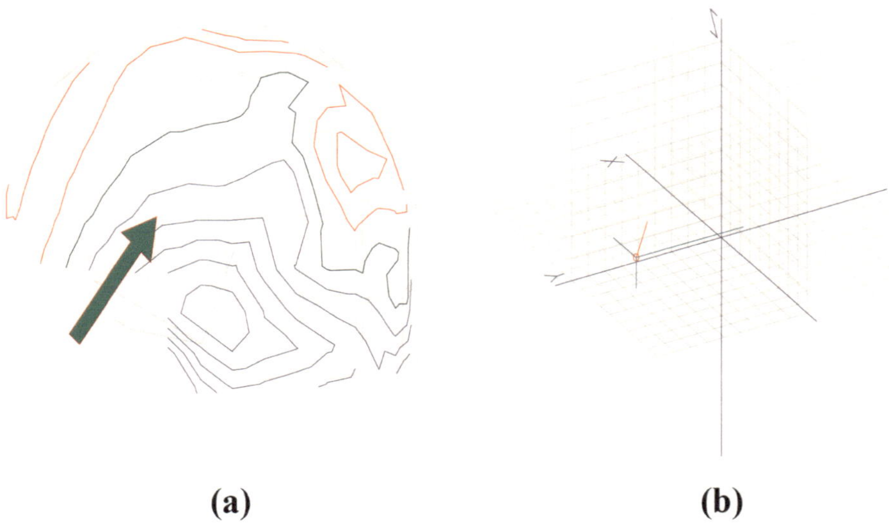

Figure 9.
An example of MEG responses to smelling "Zuko" incense rubbing into the hands and putting the hands together in subject B5. (a) Contour map of equivalent magnetic fields and an estimated current dipole (green arrow) on the head for the smelling "Zuko" incense with putting the hand in subject B5. (b) A vector of single current dipole (red line) estimated in the brain using a 3-D coordinates.

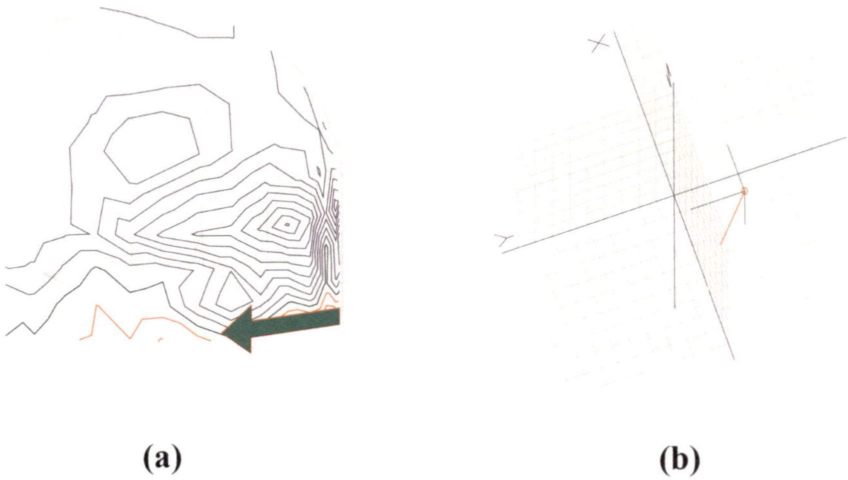

Figure 10.
An example of MEG responses to smelling "Zuko" incense rubbing into the hands and putting the hands together in subject A4. (a) Contour map of equivalent magnetic fields and an estimated current dipole (green arrow) on the head for the smelling "Zuko" incense with putting the hand in subject A4. (b) A vector of single current dipole (red line) estimated in the brain using a 3-D coordinates.

equivalent negative magnetic fields on the subject's head surface. A green arrow shows an estimated single current dipole obtained from these contour mapping by the computer.

3.1.1.4 The response for an "auditory oddball paradigm" with smelling "Zuko" incense rubbing into the hands

P300m peak of the cognitive response for a rare auditory stimulation with smelling "Zuko" incense rubbing into the hands. In this experimental task on an "auditory oddball paradigm," a subject concentrates his attention to the rare auditory pulse stimulation which was given without smelling. A subject must push the optic fiber button quickly when he caught the rare auditory tone.

In this "auditory oddball paradigm," two kinds of auditory pulse stimuli were used (1ch, rare stimulation, 1 kHz tone burst, 2ch, frequent stimulation, 2 kHz tone burst). Two auditory pulse stimuli were given to the subject in the duration of 300 ms pulse tone burst at random intervals which were controlled at the rate of 1:3 for rare stimuli (1 kHz tone): frequent stimuli (2 kHz tone).

We obtained a P300 peak response of the subject's type as an individual variation for the priority of brain laterality regarding for "auditory oddball paradigm" with smelling "Zuko" incense rubbing into the hands.

Figure 11 shows an example of P300m MEG response to an "auditory oddball paradigm" for a subject B2 with smelling "Zuko" incense into the hands. The active area in the brain was obtained with the single current dipole tracing method for this MEG experimental condition. We analyzed the estimated active areas continuously using a real-time estimation method. **Figure 11a** shows an example of P300m of MEG wave (black wave line) response to "auditory oddball paradigm" for subject B2 with smelling "Zuko" incense into the hands.

Figure 11b shows a vector of single current dipole estimated in the brain using 3-D coordinates. In this case, we obtained that active area was at the right anterior temporal area in the brain when he recognized a rare tone at the "auditory oddball paradigm" without smelling "Zuko" incense into the hands.

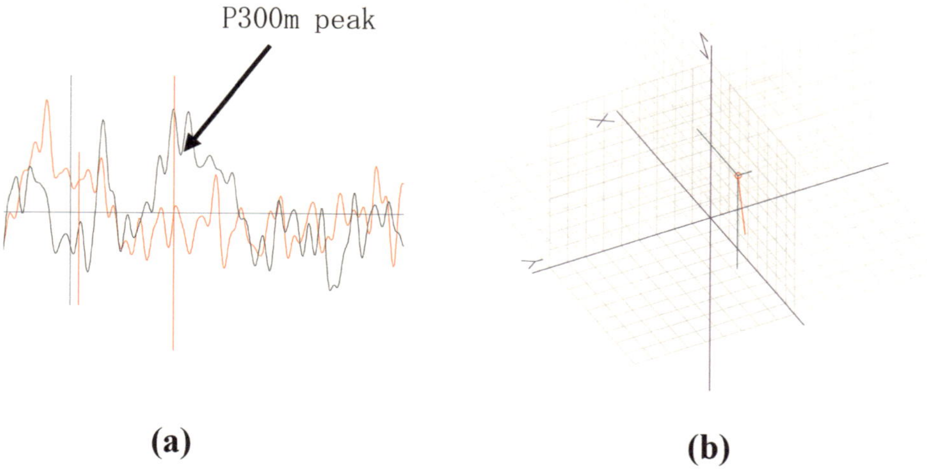

Figure 11.
An example of P300m MEG response for an "auditory oddball paradigm" with smelling "Zuko" incense in subject B2. (a) An example of P300m MEG wave (black wave line) response for an "auditory oddball paradigm" with smelling "Zuko" incense in subject B2. (b) A vector of single current dipole (red line) estimated in the brain using a 3-D coordinates.

Figure 11a shows that the value of the maximum peak height of P300m was 60.4 fT/cm and the size of the peak area was S = 32.0 $(fT/cm)^2$ as the latency time of P300m at T = 310.5 ms. **Figure 11b** shows that an active area of the cognitive P300m peak of "auditory oddball paradigm" with smelling "Zuko" incense into the hands was at the left superior temporal area in the brain.

Figure 12 shows also another example of P300m MEG response to an "auditory oddball paradigm" for a male subject B1 with smelling "Zuko" incense into the hands. The active area in the brain was obtained with the single current dipole tracing method for this MEG experimental condition. We analyzed the estimated active areas continuously using a real-time estimation method. **Figure 12a** shows an

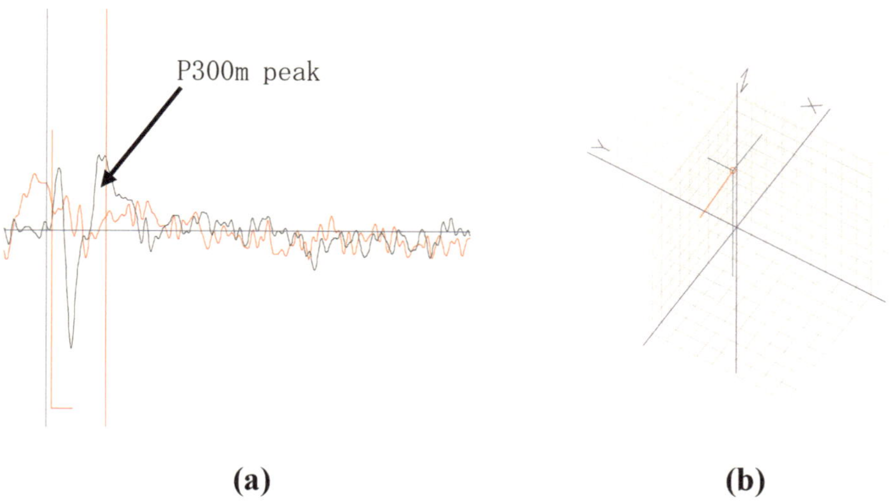

Figure 12.
An example of P300m MEG response for an "auditory oddball paradigm" with smelling "Zuko" incense in subject B1. (a) An example of P300m MEG wave (black wave line) response for an "auditory oddball paradigm" with smelling "Zuko" incense in subject B1. (b) A vector of single current dipole (red line) estimated in the brain using a 3-D coordinates.

example of P300m of MEG wave (black wave line) response to "auditory oddball paradigm" for subject B1 with smelling "Zuko" incense into the hands. **Figure 12b** shows a vector of single current dipole estimated in the brain using 3-D coordinates. In this case, we obtained that active area was at the left posterior temporal area in the brain when he recognized a rare tone at the "auditory oddball paradigm" with smelling "Zuko" incense into the hands.

From these estimations of **Figure 12**, it was obtained that the results of a cognitive P300m peak height in the brain was 26.0 ft./cm and the active wave area value of the P300 peak was S = 15.0 $(fT/cm)^2$ at the time T = 281.4 ms when a rare tone was recognized at "auditory oddball paradigm" with smelling "Zuko" incense in the MEG experiment. And it was also obtained that the cognitive P300 peak was found in left posterior temporal area.

3.1.2 The comparison of a P300m peak of MEG response with nonsmelling and smelling "Zuko" incense

From the example of a female subject B2, a cognitive P300m peak without smelling "Zuko" incense at the oddball paradigm of MEG experiment was shown in the following results of **Figure 3a**. And also a P300m peak of the same female subject B2 with smelling "Zuko" incense was shown in the following results of **Figure 11a**.

An example result of the comparison of female subject B2:

	Latency time	Peak height	S = active wave area
Without smelling	344.2 ms	26.4 fT/cm	14.3 $(fT/cm)^2$
With smelling	310.5 ms	60.4 fT/cm	32.0 $(fT/cm)^2$

From another example of a male subject B1, a cognitive P300m peak without smelling "Zuko" incense at the oddball paradigm of MEG experiment was shown as the following results of **Figure 4a**. And also a P300m peak of the same male subject B1 with smelling "Zuko" incense was shown as the following results of **Figure 12a**.

An example result of the comparison of male subject B1:

	Latency time	Peak height	S = active wave area
Without smelling	364.2 ms	11.8 fT/cm	7.5 $(fT/cm)^2$
With smelling	281.4 ms	26.0 fT/cm	15.0 $(fT/cm)^2$

3.2 Results of the statistical analysis of the alpha-amylase value

Table 1 shows the results of statistical analysis of the alpha-amylase value in the saliva of 10 subjects.

A significant difference ($P < 0.079$) was found between the mean alpha-amylase value of the condition before smelling "Zuko" incense and after smelling "Zuko" incense for female subjects (see **Figure 13**).

Figure 14 shows that it has no significant for the statistical alpha-amylase value T-tests of the comparison with habit and no habit with the hands in daily life. From these tests, we could not find a significant difference for habit/no habit with putting hands in daily life and could not also find the difference before smelling and after smelling "Zuko" incense.

Alpha-amylase value (μg/dL)	A-group (habit group)							B-group (no habit)						
Subject	A1	A2	A3	A4	A5	Average	Standard deviation	B1	B2	B3	B4	B5	Average	Standard deviation
Before experiment	4	22	31	10	3	14	12.14	6	15	28	3	3	11	10.7
After experiment	3	5	72	19	3	20.4	29.61	2	23	3	35	9	14.4	12.15
Average	3.5	13.5	36	14.5	3	17.2	21.07	4	19	15.5	19	6	12.7	11.93

(2)-1 Alpha-amylase value before smelling "Zuko" and MEG experiments.
(2)-2 Alpha-amylase value after smelling "Zuko" and MEG experiments.
The alpha-amylase value (μg/dL) is an index of the state of stress.
A-group is the subject having the habit of putting the hands in daily life.
B-group is the subject having no habit of putting the hands in daily life.

Table 1.
Results of alpha-amylase (μg/dL) in the saliva for each 10 subjects.

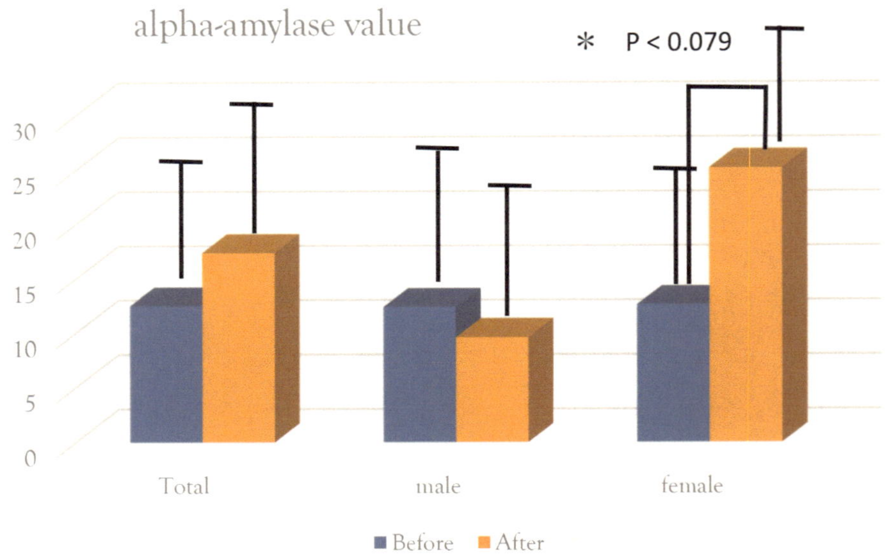

Figure 13.
Results of the comparison for sex difference of alpha-amylase value. P value shows statistical T-tests.

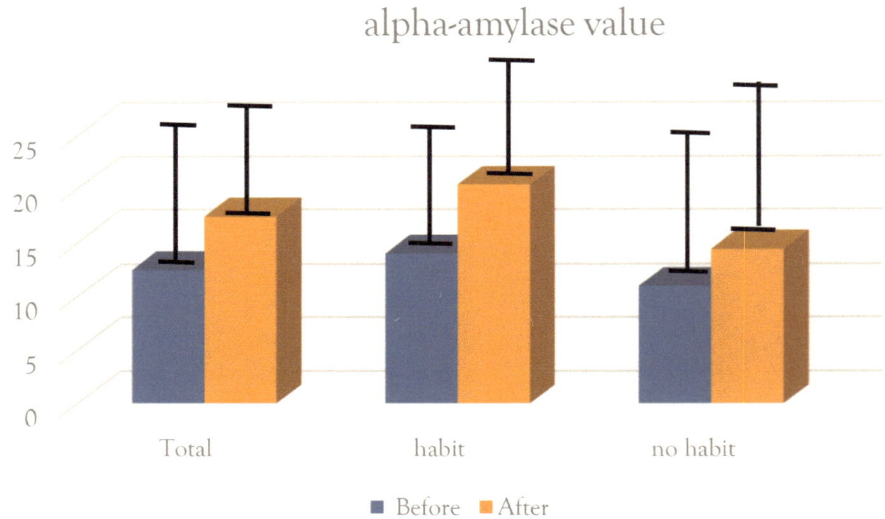

Figure 14.
Results of the statistical comparison with habit and no habit with putting the hands for alpha-amylase value.

From the individual analysis of alpha-amylase value in **Table 1**, we can find that almost all females have more stress after the experiment of smelling "Zuko" incense with putting hands and measuring MEG than before this experiment. And especially the value of subjects A3, A4, B2, and B4 were larger after the experiment than before it. So, we can find that subjects A1, A2, A5, B1, and B2 were almost no stress after the experiment than before it.

3.3 The comparison between the response of only smelling "Zuko" incense and the response of smelling "Zuko" with putting the hands together

A few typical examples of the response of only smelling "Zuko" incense were shown in 3.1.2.2 as in **Figures 5–7**.

	A-Group (Habit Group)					B-Group (No-Habit Group)				
Subject	A1	A2	A3	A4	A5	B1	B2	B3	B4	B5
Smelling "Zuko" only (laterality)	Right	Left	Left	Left	Right	Right	Right	Right	Right	Left
Smelling "Zuko" only (Activated Region)	inner temporal cortex	lateral temporal cortex	occipital cortex (visual area V1)	innner temporal cortex	inner frontal gyrus (F5 language area)	frontia region of temporal cortex	lateral temporal cortex	OFC (orbito frontal cortex)	inner frontal gyrus	inner frontal gyrus (F5 language area)
Smelling "Zuko" with putting the hands together (laterality)	Left	Right	Left	Left	Left	Right	Left	Right	Right	Left
Smelling "Zuko" with putting the hands together (Activated Region)	inner temporal cortex	lateral temporal cortex	OFC (orbito frontal cortex)	occipital cortex (visual area V1)	innner temporal cortex	inner temporal cortex	occipital cortex (visual area V1)	inner temporal cortex	lateral temporal cortex	inner frontal gyrus (F5 language area)

Table 2.
Summaries of active areas in the brain for the response of only smelling "Zuko" incense and for the response of smelling "Zuko" incense with putting the hands together.

A few typical examples of the response of smelling "Zuko" incense with putting the hands together were also shown in 3.1.3.3 as in **Figures 8–10**.

These results are summarized in **Table 2**.

3.4 The summaries of active areas in the brain for the changing from only smelling "Zuko" incense to smelling "Zuko" incense with putting the hands together

From the results **Table 2** in Section 3.3, we can summarize the active areas in the brain for changing from only smelling "Zuko" incense to smelling "Zuko" incense with putting the hands together.

Figure 15 shows the summaries of active areas in the brain for these changes.

In **Figure 15**, we draw two experimental states, for example, yellow symbol color showed the state of the habituation of putting the hands together, and blue symbol color showed the state of the no habituation of putting the hands together.

In **Figure 15**, active brain areas for the response of smelling only "Zuko" incense showed almost temporal regions in the case of habituation of putting the hands together except for two subjects A3 and A5. The response of subject A3 was shown at the left visual V1 area, and the response of subject A5 was shown at the right inner frontal area. However, active brain areas in the case of smelling only "Zuko" incense but no habituation of putting the hands together also showed almost temporal regions except for one subject B3. The response of subject B3 was only shown at the right orbitofrontal cortex.

On the contrary, active brain areas of smelling "Zuko" incense with putting the hands together showed larger change and different responses from smelling only "Zuko" incense.

In **Figure 15**, we showed these larger changing regions to the square symbols from the ellipse symbols using arrows. In the case of habituation of putting the hands, subject A3 showed larger change to the left orbitofrontal cortex from the left visual V1 area, and another subject A4 showed larger change to the left visual V1 area from the inner temporal area. These results are considerable to suggest that subject A3 and A4 may be activated especially at the orbitofrontal cortex and left visual V1 area, respectively.

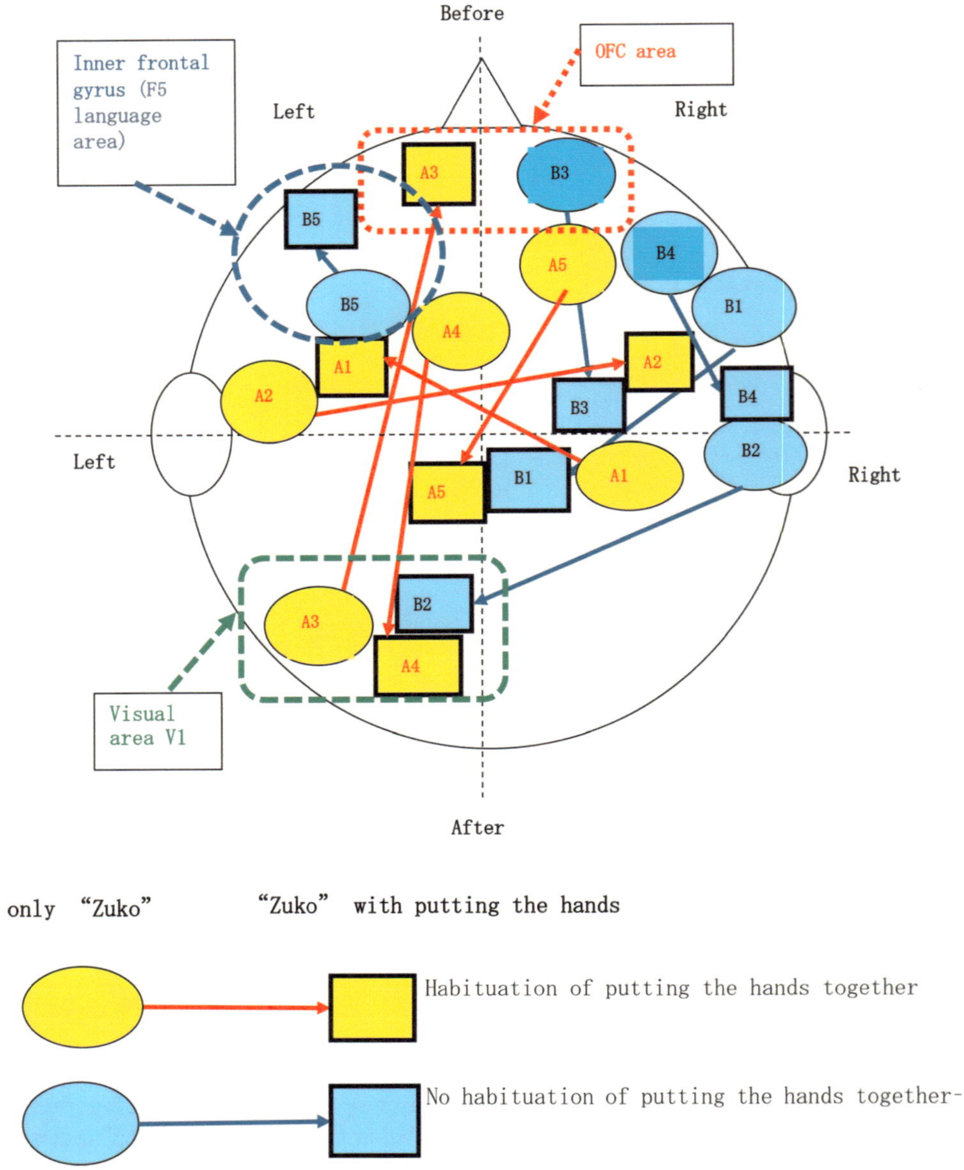

Figure 15.
The summaries of active areas in the brain for changing from smelling "Zuko" incense to smelling "Zuko" incense with putting the hands together.

As the same larger changing, in the case of no habituation of putting the hands the subject B2 showed the larger change to the left visual V1 area from right outer temporal area, the subject B5 the change to the left frontal gyrus F5 area (language area) from inner frontal area. These results are considerable to suggest that subject B2 and B5 may be activated especially at the visual V1 area and the left F5 language area, respectively, although they have no habituation of putting hands together in daily lives.

These larger change results on the brain active areas show that smelling "Zuko," rubbing into the hands, and putting the hands together activate specific brain areas more than smelling only "Zuko".

From **Figure 15**, we can find that smelling "Zuko" incense activates a few special areas, for example, orbitofrontal cortex, left inner frontal gyrus (F5 language area), occipital cortex of visual area V1, and so on.

And also we can find that smelling "Zuko" incense with putting the hands together more activates the same few special areas, for example, OFC area, left inner frontal gyrus (F5 language area), occipital cortex of visual area V1, and so on.

From these results of the comparison among the above two mode states, we can obtain large changes from control state to the state of smelling "Zuko" incense and also larger changes from the state of only smelling "Zuko" incense to smelling "Zuko" incense with putting the hands together. In these changing active areas in the brain, the common special changes was the change of laterality in the brain. **Figure 15** shows large changes for literalities in the brain with the change of active areas too. These results can make sure that Smelling "Zuko" incense activates a few special regions in the brain and raises up a few complex larger changes for activation areas in the brain.

3.5 Summary of results

3.5.1 The specific and distinct mirror neuron activities without the error activity on the hand motor system by putting the hands together

Our MEG experiments of the above results were shown by using the results of 3.1.1 and 3.1.2 in the previous paper [23].

From the previous paper [23], the response areas were obtained in superior and anterior temporal gyrus or central and caudal temporal and frontal gyrus.

Our previous MEG experiments [23] showed the distinct and objective activities of our brain on the state of simultaneous responses of putting the hands together and at the same time smelling incense odor. In this simultaneous status mode of our MEG experiments, these specific active areas were especially shown in distinct F5 language areas of the inner regions of the left frontal lobe or orbitofrontal gyrus clinically. These specific results showed the simultaneous new distinct stronger effects of both the mirror neuronal activities as the imitation without the artifacts of the simple moving error activities and olfactory activated effects.

These results show the specific new stronger effects of simultaneous responses in relation of both the mirror neuron activities and olfactory effects at the same time.

3.5.2 The mode of smelling "Zuko" incense only without putting the hands together (olfactory sensing response and visual imaging response)

The detailed responses of our MEG experiments of the above results in the mode of smelling "Zuko" incense only without putting the hands together (olfactory and visual activities) were shown in **Figures 5–7** in Section 3.1.2.2 and **Table 2** in Section 3.3. From these analyses we mainly obtained the active areas in the brain such as inner frontal gyrus, left F5 language area and left occipital gyrus (V1 visual region), and so on.

3.5.3 The mode of smelling "Zuko" incense rubbing into the hands and putting the hands together

The detailed responses of our MEG experiments of the above results in the mode of smelling "Zuko" incense rubbing into the hands and putting the hands together were shown in **Figures 8–10** in Section 3.1.2.3 and **Table 2** in Section 3.3 with almost all the subject's data. From these clinical and objective MEG measurements and analysis, we obtained the distinct olfactory active areas clearly such as the OFC frontal regions and left inner frontal region F5 (language area) and occipital regions V1 (visual area) for a mirror neuron activity in the brain, nevertheless habit (A-group) and no habit (B-group) of putting the hands in daily life. The larger active effects for smelling "Zuko" incense rubbing into the hands and putting the hands were obtained more than the previous smelling incense odor activity with putting the hands from the results of summaries in **Figure 15** in Section 3.4.

4. Discussions

4.1 A possibility for improving cognitive ability by smelling "Zuko" incense from the results of P300m responses of "auditory oddball paradigm"

We try to discuss a possibility for improving cognitive ability by smelling "Zuko" incense from the results of the following examples of P300m responses of "auditory oddball paradigm" MEG experiments.

4.1.1 The comparison of a P300m peak of MEG response with nonsmelling and smelling "Zuko" incense

Though the typical examples are the results of P300m MEG responses of only two subjects, we can find out the results as follows:

1. As a cognitive P300m response, it was shown that the result with smelling "Zuko" had shorter latency time than without smelling "Zuko."

2. As a cognitive P300m response, it was shown that the result with smelling "Zuko" had bigger peak height than without smelling "Zuko."

3. As a cognitive P300m response, it was shown that the result with smelling "Zuko" had larger active wave area S than without smelling "Zuko."

From these typical results of P300m responses, it can be considered that a possibility of the improving cognitive ability of P300 peak was shown by smelling "Zuko" incense using "auditory oddball paradigm."

4.2 Effects of stress on the comparison with before and after smelling "Zuko" incense by measuring alpha-amylase value in saliva

We can find out few effects of stress for smelling "Zuko" incense by measuring alpha-amylase value in saliva from the results of **Table 1**, **Figures 13** and **14**.

From these results of alpha-amylase value in saliva, it was shown that the following discussions were obtained:

1. This report shows the results of the statistical comparison with habit and no habit with putting the hands by using alpha-amylase value in saliva.

2. We could not find out a significant difference among the sex in 10 Japanese subjects as the statistical value of alpha-amylase in saliva.

3. We could not find out a significant difference among the habit and no habit with smelling "Zuko" incense and putting hands together in daily life.

4. In only female subjects, we found out a significant difference ($P < 0.079$) in T-tests among before and after smelling "Zuko" incense rubbing into the hands.

5. Alpha-amylase value was almost all shown as a characteristic index of stress which was more increasing up after smelling "Zuko" incense than before smelling regardless of male/female and habit/no habit with putting the hands in daily life.

From these results of measuring alpha-amylase value in saliva, it can be considered that something stress on smelling "Zuko" incense was usually given to the subject.

4.3 The meaning of smelling "Zuko" incense rubbing into the hands with putting the hands together

The meaning of smelling "Zuko" rubbing into the hands with putting the hands is as follows.

In habits of daily life, the brain of A-group peoples after smelling "Zuko" incense rubbing into the hands and putting their hands together or praying was activated at the orbitofrontal area, inner lobe of the frontal area, anterior and posterior areas in the temporal cortex, left visual area V1 in occipital cortex, and others. The brain of B-group individuals who did not has the habit of smelling incense odor or putting their hands together or praying in their daily life was also activated at the orbitofrontal cortex, inner lobe of the frontal area, left F5 language area, left visual area V1 in the occipital cortex, and anterior and posterior temporal cortex and larger changed.

Figure 15 shows that one subject's brain was activated at the F5 language area in the left inner frontal cortex. The brain for two of three subjects was activated at the right inner frontal cortex regardless of whether they have a habit of putting their hands together in their daily life or not. On the other hand, the brain for three subjects smelling "Zuko" incense with and without putting their hands together was also activated at the left calcarine sulci of the V1 visual area in the occipital cortex [36–39]. This result means the subject had a something sense of visual imaging by smelling "Zuko" incense with putting the hands together.

4.4 Smelling "Zuko" incense and putting the hands together showed larger changes than smelling incense odor with putting the hands together

We already have the results of the previous MEG experiments for smelling incense odor with putting the hands together as shown in our paper published in IntechOpen [23]. From these results of previous MEG experiments, it was obtained that smelling incense odor with putting the hands activates few specific brain areas.

On the other hand, in these MEG experiments, it was obtained that the results of smelling "Zuko" incense into the hands and putting the hands promote to excite few same specific brain areas as shown in **Figure 15** in Section 3.4.

From the results of **Tables 1** and **2**, we can find out that subject B5 obtained in orbitofrontal cortex OFC, subject A5, and B4 obtained in inner frontal area, subject A3, A4, and B2 obtained in occipital cortex V1 as an estimation active area in the brain clearly show almost all larger value ofα-amylase after smelling "Zuko" and putting the hands and MEG experiments before these experiments. These results are considered to show something stress by smelling "Zuko" incense and putting the hands for the response of subject A3, A4, B2, B3, B4, and B5 which showed large activity in a few special areas in the brain.

From the comparison with these two experimental results and analysis, we can obtain that smelling "Zuko" incense and putting the hands together showed clearly larger changes than smelling incense odor with putting the hands together. We can find larger changes in the brain, for example, from the right area to the left area for subject A5, B1, and B2 and from the left area to right area for subject A2 as shown in **Figure 15**. And we can also find out other larger changes in the brain in the same laterality, for example, from the occipital area to the prefrontal area for subject A3 and from the inferior parietal area to the occipital area for subject A4 at the left side in the brain.

These above results of larger changes show that the usage of "Zuko" incense rubbing into the hands promote to activate the brain more than smelling incense odor.

5. Conclusions

This research revealed that smelling "Zuko" incense rubbing into the hands and putting the hands together promoted to excite a few specific brain areas, for example, the orbitofrontal cortex of olfactory area, inner areas of the prefrontal cortex, left language F5 regions, occipital regions of left imaging area V1, and so on in the human brain.

A P300 response peak which was known as a kind of ERP responses in brain waves was researched as a response of "cognitive function" by using "oddball paradigm" experiment.

In this MEG experiments, P300m response using "auditory oddball paradigm" was measured both before smelling "Zuko" incense and after smelling "Zuko" incense.

In our experiments, evoked neuronal activity was recorded by the MEG and the alpha-amylase value in the subject's saliva was also measured in the stage before and after smelling "Zuko" incense and measuring the response of MEG in the brain.

From the summary of results in 3.5.1-3.5.3 in Section 3.5, we can conclude the distinct activities as follows. Both smelling "Zuko" incense only without putting the hands and smelling "Zuko" incense into the hands with putting the hands promoted to activate mainly a few specific brain areas such as the OFC frontal regions, left inner frontal region F5 language area, left inner occipital regions V1 visual areas, and so on.

As a cognitive P300m response, it was shown that the result with smelling "Zuko" had shorter latency time; the bigger the peak height, the larger the active wave area S than without smelling "Zuko." From these typical results of P300m responses, it can be considered that a possibility of improving cognitive ability of P300 peak was shown by smelling "Zuko" incense using "auditory oddball paradigm."

From these typical results of P300m responses, it can be considered that a possibility of improving cognitive ability of P300 peak was shown by smelling "Zuko" incense using "auditory oddball paradigm."

An alpha-amylase value was shown as a characteristic index of stress which was more increasing up after smelling "Zuko" incense than before smelling although male/female and habit/no habit with putting the hands in daily life. From these results of measuring alpha-amylase value in saliva, it can be considered that something stress on smelling "Zuko" incense was usually given to the subject.

From these results of measuring alpha-amylase value in saliva, it can be considered that something stress on smelling "Zuko" incense was usually given to the subject.

From an individual analysis, we can also find out that subject B5 obtained in orbitofrontal cortex, subject A5 and B4 obtained in the inner frontal area, subject A3, A4, and B2 obtained in the occipital cortex V1 as an estimation active area in the brain clearly show almost all larger value of alpha-amylase after smelling "Zuko" and putting the hands and MEG experiments before these experiments. These results are considered to show something stress by smelling "Zuko" incense and putting the hands for the response of subjects A3, A4, B2, B3, B4, and B5 which showed large activity in a few special areas in the brain.

From the above results, we consider that the F5 language area in the left frontal cortex and V1 visual area were promoted to activate by smelling "Zuko" incense rubbing into the hands with putting the hands together.

Alpha-amylase showed something stress like for smelling "Zuko" incense with putting the hands, and the specific mirror neuron and default-mode network showed activity of the special areas in the brain.

We concluded that new specific effects both in smelling "Zuko" incense into the hands and imitating the behavior of putting the hands together can be considered to promote excitation of the higher activities and to make larger changes in the brain activities dynamically in a few specific regions in the human brain.

Acknowledgements

We sincerely thank Mr. Kimiyoshi Yoshino and Mr. Masaru Yamamoto in Nippon Kodo Co. Ltd. in Japan for the subject's attendance and the supply of "Zuko" incense powder.

This study was supported by the Awards of Alzheimer's Disease in Osaka-Gas Co. and Grants for Alzheimer's Disease in Osaka Research Association in Japan.

Author details

Mitsuo Tonoike
Department of Medical Engineering, Faculty of Health Science, Aino University, Ibaraki, Osaka, Japan

*Address all correspondence to: gah00161@nifty.ne.jp

References

[1] Herrera MD, Smoke H. The Use of Incense in the Catholic Church. San Luis Obispo: Tixlini Scriptorium; 2011. Available from: www.SmellsBells.com

[2] Buttner A. Springer Handbook of Odor. Cham, Switzerland: Springer; 2017. p. 79. ISBN: 9783319269320. Available from: https://books.google.co.uk/books

[3] Takagi SF. Olfactory frontal cortex and multiple olfactory processing in primates. In: Peters A, Ones EG, editors. Cerebral Cortex. Vol. 9. NewYork: Plenum; 1991. pp. 133-152

[4] Zatorre RJ, Jones-Gotman M, Evans AC, Meyer E. Functional localization and lateralization of human olfactory cortex. Nature. 1992;**360**: 339-340

[5] Tonoike M, Maeda A, Kawai H, Kaetsu I. Measurement of olfactory event-related magnetic fields evoked by odorant pulses synchronized with respiration. Electroencephalography and Clinical Neurophysiology. 1996;**47**:143-150

[6] Sobel N, Pranhakaran v, Desmond JE, Gloverre GH, Goode RL, Sullivan EV, et al. Sniffing and smelling: Separate subsystems in the human olfactory cortex. Nature. 1998;**392**:282-286

[7] Tonoike M, Yamaguchi M, Hamada T, Kaetsu I, Koizuka I, Seo R. Odorant perception and active olfaction: A study of olfactory magnetic fields evoked by odorant pulse stimuli synchronized with respiratory cycle. In: Proceedings of 20th Annual International Conference IEEE/EMBS'98, Vol. 4. 1998. pp. 2213-2216

[8] Iacoboni M, Woods RP, Brass, et al. Cortical mechanisms of human imitation. Science. 1999;**286**:2526-2528

[9] Rizzolatti G, Fogassi L, Gallese V. Neurophysiological mechanisms underlying the understanding and imitation of action. Nature Reviews Neuroscience. 2001;**2**:661-670

[10] Rammachandran VS, Vilayanur S. Mirror neurons and imitation learning as the driving force behind "the great leap forward" in human evolution. 2005. Available from: http://www.edge.org/3rd_culture/raachandran/ramachandran_p1.html [Accessed: June 15]

[11] Raiche ME, Macleod AM, Snyder AZ, et al. A default mode of brain function. Proceedings of the National Academy of Science USA. 2001;**98**:676-682

[12] Chekassky VL, Kana RK, Keller TA, Just MA. Functional connectivity in a baseline resting-state network in autism. Neurology Report. 2006;**17**(16): 1687-1690

[13] Ilmonoiemi L. Neuromagnetism: Theory, techniques, and measurement [Ph.D. thesis]. Helsinki Univ. of Technology; 1985

[14] Sarvas J. Basic mathematical and electromagnetic concepts of the biomagnetic inverse problem. Physics in Medicine and Biology. 1987;**32**(1):11-22

[15] Tonoike NK, Tobinaga Y. Detection of thinking in human by magnetoencephalography. World Congress of Medical Physics and Biological Engineering. 2006;**14**:2617-2621

[16] Scherg M, Von Cramon D. Evoked dipole source potentials of the human auditory cortex. Electroencephalography and Clinical Neurophysiology. 1986; **65**(5):344-360

[17] Sutton S, Braren M, Zubin J, John ER. Evoked potential correlates of stimulus uncertainty. Science. 1965;**150**: 1187-1188

[18] Ruchkin DS, Sutton S. Positive slow wave and P300: Association and disassociation. In: Gaillard AWK, Ritter W, editors. Tutorials in ERP Research: Endogenous Components. Amsterdam: Elsevier/North Holland; 1983. pp. 233-250

[19] Hillyard SA, Picton TW. Electrophysiology of cognition. In: Plum F, editor. Handbook of Physiology. Baltimore: Williams and Wilkins; 1987. pp. 519-584

[20] Tonoike M, Yamaguchi M, Kaetsu I. Olfactory cognitive response using odorant odd-ball paradigm by magnetoencephalography. Journal of Temporal Design in Architecture and the Environment. 2003;**3**(1):43-53

[21] Chatterton RT Jr, Vogelsong KM, You-Cai L, Ellman AB, Hudgens GA. α-Amylase as measure of endogenous adrenergic activity. Clinical Physiology. 1996;**16**:433-448

[22] Speirs RL, Herring J, Cooper WD, Hardy CC, Hind CRK. The influence of sympathetic activity and isoprenaline on the secretion of amylase from human parotid gland. Archives of Oral Biology. 1974;**19**:747-751

[23] Tonoike M, Hayashi T. Simultaneous smelling an incense outdoor and putting the hands together activate specific brain areas. In: "Neuroimaging–Structure, Function and Mind" Ed. by Sanja Josef Golubic, pp. 71–100. IntechOpen. 2019

[24] Koenker RJ. Goodness of fit and related inference processes for quantile regression. Journal of the American Statistical Association. 1999;**94**: 1296-1310

[25] Cichy RM, Khosia A, Pantazis D, Torralba A, Oliva A. Comparison of deep neural networks to spatio-temporal cortical dynamics of hur-recognition reveals hierarchical correspondence. Scientific Reports. 2016;**6**:27755

[26] Sato M, Miyawaki Y. Spatial spreading of representational geometry through source estimation of magnetoencephalography signals. In: 2 Pattern Recognit Neuroimaging PRNI 2017. 2017. DOI: 10.1109/PRNI.2017.7981509

[27] Kurose Y, Omori Y. Bayesian analysis of time-varying quantiles using a smoothing spline. Journal of the Japan Statistical Society. 2012;**42**(1):23-46

[28] Yao J, Dewald JPD. Evaluation of different cortical source localization methods using simulated and experimental EEG data. NeuroImage. 2005;**25**:369-382

[29] Phillips C, Mattout J, Rugg MD, Maquet P, Friston K. An empirical Bayesian solution to the source reconstruction problem in EEG. NeuroImage. 2005;**24**:997-1011

[30] Stone JV. Independent Component Analysis: A Tutorial Introduction. Cambridge, Massachusetts: MIT Press; 2004. ISBN: 978-0-262-69315-8

[31] Chatterton RT Jr, Vogelsong KM, Lu YC, et al. Salivary alpha amylase as a measure of endogenous adrenergic activity. Clinical Physiology. 1996;**16**: 433-448

[32] Skosnik PD, Chatterton RT, Swisher T, et al. Modulation of attentional inhibition by norepinephrine and cortisol after psychological stress. International Journal of Psychophysiology. 2000;**36**:59-68

[33] van Stegeren A, Rohleder N, Everaerd W, et al. Salivary alpha amylase as marker for adrenergic activity during stress: Effect of betablokade. Psychoneuroendocrinology. 2006;**31**: 137-141

[34] Dale AM, Liu AK, Fischl BR, Buckner RL, Belliveau JW, Lewine JD, et al. Dynamic statistical parametric mapping: Combining fMRI and MEG for high-resolution imaging of cortical activity. Neuron. 2000;**26**:55-67

[35] Iwaki S, Bonmassar G, Belliveau JW. Dynamic cortical activity during the perception of three-dimensional random-dot motion. Journal of Integrative Neuroscience. 2013;**12**: 355-367

[36] Zhou W, Jiang Y, He S, Chen D. Olfaction modulates visual perception in binocular rivalry. Current Biology. 2010;**20**:1356-1358

[37] Calvert GA, Campbell R, Braer MJ. Evidence from functional magnetic resonance imaging of crossmodal binding in the human heteromodal cortex. Current Biology: CB. 2000;**10**: 649-657

[38] Calvert GA. Crossmodal processing in the human brain: Insights from functional neuroimaging studies. Cerebral Cortex. 2011;**11**:1110-1123

[39] Davis MH. Measuring individual differences in empathy: Evidence for a multidimensional approach. Journal of Personality and Social Psychology. 1983; **44**:113-126